THE
KETO RESET
DIET

THE KETO

REBOOT YOUR METABOLISM IN 21 DAYS AND BURN FAT FOREVER

HARMONY
BOOKS · NEW YORK

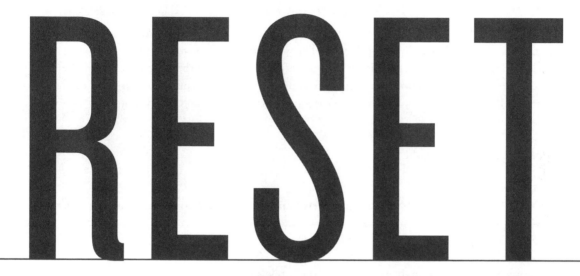

RESET DIET

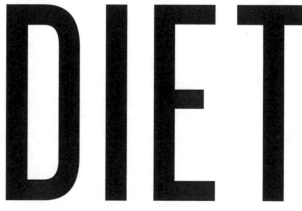

MARK SISSON
WITH BRAD KEARNS

The material in this book is for informational purposes only and is not intended as a substitute for the advice and care of your physician. As with all new diet and nutrition regimens, the program described in this book should be followed only after first consulting with your physican to make sure it is appropriate to your individual circumstances. The author and publisher expressly disclaim responsibility for any adverse effects that may result from the use or application of the information contained in this book.

Published in the United States by Harmony Books, an imprint of the Crown Publishing Group, a division of Penguin Random House LLC, New York.
crownpublishing.com

Harmony Books is a registered trademark and the Circle colophon is a trademark of Penguin Random House LLC.

Library of Congress Cataloging-in-Publication Data
Names: Sisson, Mark, 1953–, author.
Title: The keto reset diet : reboot your metabolism in 21 days and burn fat forever / Mark Sisson.
Description: First edition. | New York : Harmony Books, [2017]
Identifiers: LCCN 2017022962 | ISBN 9781524762230 (hardback) | ISBN 9781524762247 (ebook)
Subjects: LCSH: Reducing diets. | Ketogenic diet. | BISAC: HEALTH & FITNESS / Diets. | HEALTH & FITNESS / Weight Loss.
Classification: LCC RM222.2 .S558 2017 | DDC 613.2/5—dc23
LC record available at https://lccn.loc.gov/2017022962

Printed in the United States of America

Design by Elina Nudelman
Photographs by Andrew Purcell
Jacket design by Jenny Carrow

10 9 8 7 6 5 4 3 2 1

First Edition

DEDICATED TO MY WIFE, CARRIE, WHO OFFERS INSIGHTS INTO LIFE I COULD NEVER HAVE DISCOVERED ON MY OWN

CONTENTS

|||

Going Keto

Introduction

THE KETO TO A LONG, HAPPY, HEALTHY LIFE

THE *Keto Reset Diet* is going to help you reprogram your genes back to the original human factory setting of being *fat- and keto-adapted* (a term that appears throughout the book—let's nickname it "keto"). Keto is a state of *metabolic efficiency* where you are able to burn stored energy in the form of body fat and ketones, and not be dependent upon regular high-carbohydrate meals to sustain your energy, mood, or cognitive focus. When you conduct the 21-Day Metabolic Reset and transition away from carbohydrate dependency, then go keto, you will normalize your appetite hormones so that you are almost never hungry. This happens very quickly, and it's an absolutely stunning revelation. It's like discovering a hidden superpower that stabilizes your energy, mood, and brain function all day long, because you have readily available stored energy to burn—even if you skip meals.

You'll enjoy delicious, nutrient-dense meals and snacks that are deeply satisfying in a way that a carb binge never will be. This means you never have to worry about adding excess body fat, blowing your "diet" and tail spinning, or falling victim in your later years to diet-related diseases. You become what I affectionately call a fat-burning beast, and you'll stay this way for the rest of your life.

I'm eager to share this journey to keto with you because my own journey to keto represents the culmination of a long career in the health and fitness world, and a long quest to discover the truth. While the truth is that personal preference and dietary flexibility will always trump any regimented dietary protocol, it's also important to acknowledge that keto is the default human metabolic state, because it was the only way humans were able to survive the withering selection pressure of human evolution. I sincerely believe that *The Keto Reset Diet* journey we are about to commence could represent the greatest breakthrough in the history of nutritional science—and the history of dieting (finally!)—to promote successful long-term fat loss and weight management.

My passion for nutrition, fitness, and healthy living dates back to my teenage years. Yes, I was one of those weird kids running to and from school, sometimes in snowstorms (I'm known as a Malibu dude today, but I grew up in Maine), to prepare for high school distance running. I devoured nutrition texts instead of comic books. After college, I ditched plans of medical school to train for the U.S. Olympic team for the marathon. I ran over 100 miles a week for ten years, once placing fifth in the USA national championships.

After trashing all my joints from extreme running, I moved over to triathlons and took fourth at the famed Hawaii Ironman competition. I could perform great endurance feats and had a lean, toned physique, but on the inside I was in horrific shape. I suffered from chronic inflammation, tendonitis, osteoarthritis, and IBS, and I definitely had what we now identify as leaky gut syndrome. I caught six upper respiratory infections each year, and I was not fit for anything except moving straight ahead for hours on end. I thought my strict low-fat, high-carb diet was making me healthy, but—in tandem with my chronic training—it was significantly accelerating the aging process in my body. Before I was 30 years old, I had crashed and burned out of elite racing and turned my attention to helping others as a coach and personal trainer.

My athletic successes were gratifying and character building, but it was my struggles and failures that shaped the defining mission of my career: to help others enjoy healthy, fit, happy, and long lives without the pain, suffering, and sacrifice we have come to believe, erroneously, is necessary.

Today, breaking scientific developments in epigenetics and evolutionary biology validate a simple premise: the secret to lifelong health and peak performance is in modeling the lifestyle behaviors of our hunter-gatherer ancestors. This promotes optimal gene expression and counteracts the many health-compromising forces of fast-paced, fast-food modern life. With the primal/paleo/ancestral health movement in full bloom, and conventional wisdom getting challenged and recalibrated each day, it feels like we are finally on track to eventually manage the epidemic disease patterns of metabolic syndrome, Type 2 diabetes, cancer, and heart disease that are directly linked to adverse dietary and lifestyle practices. And yet the primal baseline of ditching grains, sugars, and industrial oils and of avoiding chronic exercise are just scratching the surface of the potential to transform your life through ancestral living in general, and keto in particular.

Ketogenic eating can also protect against assorted inflammatory conditions that lead to dysfunction and disease; dramatically improve immune and cognitive function; minimize the risk of today's epidemic heart disease, cancer, and cognitive decline; and enable phenomenal breakthroughs in athletic performance and recovery, both for endurance efforts and strength and power. These are some big claims, I know, but the research and case studies prove that if you follow the correct approach to going keto (as we'll do in this book), the results will surpass anything you've ever experienced before.

While keto is the key to health transformation, the booming popularity of keto has also made it the latest fad diet, replete with marketing hype, oversimplification, misinformation, and promoters misinterpreting the foundational science and proven strategies. I'd like to help you avoid the hazards of most fad diets; that's why I'm sharing my unique program in this book. *The Keto Reset Diet* will protect you from the pitfalls of many of these questionable programs. Instead, you'll follow a thoughtful, proven two-step approach that is flexible, highly customizable, effective, and intuitive instead of regimented.

With the plan I've created, you reprogram your genes to make fat and ketones your preferred fuel, instead of the carbohydrates that modern humans have become dependent upon owing to ill-advised food choices, coupled with overly stressful exercise and lifestyle habits. The *Keto Reset Diet* will make this happen at the deepest level of gene reprogramming, so that it lasts for the rest of your life. As I'll detail shortly, this is a refreshing contrast to the typical quick-fix weight-loss programming that often has adverse rebound consequences. *The Keto Reset Diet* blends cutting-edge information from numerous research and clinical experts with anecdotal evidence from keto devotees ranging from ordinary health enthusiasts to some of the world's elite athletes. I'll also share the breakthrough science and expert recommendations for how to avoid common mistakes and ensure success.

The Two Steps to Going Keto

The ultimate objective of the two-step plan I've developed is to build what I like to call *metabolic efficiency* or *metabolic flexibility*—being adept at burning stored energy in the form of fat and ketones instead of relying primarily on carbohydrates you consume at regularly timed meals. The first step in the process is the 21-Day Metabolism Reset to kick your dependence on dietary carbohydrates (which is the essence of metabolic *inflexibility*) and boost your fat-burning metabolism. During the first week of the Reset, you'll learn the best way to ditch grains, sugars, and refined vegetable oils; and you'll also discover the nutrient-dense, high-fat, low-carb primal/paleo foods with which to replace them. During the second week, you'll focus on the supportive lifestyle behaviors that are essential to succeed with dietary transformation. These include optimizing your exercise patterns, dialing in your sleep, and implementing effective stress-management techniques. In your final approach to the 21-day mark, you'll put it all together—thereby escaping carbohydrate dependency once and for all, and plunging headlong into the world of fat adaptation.

This 21-Day Metabolism Reset alone is quite likely to transform your health for the rest of your life. When you kick carb dependency, you will escape from the epidemic metabolic syndrome disease patterns (e.g., obesity, Type 2 diabetes, and heart disease), and you set the stage once and for all to reduce excess body fat without having to worry about its coming back, as happens when you normalize an extreme diet or back off on exercise now and then. You will likely notice immediate weight loss, largely owing to a reduction in inflammation and the ensuing fluid retention in cells throughout the body (caused by the inflammatory effects of high-carbohydrate eating) and also because you will unlock stored body fat to burn for energy around the clock. It's not uncommon for devoted enthusiasts to drop 10 to 15 pounds total, including 3 to 6 pounds of excess body fat, during a 21-Day Metabolism Reset.

Your journey toward becoming fat- and keto-adapted continues in the final section of this book. First, you'll make some final launch preparations to fine-tune your metabolic fitness, and even take a midterm exam of sorts to ensure you are ready for your initial foray into nutritional ketosis. Then, you'll go keto, dropping your carb consumption to less than 50 grams a day and also likely lowering your protein to less than you typically consume, while also emphasizing nutritious, natural fats as your main calorie source. Your foray into nutritional ketosis should last for at least six weeks. Then, with your newly minted degree in fat- and keto-adaptation, you can consider and experiment with assorted long-term options, including going back into nutritional ketosis any time in the future to shed excess fat, protect against disease, and enhance cognitive and athletic performance.

Being fat- and keto-adapted means that you can veer off the plan now and then—a departure from ideal food choices—and not tailspin into a month-long sugar binge. When you have this esteemed metabolic flexibility, you can wake up the day after eating cake by the ocean, or even a bunch more stuff on a week-long cruise, and get right back into the groove—whether through fasting, a string of keto-aligned meals, or even strategic use of ketone supplements. In contrast, consider what happens to a carb-dependent, metabolically inflexible dieter going for a cutthroat calorie-restriction cleanse: there's fatigue from a lack of the usual steady supply of dietary carbohydrates (since you are inefficient at burning body fat), sugar cravings that will ultimately be impossible to resist, and eventual burnout from an overstimulation of the fight-or-flight response that's triggered by calorie restriction when you are not fat-adapted.

> **Having *metabolic flexibility* means you can depart from ideal food choices now and then, and then get right back into the groove.**

If you're worried about your chances of succeeding with keto, realize that your diet is only as good or as bad as your last meal—or last week or month of meals. No matter who you are and what your starting point is—even if you are battling obesity or Type 2 diabetes—you can take baby steps in the right direction each day and experience immediate, discernible benefits. If you complete the 21-Day Metabolism Reset and lose the book after that, your life still will be transformed. You will feel more alert and less hungry while at work, less exhausted after workouts, and less fried after a hectic day. These benefits occur because you are finally giving your body a break from the lifelong, high-stress roller-coaster ride of a high-carbohydrate, high insulin–producing eating pattern that promotes inflammation and oxidative damage throughout the body.

Taking that initial step of getting the junk out of your diet is a huge deal! But that only scratches the surface for the absolutely life-transforming benefits of being fully fat- and keto-adapted. That's what this book is all about—heading toward fabulous new frontiers with absolutely, positively no turning back. This time, you are going to do things the right way, once and for all. This new mindset differs, though, from thinking that you can reach for keto to work like a magic pill that slims you down for your bikini vacation or bridesmaid gig. Instead, with this approach, you won't find that annoying weight gain happening in the first place (even if you cut back on exercise); that's because your body has become exceptional at burning stored body fat for energy around the clock.

In *The Keto Reset Diet,* you'll be guided every step of the way to do things right, to proceed at a sensible pace, and to never struggle, suffer, or backslide, like so many ill-prepared and misinformed enthusiasts. You'll learn exactly which foods to eliminate from your diet and why; you'll have a wide array of delicious keto-approved foods to choose from; and you'll find out how exercise, lifestyle, and stress management fit into the picture. I provide a meal plan for your 21-Day Metabolism Reset, some fine-tuning exercises to get you ready for keto, and a 21-day Keto Meal Plan that you can follow to the letter, or borrow from here and there, during your nutritional ketosis effort. I've also included more than 100 recipes to make going keto not just a metabolic transformation but also a celebration of delicious dining.

THE
KETO RESET
DIET

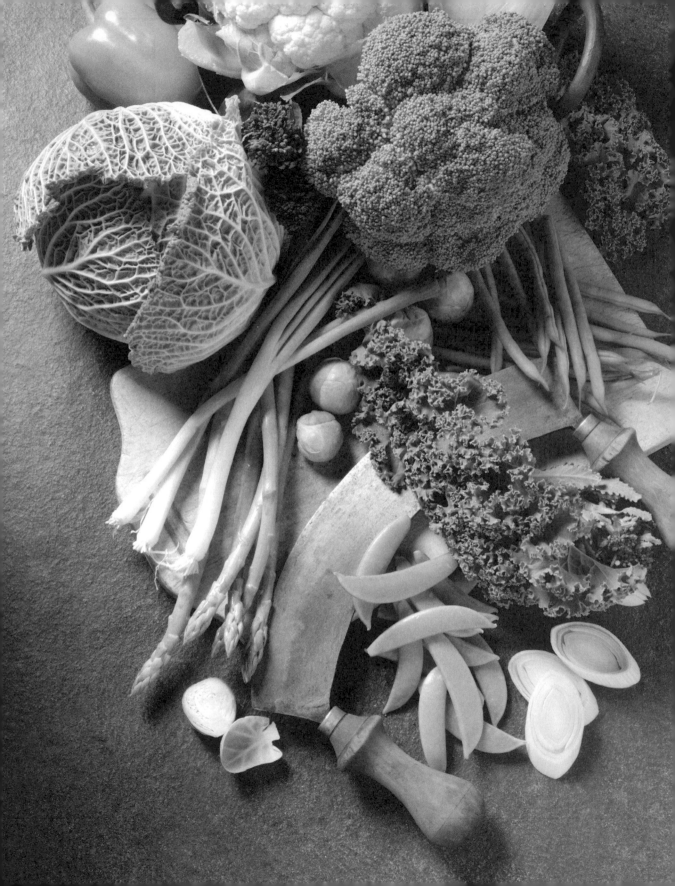

Building the Metabolic Machinery

CHAPTER 1

The Keto Reset Diet 101— What, Why, and How

I'VE been familiar with the ketosis aspect of ancestral eating for nearly two decades, but I always considered keto to be an extreme and temporary practice, perhaps suitable only for brief periods of fasting for aggressive fat reduction or as a last-ditch strategy for the obese to right the ship and protect against a medical catastrophe. In the past few years, though, there has been renewed interest in keto, both in the sciences and among the most adventurous in the ancestral health movement, as a strategy with broad application to promote the esteemed goal of *metabolic flexibility*.

Inspired by the thought leaders whom you'll meet in this book, I started fooling around with keto several years ago, and I noticed some immediate, discernible benefits, especially increased mental clarity and reduced hunger. As my writing partner, Brad, and I maintained states of nutritional ketosis for sustained periods of time during the research and writing of this book, we both experienced significant health and athletic performance breakthroughs. Indeed, *The Keto Reset Diet* book is powered by ketones! As I'll detail throughout the book, regulating appetite and developing the ability to survive—and thrive—on fewer calories is key to optimum health and maximum longevity. Owning this insight, though, requires a massive shift in mindset from the flawed "furnace will burn" thinking that represents one of the most destructive concepts in conventional dietary and exercise wisdom (details in Chapter 2).

What Is Keto?

"Keto" is a catch-all nickname for anything pertaining to the metabolic state of *ketosis*, the burning of *ketones,* a.k.a. *ketone bodies,* or the dietary macronutrient composition (ultra-low-carb, moderate-protein, high-fat) that promotes the attainment of this delicate metabolic state. Ketones are a source of caloric energy in the body that are used by the brain, heart, and muscles in the same manner as is glucose (sugar). They are produced in the liver as a by-product of fat metabolism when—owing to extreme restriction of dietary carbohydrates—insulin, blood sugar, and liver glycogen levels are very low. Most people go through life never getting anywhere near this state, and never experiencing the almost magical effects of this natural superfuel. Ketones and fat (since the burning of these two caloric energy sources always go hand in hand) help minimize the inflammation and oxidative damage that come from eating the modern grain-based high-carbohydrate diet. Keto awareness arises from the primal/paleo/low-carb dietary movement that has become wildly popular over the past decade, but it is more specific with respect to required dietary macronutrient ratios; and it can be even more effective for weight loss, disease protection, and peak cognitive and athletic performance than a standard low-carb diet.

By comparison to the Standard American Diet (SAD), the modern ketogenic diet is very high in natural nutritious fats, moderate in protein, and ultra-low in carbohydrates.

Out on the street (which I guess today means the Internet), terms like "keto," "ketone-burning," "ketogenic," and "ketotic" are used indiscriminately to describe the burning of ketones for energy and the pursuit of (or existence in) a fat- and keto-adapted state. You'll learn about the differences along the way in this book, but it's particularly important to understand the distinction between *ketosis* (a metabolic state quantified by blood or breath meter values) and *ketoacidosis*. The latter is a potentially life-threatening condition that almost always occurs only in Type I diabetics who can't produce insulin or in alcoholics with poorly functioning livers (insulin immediately shuts down ketone production; that's why a high-carb meal knocks you out of ketosis).

Unfortunately, ketoacidosis is often confused with ketosis, even among nutrition and medical professionals who should know better but have only vague exposure to the concepts related to ketone production in the liver. Owing to this common misconception, you may encounter inaccurate Internet articles from dieticians, and even doctors, who react to anything "keto" with alarm because of the severity of ketoacidosis.

The exact definition of *ketosis* is that of being in a metabolic state whereby your body is accumulating ketones in the bloodstream faster than they are being burned. Being in ketosis may not be indicative of your ability to burn ketones for fuel, however. People who have an acute illness or who are on calorie-restricted crash diets while carbohydrate dependent can get into a state of ketosis in a few days, but they may not be burning ketones for energy. Instead, they excrete these valuable energy sources in their urine and breath as they remain addicted to carbohydrates.

If you have done the work to escape carbohydrate dependency and trend toward fat burning, being in ketosis may indeed be representative of your ability to manufacture and burn ketones for energy. Consequently, *fat- and keto-adapted* is the best term to describe eating and living in a state where you are enjoying the benefits of burning fat and ketones as your preferred fuel sources. When you are fully adapted, your muscles burn mostly fat for fuel, while the ketones produced by the liver are prioritized for use by the brain. The brain is a huge energy-demand organ (it's around 2 percent of your total bodyweight, but the brain burns 20 to 25 percent of your daily calories!) that cannot burn fat and must burn either glucose or ketones.

Experts suggest that maintaining a state of nutritional ketosis requires a dietary macronutrient composition of approximately 65 to 75 percent fat, 15 to 25 percent protein, and 5 to 10 percent carbs. With carb intake, experts recommend a hard limit of 50 grams per day for active folks, and 20 grams per day for the inactive. To adhere to the stringent ketogenic carbohydrate intake limit and obtain maximum benefits, you must completely eliminate all forms of sugars, sweetened beverages, and grains from your diet, and even pass on starchy tubers like sweet potatoes. Eating an energy bar or enjoying a fresh-squeezed juice (even a modest 8-ounce glass) can bump you out of ketosis for 24 hours and possibly much longer.

Testing for Ketosis

The metabolic state of ketosis can be quantified with established parameters for blood, breath, or urine testing. Urine test strips are cheap and notoriously inaccurate—don't bother with them. Someone celebrating the darkening of a urine test strip into ketosis color is likely excreting lots of ketones instead of burning them. Breath test technology came to market in early 2017 and is believed to deliver accurate results with an expensive (about $300 for Ketonix brand made in Sweden) portable and reusable device. Handheld blood meters are also accurate. They work just like the glucose meters (popular with diabetics), whereby you prick your finger and apply a droplet of blood to a test strip. Precision Xtra is a good blood meter you can order online for ~$30; single-use testing strips are $2–$4 each—not cheap!

A blood ketone value of 0.5 millimoles per liter (mmol/L) represents the beginning of a mild state of nutritional ketosis. Therapeutic benefits of ketone burning improve up to a level of 3.0 mmol/L, although most enthusiasts are happy to land in the range of 0.5 to 1.5 mmol/L. It's pretty difficult to sustain levels higher than 3.0 mmol/L (e.g., you'd have to engage in long-term severe calorie restriction/starvation or slam an excessive amount of exogenous supplemental ketones), and there do not appear to be any additional benefits at higher levels. (Note: Ketoacidosis occurs when blood levels rise to above 10 mmol/L—virtually impossible to attain if you have normal liver function.) We'll discuss testing in later chapters, including the idea that numbers may not be an accurate indicator of your keto fitness. It's likely that you may be better off with subjective evaluations of how well you can think and perform when you skip a meal or adhere to a moderate-protein, ultra-low-carb keto-style eating pattern. Feeling great without regular high-carb meals is a sign of being fat- and keto-adapted, and the ultimate goal of the *The Keto Reset Diet* journey.

Practically speaking, 50 grams of daily carbs afford substantial consumption of vegetables, along with small amounts of incidental carbohydrates from nuts, seeds, and their butters, high-cacao percentage dark chocolate, and perhaps occasional servings of fresh seasonal berries. If you are a high-calorie–burning athlete or very carefully space your carbohydrate intake to consume no more than 10 to 15 grams (40–60 calories) at any one sitting, experts believe that you may be able to consume a bit more than 50 grams per day and still remain in the metabolic state of nutritional ketosis. By the way, I'm talking gross carbs, not net—mainly for simplification. We'll discuss the difference in Chapter 6.

If you're familiar with extreme carb-restriction weight-loss diets like Atkins, *The Keto Reset Diet* has comparable macronutrient guidelines and a shared goal of lowering insulin to mobilize stored body fat for energy. However, *The Keto Reset Diet* places greater emphasis on choosing the most nutrient-dense sources of fats, protein, and carbs, as well as avoiding unhealthy processed foods—even if they might meet ketogenic macronutrient standards. On the carbohydrate front, *The Keto Reset Diet* allows for and encourages varied and abundant intake of fresh, colorful vegetables even during the most hard-core keto phases. Consequently, *The Keto Reset Diet* should be viewed as a healthy lifelong eating strategy rather than a rigid weight-loss protocol.

Keto Delivers Fasting-Like Benefits Without Having to Starve!

Ketogenic eating allows you to benefit from the extraordinary (and long scientifically validated) metabolic efficiency, general health, and longevity benefits of fasting, but without having to actually starve yourself. When you are starving, engaging in a purposeful fast, or adhering to a nutritional ketosis eating pattern, your cells prefer to burn fat and ketones. Fat and ketones burn efficiently and quickly in the body—they have been the preferred human fuels in our body for 2.5 million years of our hunter-gatherer existence.

On the other hand, the high-carb, high-insulin–producing Standard American Diet (SAD) causes you to burn glucose, a.k.a. sugar—the primary human fuel since the cultivation of grains and the consequent advent of civilization around 10,000 years ago. Glucose burns quickly and easily, but it also burns dirty via the excessive production of free radicals. Free radicals are the driving force behind inflammation, cancer, and accelerated aging. They are an inevitable by-product of living life—burning calories, breathing air, or absorbing sunlight—so you can't avoid them, but concerns arise when free radical production is excessive. This happens when you introduce stressors like high-carbohydrate eating, excessive exercise, or adverse lifestyle behaviors such as smoking, alcohol or drug use, or having stressful personal relationships.

The reason glucose burning generates more free radicals is that, unlike fat and ketones, glucose doesn't require oxygen to burn. When you burn glucose without oxygen, you bypass the protective benefits of mitochondria, the energy-producing power plants located inside each cell. The more mitochondria you have and the better they work, the more protection you have against free radicals when you burn calories. You can consider fat and ketones the big logs in a campfire. Heat them up carefully and they keep you warm for hours—not much smoke. Glucose is like kindling—burning quickly with lots of smoke. Thus, if your metabolic machinery is carbohydrate dependent (because you consume too many carbs and produce too much insulin—which keeps body fat locked away in storage), you don't have the big logs to burn, instead having to continually stoke your fire with twigs—that is, eating regular high-carbohydrate meals and snacks to prop up sagging blood sugar levels.

This concept that your body operates much more efficiently when starving, fasting, or eating keto is critical to consider in today's age of chronic overfeeding and excess insulin production (a.k.a. *hyperinsulinemia*). It may feel satisfying at some level to be a glutton (no offense, but anyone who eats breakfast, lunch, and dinner each day is a glutton from an evolutionary perspective), but overfeeding drives accelerated aging and increases disease risk. When we have chronic caloric abundance, we not only (most likely) get fat but our bodies also accelerate cell division instead of being frugal and efficient with the cells we have. Why bother being efficient (repairing and recycling existing cells) when more calories (that can help make new cells) are coming down the pipe every few hours?

Accelerated cell division is great for infants trying to triple their bodyweight in one year, adolescents trying to grow to their full height, or bodybuilders trying to develop huge guns. For the rest of us, accelerated cell division is the essence of accelerated aging. Even in people with lucky genetics who are not predisposed to accumulating excess body fat, bad stuff is likely happening inside when you exist in carbohydrate dependency. If you are flaunting your slim figure and thinking you're immune to the ravages of accelerated aging, you may want to test your blood for signs of metabolic dysfunction and elevated disease risk, like the triglyceride-to-HDL ratio (1:1 is optimal; over 3.5-to-1 is dangerous), inflammatory markers like C-reactive protein and Lp2A, and metabolic markers like fasting blood glucose and fasting blood insulin. In the endurance athletic world, it's disturbingly common to see elite performers coming up with dysfunction and disease of the cardiovascular system, despite being physical marvels. These are the ravages of oxidation and inflammation from overtraining and overconsumption of carbohydrates.

In contrast to being overfed and inflamed, becoming metabolically efficient (through low-carbohydrate eating in general, and especially through Intermittent Fasting and nutritional ketosis) optimizes *autophagy,* the natural cellular detoxification process whereby cellular material is recycled, repaired, or destroyed (*autophagy* means "self-eating"). Dr. Colin Champ, author of *Misguided Medicine,* explains: "Autophagy makes us more efficient machines to get rid of faulty parts, stop cancerous growths, and stop metabolic dysfunction like obesity and diabetes." Fasting and ketogenic eating are especially helpful to promote autophagy in the brain, and thus protective against today's increasingly common conditions of cognitive decline and disease.

> **Overfeeding is the essence of accelerated aging; metabolic efficiency is the essence of longevity.**

The scientists, medical professionals, and athletes on the ground floor of the keto movement can barely contain their excitement: the research continues to validate the theory that ketogenic eating offers everything from the most reliable way to reduce excess body fat; enhance neurological function and protect against diseases of cognitive decline; slow the rate of inflammation and oxidative damage that represent the essence of the (accelerated) aging process; help prevent seizures and halt the growth of cancerous tumors; and improve athletic performance for both strength/power athletes and endurance athletes.

The Keto Reset Diet Is Not a Shortcut Program

While rapid weight loss can be easily achieved with an extreme and regimented program, the goal with the more deliberate process outlined in *The Keto Reset Diet* is to make sure that you don't fail or backslide after three days, 30 days, three months, or 30 months. The speed of your progression toward full-blown keto depends upon your current personal starting point with your health and fitness, and how well you respond to the dietary and lifestyle recommendations. One thing is for sure: you're not going to fail from lack of preparation. If you're not ready, you'll know why you're not, and you'll learn exactly what action to take to get ready. We're in this together for the long haul, and you'll have an understanding, supportive, patient, and focused coach in your corner the entire time.

What's more, nothing here is going to be a struggle, because that's a sure setup for failure. Unlike so many programs that shove a rigid agenda down your throat and disregard intangibles like "Are we having fun yet?," *The Keto Reset Diet* will feel like fun, it will be sensible, and it will be doable at all times. To succeed with long-term diet and lifestyle transformation, it's essential to enjoy every step of your journey, and to never struggle or suffer in the name of health. Suffering is as unhealthy to your psyche as junk food is to your body.

This is one way that *The Keto Reset Diet* differs from the all-too-popular "hack" approach—where results are obtained via enticing shortcuts instead of honoring the laws of nature, the realities of hectic modern life, and the long-term consequences of a shortcut strategy. My 21-Day Metabolism Reset will ease you into an effective plan that will help transform your body naturally. If you are able to lose weight following one of those typical ill-prepared, poorly designed keto shortcut plans, it will largely come from an extreme overstimulation of fight-or-flight hormones. Pumped up for your challenge (perhaps fueled by anger, frustration, desperation, vanity, or other tenuous extrinsic motivators), you can restrict carbs and total calories with tremendous willpower, exercise like crazy at those 6 A.M. workouts, and temporarily feel pumped full of extra energy thanks to a cocktail of powerful adrenaline-like adaptive (conferring a fitness or metabolic benefit) hormones, especially cortisol.

You can perform like a champ to meet extreme demands and "watch the fat melt away" for a few weeks or a few months, if you are particularly bull-headed and lucky enough to not fall apart sooner. Then one day the buzz wears off and you wake up and realize, "This sucks. I'm fried." The fight-or-flight hormonal processes that you've egregiously abused become exhausted, and you have arrived at the familiar destination of burnout.

Regardless of your impressive willpower and type-A personality gold-level membership card, you start producing lower than healthy baseline levels of these important endocrine hormones, and you find yourself in a PTSD-like haze: your appetite goes haywire and all the fat you lost—and then some—comes back quickly. You wake up feeling unmotivated, lethargic, and craving sugar, and you go to bed the same way. These are the laws of nature, balance, and karma kicking in.

This disturbingly familiar story is the dirty little secret of the diet and fitness industry. The popularity of clean eating and active living is currently at an all-time high, but if you look more closely, you'll see massive attrition and turnover rates with gym memberships, personal trainer clientele, and on the starting lines of endurance events. The chaos, confusion, and dead ends in the diet and fitness game are such that the average fitness enthusiast's dusty bookshelf is a graveyard of false hopes and false promises.

This will not happen with *The Keto Reset Diet*. What we are going for here is not just a quick-fix cleanse or a detox, but something much deeper: a reprogramming of your genes and a long-term recalibration of your appetite and metabolic hormones in the direction of fat- and ketone-burning and away from carbohydrate dependency.

The rebuilding of your metabolic machinery is no small task; it requires a broader approach than just modifying the macronutrient content of your diet. Being a fat- and ketone-burning beast (which is who you will be at the end of this journey) requires a big-picture approach of optimal eating, exercise, movement, sleep, and stress-management practices. That's why you will be introduced to supportive lifestyle elements in week 2 of your 21-Day Metabolism Reset (exercise, sleep, and stress management), and emphasize them in concert with your dietary transformation.

One of the important, key aspects of this plan that differs from shortcut programs is that you'll build the metabolic machinery to become fat- and keto-adapted. While other programs might offer you short-term results by getting you into ketosis, they won't have the long-term benefits that come with being fat- and keto-adapted, and they can come with elevated risk of fight-or-flight burnout. We'll be discussing cortisol and the stress response in relation to diet, exercise, and lifestyle factors frequently throughout the book, so please absorb the message in the sidebar!

The Rise and Fall of Cortisol

Cortisol—the most prominent fight-or-flight hormone—is secreted by the adrenal glands in response to environmental stimulation (a.k.a. stress) perceived by the brain. One of these stressors is low blood sugar, a fundamental problem for people who are not fat- and keto-adapted. When you sugar-crash, the brain frantically tells the adrenals to secrete cortisol, which prompts the conversion of lean muscle tissue into glucose to keep you humming along until you find some carbs to slam down. Cortisol's prominent role in regulating blood sugar is just one of its many critical functions. It influences a full 20 percent of the human genome, including profoundly impacting immune function, inflammatory processes, metabolism, and cognitive function. Optimal cortisol production helps you optimize all of the aforementioned mechanisms. However, when you chronically overproduce cortisol due to incessant high levels of stress, including sugar-crash urgencies, chronic training patterns, insufficient sleep, hectic daily schedules, or difficult personal or work relationships, you are headed toward the uniquely modern affliction of burnout. Having so abused your delicate and powerful fight-or-flight mechanisms, your adrenal glands are no longer able to keep up with your bare minimum energy and metabolic requirements.

When the fight-or-flight response wears out, you feel exhausted waking up, have difficulty controlling blood sugar, mood, and energy levels throughout the day, experience drastically diminished workout performance and immune function, suffer from system-wide inflammation, have diminished cognitive function and elevated risk of cognitive decline, have dysregulated appetite and fat-storage hormones, and display a generally very poor tolerance for all forms of life stress. You go from wired—for weeks or months on a tenuous cortisol high—to fried, often in a disturbingly abrupt manner. Burnout is a bummer when you are trying to shake a lingering illness or improve your performance as an athlete, but is also a fundamental driver of accelerated aging in general in today's overstressed, carbohydrate-dependent society.

When you become fat- and keto-adapted, the stress of having to constantly balance blood sugar goes away. Then, you can optimize your production of cortisol to support stable energy levels and have a ready reserve of cortisol for those brief fight-or-flight peak performance efforts that your genes are designed to deliver.

Going Keto the *Right* Way

Regardless of how unfortunate your current starting point is, going keto is within your reach, and it can happen quickly—*if* you commit to the correct approach from the outset. You may have heard some buzz about how strict and difficult keto is, and how many people try and fail. I contend that these complaints and fallout are largely due to a flawed approach by people who are ill-prepared. Many fail because they rush through the progression away from carb dependency; they don't actually cut carbs enough to produce ketones; they exercise in chronic patterns while they are not yet fat-adapted and run out of energy; or they don't adequately increase intake of water, sodium, and other important minerals and electrolytes (because—seriously—you become less bloated and inflamed when you go keto; more on this later). In these unfortunately common follies, people have trouble stabilizing energy, mood, concentration, and appetite, and they bail out before the true metabolic flexibility benefits of keto kick in.

When you transition away from carb dependency toward fat- and keto-adaptation, you are rarely hungry. This could be the most life-altering benefit of going keto.

While the benefits of being fat- and keto-adapted are life-changing, it's important to respect the seriousness of your decades-long existence in carbohydrate dependency. It started from the moment you were weaned off breast milk (the healthiest food in the history of humanity—and high in fat, by the way!) and started on the Standard American Diet (SAD). A high-carbohydrate/high-insulin-producing SAD diet shuts off fat burning and creates a dependency on regular carbohydrate-based feedings for energy. Before you mess around with keto or any other dietary transformation, you have to ditch all foods containing grains (yes, even whole grains!), sugars, and refined vegetable oils.

Ditching grains, sugars, and refined vegetable oils is no small task, because decades of SAD eating has likely resulted in mild to extreme metabolic damage in your body—especially if you've engaged in yo-yo dieting, followed extreme fitness pursuits, or have familial genes that predispose you to fat storage. Metabolic damage is evidenced by difficulty getting rid of excess body fat even when you cut calories; leaky gut syndrome and related digestive and/or autoimmune conditions (traced strongly to grain consumption); thyroid or adrenal dysfunction; metabolic syndrome blood markers (especially high triglycerides); other blood risk factors for diabetes or cardiac disease; or generally feeling hungry, moody, fatigued, or fried too often in daily life. If these symptoms hit home, your initial 21-Day Metabolism Reset out of carb dependency and into fat- and keto-adaptation might take a bit longer than 21 days, requiring you to exercise some patience and extend your timeline. Becoming fat- and keto-adapted is also more difficult the older you get, because the negative effects of high-carbohydrate intake worsen with age.

> **If you've sustained metabolic damage from decades of high-carb eating, your initial 21-day transformation out of carb dependency and into fat- and keto-adaptation might take a bit longer.**

If you are already lean and fit and eat a nutritious low-carb diet, or are willing to really work hard to optimize diet, exercise, sleep, and stress management during your 21-Day Metabolism Reset, you can expect your transition to keto to be smooth and graceful. The great thing about *The Keto Reset Diet* approach is that each step leverages your success in previous steps. You'll know when you're ready to proceed and when you aren't (yep, you'll have an actual midterm exam to take along the way!), and you won't ever try something that you are not ready for. Furthermore, you never have to struggle or suffer in the name of going keto, never have to eat any foods you don't like, and can emphasize the foods that you enjoy most—within the parameters for fat- and keto-adapted eating, of course.

I especially appreciate the dynamics of keto because I'm a guy who loves to eat, loves to enjoy my life, and hates to be a slave to food or clockwork meals to fuel my busy days. I can't be bothered following a regimented diet, and I never eat anything I don't absolutely love—seriously! If I'm traveling and am faced with airport or roadside junk, I prefer to engage in Intermittent Fasting (IF); this affords a great opportunity to fine-tune my fat- and keto-adapted metabolic machinery. By the way, fasting and ketone burning help me completely eliminate jet lag from my travel experience; I travel a ton and I'm not kidding, it really works—*if* you have the right metabolic machinery.

Whatever pitfalls and detours you've had on your journey toward healthy eating and healthy living, you can put your fears aside and jump in with full enthusiasm and commitment to *The Keto Reset Diet;* that's because this really is the original human eating strategy. It is your destiny and your birthright to burn fat and ketones, and kick sugar once and for all. While it might take a bit of discipline and discomfort to wean yourself off carbs at the outset, you will build momentum with every single keto-aligned meal, every skipped meal, and every lifestyle behavior you exhibit in the name of health and balance.

This momentum will come in the form of immediate, discernible benefits of becoming fat- and keto-adapted. Mainly, you'll notice a regulation of your appetite such that you feel alert, well nourished, and rarely hungry—and rarely bothered by the strict keto standards. This insight can be comforting if you're worried about whether you have enough willpower to adhere to keto. Honestly, it's best to forget about such nonsense! Lindsay Taylor, Ph.D., a behavioral psychologist and keto enthusiast who did much of the recipe preparation and testing in this book, reminds us that willpower is a fragile and easily depleted resource. "The more you enlist willpower to regulate your behavior, the more likely you will drain the tank and succumb to temptation," explains Taylor. This concept is highly validated by respected studies in behavioral psychology. Besides, major dietary overhaul is such a big-ticket item (often loaded with emotional baggage like the scars of past failures, negative self-talk, peer pressures and judgments—and gosh knows what else) that willpower is not a strong enough weapon to win the battle.

Instead, with *The Keto Reset Diet* you are going to let success come to you naturally, by reaping the hormonal, cognitive, and metabolic benefits of fat- and keto-adapted eating patterns. Before you get flustered about this sounding too good to be true, let's admit that we are getting into some tricky business here with this keto thing. For starters, keto has reached crazy-fad status, and with that distinction comes a lot of baggage and potential pitfalls. If you google "keto diet," you'll get bombarded with a dizzying amount of multimedia information, some of it excellent (we'll introduce you to some of the most respected thought leaders shortly) and some of it highly questionable.

Simply exposing yourself to this information overload can create stress, anxiety, and potential booby traps. Consequently, my goal with this book is to help guide you in the manner of a personal coach. While I have a strong understanding of the health sciences, have been deep in the trenches of the evolutionary health scene since the very beginning, and have consulted the world's leading scientists and medical experts extensively to prepare this book, at my core I'm a competitor and a coach. This is great, because no one can smell bullshit or hype better than a high-level competitor; athletes know that there is no substitute for hard work and that the hack mentality is for posers.

I'll navigate you away from ill-advised hacks and shortcuts, point out potential hazards before they take you down, and encourage you to trust yourself, believe in yourself, and treat yourself with kindness so that you not only succeed from a metabolic and body composition perspective but also learn and grow as a person from the experience of taking on a challenge, carrying out the necessary commitments, and transforming your health.

True self-satisfaction comes from pursuing life goals that are natural, enjoyable, and easy to maintain.

Before you jump into your 21-Day Metabolism Reset, I want you to gain a full understanding of the scientific and evolutionary underpinnings of keto, and contrast our genetic factory setting with the disastrously flawed and dangerous approach that is the

Standard American Diet. I want you to get excited about and deeply committed to this journey by learning of the assorted life-altering benefits of keto for weight loss, brain function, immune function, disease protection, and athletic performance. We'll cover these topics in the next two chapters, and then proceed to hit the ground running with your 21-Day Metabolism Reset in Chapters 4, 5, 6, and 7. After your 21-Day Reset, you will turn a page in the book, and in your life, and go keto in the final section of the book.

A Kinder, Gentler Approach to Diet and Lifestyle Transformation

I'm all about taking action and generating results, whether with fitness, business, or personal life goals. However, as I reflect on my life journey to date, I've only achieved true self-satisfaction—the only kind of success that matters—when my approach has been *natural, enjoyable, and easy to maintain* (shout-out to my friend Johnny G, creator of the Spinning indoor cycling program, for creating this definition—and living by it!). Under no circumstances should your keto journey turn into a high-stress rush job, nor entail any form of struggling or suffering.

If you're impatient to succeed and think that you can force progress through the application of type-A focus and discipline, you may in fact succeed in the short term (like millions of ill-fated dieters), but you may suffer and struggle too much from fluctuating energy, appetite, and mood. Over time, this will erode your resolve, not to mention your enjoyment of life. Consequently, you will be at high risk of backsliding at some future date. I can't count the number of ambitious peak performers I've counseled who plunge with great energy and enthusiasm into a dietary transformation and adhere for a period of days or weeks. After a while, things get a little quieter from their emails, texts, and Instagram meal photos. Eventually, I'm compelled to reach out to them and hear about the hot fudge sundaes and wet burritos that have returned to the scene.

I prefer that you view this keto journey as a lifestyle modification and gene reprogramming exercise that will last forever, and that you be kind and patient with yourself along the way. If you have a fair measure of metabolic fitness, you can make phenomenal progress during your initial 21-Day Metabolism Reset, and then experience truly life-changing breakthroughs from nutritional ketosis, whether you use it as an occasional tool for targeted benefits or implement keto as long-term dietary baseline.

If you have to take longer than 21 days to repair metabolic damage and really, truly ditch carb dependency once and for all, rejoice that you are making progress each day—even if it's taking longer than you hoped. If you experience minor setbacks or even major backslides, have some compassion for yourself. I'm talking real compassion, which is radically different from having ready-made excuses and rationalizations. Accept your imperfections, let go of what's happened in the past, and don't worry about the future. Just do the best you can each day and enjoy the heck out of the journey.

CHAPTER 2

Metabolic Efficiency: The Ultimate Goal for Weight Loss, Health, and Longevity

BEFORE you tackle the progressive, actionable steps to fat- and keto-adaptation, it's critical that you gain a basic understanding of the science and evolutionary underpinnings of ketone burning, and also explore the numerous specific benefits of it, especially in contrast to the adverse health consequences of burning the cheap and dirty fuel that is glucose. Before we get deep into the science and benefits, I want to propose a critically important shift in your belief system about the role of food in your life. These could be the two most life-changing insights in the entire book:

- **Going keto will virtually eliminate hunger**, and the accordant fluctuations in energy, mood, and concentration levels that you struggle with in your busy day.

- **Going keto will make you metabolically efficient such that you can survive, and thrive, on fewer calories** over the course of your lifetime. This may boost your longevity more than any other single lifestyle practice.

Right about now, you might be thinking that a life of fasting, skipping meals, and swearing off desserts, sweetened beverages, and even the grain-based comfort foods that are cultural centerpieces around the world might not seem like much fun; or that eating less food can't actually bring more health and even more enjoyment of food. After all, we've been programmed to believe—incorrectly—that building a fast metabolism (by exercising like crazy and taking care to eat regular meals and frequent snacks) is the key to weight control and high-energy living. It is indeed time to completely reframe your beliefs about the role of food in your metabolic function, and start to consider an empowering new philosophy of enjoying more (energy, concentration, peak performance) from less (total calories, and especially way fewer carbohydrate calories).

> **Building a fast metabolism as a health goal is completely flawed—accelerated metabolic function accelerates aging.**

Serious exercisers have long had the ethos of: "If the furnace is hot enough, anything will burn." If you put in the hard miles or hours, you earn a free pass at the buffet table to eat as much as you want. Believe me, I worshipped the party line! Decades after writing my first training book, I still take ribbing for my description of the evening meal that fueled my best-ever marathon race the following day: three beers, a bag of frozen peas, and a half-gallon of rocky road ice cream. Oh, and a joint for dessert—pretty much all that was around my bachelor pad on that occasion.

Today, we've made embarrassingly little progress on the "furnace will burn" mentality to the extent that even serious athletes who train 10 or 20 hours a week still carry an extra 10 or 20 pounds of body fat. One disturbing study revealed that 30 percent of the participants in the Cape Town (South Africa) Marathon were classified as overweight or obese. This is about the same percentage of the world's population in general, meaning the physical appearance of the participants in a 26.2-mile marathon race is indistinguishable from that of the spectators. Something's wrong with that picture!

The counterintuitive idea that exercise doesn't contribute directly to weight loss has now been scientifically validated, and is known as the *compensation theory*. Calories burned during workouts stimulate a requisite increase in appetite, along with generally increased laziness and diminished dietary self-discipline throughout the day because of your workout. If you've ever done a lively 40-minute Spinning class (burns ~600 calories) and then dropped by Jamba Juice to grab a large Banana Berry Smoothie and a small Kind Fruit&Nut bar afterward (delivers around 600 calories, including over 100 grams of carbs), you have actualized the compensation theory. Compensation happens both consciously ("I ran 10 miles this morning, so I deserve a hot fudge sundae tonight") and subconsciously—defaulting to elevators instead of stairs; reaching again and again into the abyss of the ice cream pint container until it's empty; or spending your leisure hours sprawled out on the couch as a consequence of exhausting workouts. The more strenuously or chronically you train, the more you may eat and the lazier you may feel when not working out.

> **Going keto allows you to thrive on fewer calories; this may boost your longevity more than any other practice.**

Born to Burn Fat

Losing excess bodyweight is simply not about balancing calories consumed with calories burned but, rather, about what I like to describe as *metabolic efficiency, metabolic flexibility,* or *hormone optimization*. These are all just fancy ways of saying that you will reprogram your genes to burn fat and ketones instead of sugar as your primary fuel source; and optimizing your appetite and satiety hormones so that you are rarely hungry and can subsist just fine when you skip meals. Furthermore, when you ditch the nutrient-devoid grains, sugars, and bad oils (some estimates suggest that two-thirds of the total calories in the Standard American Diet come from these "edible food-like substances," as author Michael Pollan likes to say) in favor of nutrient-dense primal fare (meat, fish, fowl, eggs, vegetables, fruits, nuts and seeds, and moderate amounts of high-fat dairy and high-cacao dark chocolate), your meals and snacks deliver satisfaction at the deepest hormonal and cellular levels. Wholesome, nutrient-dense foods give your brain's appetite center what it's been searching a lifetime for!

In carbohydrate dependency, you will have to eat significantly more calories over the course of your lifetime, because you can't burn stored energy well. You'll also require a fairly rigid schedule of external feedings to sustain energy, which fosters the aforementioned accelerated cell division, oxidation, inflammation, and a significant speeding up of the aging process that we unfortunately view as normal today (i.e., our organisms are built to live to 120, but we're content to make it to 80). When you recalibrate your metabolic machinery to become fully fat- and keto-adapted, as you will do with your 21-Day Metabolism Reset followed by your foray into nutritional ketosis, you will be able to gracefully burn stored energy whenever you need it, almost never feel hungry, avoid the mood and energy level swings that come from being on the glucose-insulin roller coaster, and avoid the patterns of disease and decline caused by overfeeding.

When you become metabolically efficient through fat- and keto-adaptation, life gets more awesome because food finally becomes one of the great pleasures of life that it's intended to be. You'll be able to groove with a pattern of eating when you're truly hungry, and enjoy the heck out of rich, deeply satisfying and nourishing meals and snacks (flip to Chapter 12 to get a sneak preview of over 100 delicious keto meals). Also, you'll break free of the destructive psycho-emotional consequences of having your moods and energy levels beholden to readily available meals and snacks. This is absolutely huge for anyone who has struggled with calorie obsession, willpower shortcomings, or body image. If you don't cop to having issues in these areas, I'd argue that just about every one of us has an unhealthy relationship with food at some level. Besides, developing the ability to generate and sustain energy without food is empowering and liberating for anyone.

Inside your fat- and keto-adapted body, more good things are happening. You burn fuel with great efficiency (and minimal free radical production), autophagy keeps your cells safe and high-functioning, and you produce only the minimal amount of insulin necessary to deliver needed nutrients to muscles and organs throughout the body.

Does Your (Metabolic) Factory Really Need That Cheesecake?

In contrast to the intense and deeply satisfying cellular nourishment provided by wholesome foods, processed foods and sweets deliver an intense initial burst of pleasurable flavor going down the hatch—and that's it. The ensuing glucose spike, insulin flood, oxidative stress, inflammatory and autoimmune responses throw you unceremoniously out of homeostasis. Your systems react with alarm to get things back in order, but crying wolf too often leads inevitably to burnout. Over time, you trend toward the epidemic conditions of metabolic syndrome, Type 2 diabetes, cancer, and cognitive diseases that are now being strongly associated with junk-food consumption. Also, the more you indulge, the less you may notice the destruction caused by a crappy diet. You become desensitized to carbs in the same manner as a smoker or heavy drinker is desensitized to regular ingestion of these toxins. Your baseline is lousy but you don't know any better, because it's all you've ever known.

Believe me, I know as well as anyone else how delicious a hot fudge sundae, cheesecake, French toast, or other wonders of Americana taste—and how they serve as a cathartic release from the stress of daily life. In my case, because I cleaned up my diet and reprogrammed my genes away from carbohydrate dependency in 2002, my complete lemony cheesecake experience today includes not only the delicious bites going down but also the ensuing Lemony Snicket Series of Unfortunate Events: gas, bloating, headache, a fluttery heartbeat, and difficulty falling asleep.

While it might seem frightening to consider ditching your go-to indulgences forever and ever, some good things happen when you elevate your commitment to clean eating. First, your perspective broadens to the big picture of unfortunate events, adding a little more reason and deliberation to the impulsive decisions that allow grain staples, exotic sweetened beverages, and desserts into your diet. Second, when the time is right and you make the thoughtful decision to indulge, you discover that a little goes a very long way. Owing to your heightened standards and sensitivity, sweet stuff tastes so much sweeter that you're all good after a couple bites or sips.

Lifespan Is Graded on a Curve

The metabolic efficiency attributes of fasting and fat- and keto-adaptation are extremely important for health and longevity—something that has become a crusade for longevity physician Peter Attia, M.D., who practices in San Diego and New York City, and is an accomplished ultra-endurance swimmer and cyclist known for performing extreme metabolic self-experiments, which he chronicles in detail at eatingacademy.com. Attia maintained a state of strict nutritional ketosis for over three years (*averaging* 1.8 mmol/L over his hundreds of measurings), and showed the power of diet to transform fuel substrate utilization (ratio of carbs to fat burned) during endurance exercise. Attia explains that his all-time dream longevity strategy would be to produce an optimally minimal amount of insulin to keep your cells nourished with energy. Consequently, you spare your system the oxidation, inflammation, and accelerated cell division characterized by hyperinsulinemia (chronically high levels of insulin in the bloodstream). Attia's fondness for optimally minimal insulin levels aligns with the truth that across all species, the individuals who produce the least amount of insulin generally live the longest.

While insulin patterns are essentially impossible to measure outside of long-term confinement to a hospital bed, you can get an idea of your insulin fitness by conducting a glucose tolerance test that is often given to those with, or at high risk for, diabetes. Here, you measure fasting blood glucose levels, drink a disgustingly sticky substance that is pure glucose, and then take further glucose readings at regular intervals. In daily life, what you are looking for is a moderate fasting glucose level and a tight regulation of glucose after meals. Attia had a continuous glucose monitor surgically implanted in his abdomen to deliver real-time glucose values to his smartphone. He maintains a baseline fasting glucose in the mid-80s and a standard deviation of around 10. For reference, an acceptable fasting baseline level is 100, and it's undesirable to exceed 125, even after meals. Failing a high-tech implant or a physician-ordered test, you can get a portable handheld glucose and ketone monitor on the Internet and start tracking your values to quantify the benefits that will be obvious: rarely feeling hungry, skipping meals and still feeling great, and so forth. We cover tracking and testing in detail in the Appendix.

The essence of longevity is to thrive, hormonally and metabolically, on as few calories as possible without feeling hungry. Chronic overfeeding and excess insulin production are the essence of accelerated aging.

If you are interested in living a long healthy, happy life, you may want to reframe your perspective away from "How many calories can I stuff down without getting too fat?" to something more along the lines of "How can I become more metabolically efficient, so I can thrive, and achieve total dietary satisfaction, on a minimal amount of calories?" Ketogenic eating can be extremely satisfying owing to the high fat content and the moderation of your appetite hormones such that you are less hungry and can actually thrive, hormonally and metabolically speaking, on fewer calories without feeling hungry. This is the essence of optimum health, stable energy, low body fat, maximum enjoyment of life, and longevity—with no sacrificing or suffering.

Perhaps you are of the mindset that life is short, so you might as well enjoy as much food, fun, and laughter as you can before your time is up? Well, the latter two promote longevity just like keto! However, when you are constantly well-fed to overfed (because, remember, you suck at burning stored energy, so you are highly reliant on regular meals to keep the flame burning), and stimulate chronically excessive insulin production (because your regular feedings are high in carbohydrate, per conventional wisdom recommendation for a "heart healthy," "high energy" diet), this represents the essence of accelerated aging and increased disease risk.

Chronically high glucose and insulin promote a condition known as *systemic inflammation,* which health experts are increasingly realizing represents the root cause of virtually all forms of disease and dysfunction in the body, particularly autoimmune conditions, heart disease, and cancer. A high glucose–high insulin eating pattern also causes mitochondria to atrophy and/or become dysfunctional, leaving you more vulnerable to oxidative damage from free radicals; and triggers a chemical reaction known as *glycation,* whereby excess glucose molecules bind to important structural proteins throughout the body and inflict long-term damage. The body's longest lasting cells—brain, cardiovascular system, eyes, kidney, and skin—are the most vulnerable to glycation. This is why diabetics (they are poor at regulating glucose) frequently have vision and kidney problems, and why wrinkles are reflective of aging. Hardened arteries and the senile plaques and neuro-fibrallary tangles of Alzheimer's disease are also reflective of the damage caused by glycation.

Jamba-Fasting, Mon!

The metabolic efficiency of fasting and keto is important to keep in mind in light of the incredible popularity these days of "green" juices and smoothies. When you squeeze liquid out of fresh fruits and veggies, you will indeed get a ton of antioxidants, phytonutrients, and vitamins, but you will also get an offensive bomb of sugar, and a consequent surge of insulin. As you know, the glucose and insulin will dysregulate your appetite and fat-storage hormones in the hours afterward. If you make green drinks a daily habit, the lauded micronutrient benefits may be snuffed out by the glycation, oxidation, and inflammation caused by slamming your system with too much glucose and insulin regularly.

Fasting quietly at home might not be as sexy as stopping by the lively juice bar to enjoy a morning shot with like-minded health enthusiasts, but fasting reduces inflammation, increases internal antioxidant production, and generally helps you burn caloric energy with less free radical production. Instead of a green sugar bomb, consider obtaining your plant nutrients from whole-food sources. This will minimize the glucose spike, allow you to enjoy the benefits of prebiotic fiber, and activate more digestive enzymes, because you are chewing your food. If you really want to obtain a concentrated source of green nutrition, at least prepare a smoothie with a better macronutrient balance than the high-carbohydrate store offerings. Use full-fat coconut milk as your liquid, throw your kale, spinach, or other favorite greens in the blender, add a bit of whey protein powder, and consider tossing in a high-fat avocado (after all, it's green!). This will give you a more nutritionally balanced and satisfying meal experience.

Another option is to enjoy a ketone supplement as a stand-in for your nutrient-dense green drink. If you just mix one of the powdered products (an overview of ketone supplements is provided in the Appendix) in warm or cold water to start your day, you enjoy a potent anti-inflammatory and neuro-enhancing effect.

The Evolution of Ketone Burning

Our ability to effortlessly manufacture and burn internal sources of energy was a key component of survival for 2.5 million years of human evolution. When our ancestors lacked a consistent supply of dietary calories (which was often), they were able to easily burn stored body fat as their main source of energy, fuel their brain function with ketones instead of glucose, recycle amino acids to build or maintain muscle, and even convert certain amino acids into glucose when they needed a quick emergency energy source, via a process called *gluconeogenesis*. Latin for "making new sugar," gluconeogenesis is a metabolic process, occurring mostly in the liver, that results in the generation of glucose from ingested or stored amino acids. It is a fundamental component of the fight-or-flight response (along with assorted other stress hormones that temporarily elevate the function of all body systems), that kicks in when we have to run for our lives—or any modern-day peak-performance equivalent (think: presentation in front of the boss, argument with a loved one, traffic jam making you late to the ballgame, the baby crying before bedtime, and all the other chronic situations in our hectic daily schedule).

Besides the triggering of gluconeogenesis as a response to stressful life events, we also make sugar too frequently because we are terrible at burning fat. When we get the energy/concentration/mood decline and the appetite spike between (high-carb) meals, and the fat is locked away in storage due to hyperinsulinemia, we either seek more quick-energy carbs to eat or we trigger gluconeogenesis to fuel brain and muscles that are starving—literally, because insulin levels are too high to allow access to stored body fat or for the liver to generate ketones. Obviously, the fight-or-flight response is designed for use in emergencies only; and glucose, as a scarce and dirty-burning fuel, was never meant to be a prominent human fuel source day after day. Abusing the delicate fight-or-flight survival mechanisms and suffering blood sugar swings throughout the day are stressful and destructive to health in many ways, and result in the familiar condition known as burnout. Over the long term, being a carbohydrate-dependent sugar-burner has serious inflammatory, oxidative, catabolic, immune-suppressing, and accelerated aging effects.

> **Glucose is a scarce and dirty-burning fuel; it was never meant to be the predominant human fuel source.**

Our ancestors knew none of these carb dependency troubles because they would not have survived routine periods of mild or severe famine periods as sugar-burners. Consider that dietary carbohydrate availability and intake in primal times were only fractions of today's norms; that we can only store 400 to 600 grams of glycogen (the storage form of glucose) in the liver and muscles (by comparison to the pounds of fat and tens of thousands of fat calories even the leanest humans have in storage); and that there are assorted adverse health consequences to being a sugar-burner. Our *Homo sapiens* genes are programmed to use gluconeogenesis-derived glucose as emergency fight-or-flight fuel, or to occasionally binge on dietary carbs (i.e., fruit in narrow ripening seasons). Yes, we really did evolve a sweet tooth, and an efficient system of converting carbs into fat and storing them—to help us fatten up in preparation for the scarcity of calories in the winter, and then access and burn stored sources of energy (i.e., fat and ketones) for as long as necessary.

It's a scientific fact that carbohydrates are not required for human survival, and that humans can and have survived for long periods eating little to no carbohydrates. That said, there are many wonderful benefits to eating nutritious sources of carbs—namely, abundant intake of fresh, colorful, high-antioxidant vegetables; sensible intake of seasonal fruits and starchy vegetables like sweet potatoes; and responsible consumption of incidental carbs present in nutritious foods like nuts and seeds, high-fat dairy products, and high-cacao percentage dark chocolate.

Often, our ancestors weren't so fortunate as to obtain sufficient nutritious carbohydrate sources, but they needed a steady supply of glucose to preserve sharp cognitive function—a matter of life or death in primal times. Consequently, we evolved a reliable and efficient backup source of glucose-like brain fuel in the form of ketones, which we manufactured and burned any time dietary carbohydrate and insulin levels were low.

Our preference for fat- and ketone-burning is hardwired into our genetics and available for our enjoyment any time we want to tap into it, but we have unknowingly rejected the legacy of our ancestors in favor of carbohydrate dependency—and all the health and waistline complications that go along with it. Fat- and ketone-burning went out of style in conjunction with the gradual advent of grain-based civilization, which started in modern-day Egypt around 7,000 years ago and occurred independently around the globe, up until North America finally became civilized around 4,500 years ago.

After a couple million years of existence as hunter-gatherers, we suddenly transitioned into a civilized life based on the cultivation of grains and later livestock. The introduction of agriculture afforded humans a long-term, reliable source of calories, so we could live in permanent settlements, develop specialized labor, and progress inexorably toward an ever more advanced society. This represented the most dramatic lifestyle shift in the history of humanity.

While civilization represented progress in comparison to the primitive and often harsh existence of primal hunter-gatherers, it has actually come at great expense to human health. For the past 7,000 years, humans have lived in a state of carbohydrate dependency, which is a severe affront to our genetic factory setting as fat-burning hunter-gatherers. A grain-based high-carbohydrate diet basically overrides the elegant and highly efficient fat- and keto-adaptation of our ancestors, and forces us to rely on external sources of calories for energy.

This may be review, but you need to "own" this story: The ingestion of carbohydrates, especially the refined grains and sugars that are so prominent in the modern diet, causes a spike in blood sugar and a temporary energy boost. Then, because a glucose overdose is toxic in the bloodstream, insulin floods the bloodstream to remove any glucose you don't burn immediately and stores it as either glycogen (in the liver and muscle tissues) or in the fat cells as triglyceride (the storage form of fat). When insulin removes glucose from your bloodstream and transports it into storage, you experience the familiar sugar crash and a craving for quick-energy carbohydrates. You have plenty of fat energy locked away in storage, but a high-insulin-producing diet prevents you from being able to access it. Instead, you become reliant on your next snack or meal for energy, and you exist in a state of carbohydrate dependency.

A high-carbohydrate, high-insulin-producing diet leads to daily fluctuations in energy, appetite, and mood; lifelong insidious accumulation of excess body fat (because you are bad at burning fat and are really good at storing fat, due to chronically excessive insulin production); a state of chronic inflammation in the body; and widespread cellular damage from glycation. Chronic inflammation, glycation, and oxidative damage are the essence of epidemic disease and accelerated aging in modern life.

> **Chronic inflammation, glycation, and oxidative damage are the essence of epidemic disease and accelerated aging.**

The good news is that you can recalibrate your metabolic machinery to become fat- and keto-adapted in a relatively short time, even if you have spent decades in carbohydrate dependency. It requires a careful and patient approach through the progressions laid out in this book, but everything is customizable (especially your pace proceeding toward going keto) to ensure that you will not only succeed with major dietary transformation but that you will enjoy every moment of it.

Keto vs. Carbo . . . Whoa!

By the time you read this book, I'm confident that you will have a strong understanding of the science and the metabolic flow of fat- and ketone-burning versus carbohydrate dependency. It's especially important to understand what's happening in your liver, the control tower for energy processing and distribution throughout your body. The liver secretes bile to help break down fats in the small intestine; detoxifies the bloodstream from alcohol, drugs, or other harmful substances; converts excess ingested carbohydrates into fat and processes excess ingested protein into glucose for energy or into the waste product ammonia; and manufactures ketones under the special circumstances of fasting or keto-aligned eating.

Dr. Peter Attia calls the liver the "ergostat appetite organ," meaning that the liver is sensing what nutrients you need in your bloodstream at all times and is delivering just the right amounts. It's sobering, literally, to reflect on the liver's exquisite regulation of blood glucose within an incredibly tight range at all times. Our optimal circulating glucose level is only around 5 *grams* (a teaspoon) within a total blood volume of around 1.5 *gallons* (5.5 liters) of blood. If the liver were to screw up and dump too little or too much glucose into the bloodstream, you'd quickly drop to the ground and lapse into a diabetic coma from hypoglycemia or hyperglycemia. The constant life-or-death peak performance delivered by your liver might make you think twice about consuming excessive carbohydrates or alcohol, for these agents are confirmed to tax the liver and wear it out over time.

In the typical, modern human carbohydrate-dependency eating pattern, your liver will fight valiantly under adverse circumstances to keep your energy balanced—until finally it succumbs to insulin resistance (your cells become resistant to the signaling of insulin, owing to chronically excessive levels) and you end up with Type 2 diabetes. In a fat- and keto-adapted eating pattern, you allow your liver to really shine. Energy to the brain and body is readily available, and there is no wasted energy or inflammation from excess caloric intake and hormonal imbalances. Let's compare and contrast what happens in the liver with a carbohydrate-dependency eating and lifestyle pattern versus a fat- and keto-adapted eating and lifestyle pattern. Yes, "lifestyle" gets a plug here, too, because chronic exercise, insufficient sleep, and a high-stress daily routine can push you into carb dependency nearly as much as can your food consumption.

Carb-Dependency Pattern

The liver is overwhelmed each day with excess glucose ingestion (and often too much protein as well), prompting excess insulin production (which overwhelms the pancreas, too.) Here's the accordant metabolic chain of events:

1. Liver glycogen stores (around 100 grams) are usually full. Muscle glycogen stores (around 500 grams) are usually full, too; if they're not full after a tough workout, they get refilled quickly from a carb addict's recovery feasts and snack binges over the course of the day.

2. Some of the carbs you eat are burned immediately by the brain and muscles, while the rest are quickly removed from the bloodstream, converted into triglycerides in the liver, and transported into fat cells for storage.

3. Excess protein is either converted into glucose or excreted, stressing the liver and kidneys and overstimulating growth factors (details shortly).

4. Low blood glucose levels (insulin took all those carbs out of your bloodstream, remember?) trigger intense cravings for food, particularly sugar. Meanwhile, elevated insulin levels prevent triglycerides from being mobilized into free fatty acid energy.

5. The cycle repeats with a pit stop for quick-burning, low-octane glucose, with the excess being locked away in fat cells and unavailable for use. *Ketones?* Didn't they sing a hit song in the 50s?

Fat- and Keto-Adapted Pattern

Fasting or high-fat, moderate-protein, very low carbohydrate eating patterns have glucose, insulin, and liver glycogen levels optimized. Here's the accordant metabolic chain of events:

1. Carb intake is ultra-low, in comparison to carbohydrate-dependent eating patterns. Protein intake is optimized—just enough to maintain homeostasis and lean body mass, with no excess.

2. With fat (either consumed or from storage) being the most prominent metabolized fuel, ketones (and a little bit of glucose) are manufactured in the liver as a by-product of fat oxidation (burning fat for energy). Ketones and glucose serve the high caloric demands of the brain. Muscles burn mostly fatty acids, some ketones, and a little glucose (from their stored glycogen).

How Did Low-Carb, and Then Keto, Get So Popular?

When I started blogging at MarksDailyApple.com in 2006, the concept of primal/paleo/low-carb eating was completely fringe and wacky—dismissed out of hand by medical and diet experts as flat-out dangerous. After decades entrenched in conventional wisdom, everybody from school kids to registered dieticians to personal trainers to family doctors could recite the mantras that fat and cholesterol were our mortal enemies, and that a grain-based, high-carbohydrate diet was the key to peak performance, weight control, and a long, healthy, happy life. Pioneers in the evolutionary health scene like Dr. Boyd Eaton (author of *The Paleolithic Prescription,* 1988), Dr. Loren Cordain (author of *The Paleo Diet,* 2002), and Dr. Art DeVany (early 2000s blogger and author of *The New Evolution Diet*, 2011) were excitedly uncovering and communicating the secrets of our hunter-gatherer past and our human genetic "factory setting" as fat-burning beasts, but only a select few were listening. Fortunately, the most open-minded among us, along with perhaps the most desperate among us (those particularly sensitive to assorted health consequences of eating gluten, sugar, and refined polyunsaturated vegetable oils), started to succeed wildly by rejecting the Standard American Diet in favor of an evolution-based eating strategy—namely, eating abundant plants (vegetables, fruits, nuts, and seeds) and animals, including the high-fat, high-cholesterol animal products we'd been admonished to stay away from (high-fat meats, including organs, along with eggs, butter, and bacon).

While the photos, videos, and social media blasting of early primal/paleo adopters came into mainstream prominence, respected scientific and medical evidence (Framingham Heart Study, Nurses Health Study, and many more studies presenting large-scale, bulletproof evidence) accumulated. Refined carbohydrates (grains and sugars) and refined high polyunsaturated vegetable oils were correctly identified as the mortal enemy of modern society and the proximate cause of obesity, heart disease, and many other mild to serious health complaints.

Leaky gut syndrome, previously not acknowledged in mainstream medicine, has become a prominent topic of discussion and study. In sensitive people, ingestion of gluten and other toxic lectin proteins can damage the delicate brush borders (*microvilli*) that line our small intestines. This allows larger, undigested protein molecules to enter the bloodstream (via the "leaky gut," a.k.a. intestinal permeability) and trigger an inflammatory autoimmune response. People struggling with digestive disturbances like gas, bloating, irritable bowel syndrome, colitis, constipation, Crohn's disease, and celiac disease, as well as inflammatory autoimmune conditions throughout the body, such as arthritis, asthma, acne, polycystic ovarian syndrome, and even autism and ADHD, have ditched grains (especially those containing gluten) and have experienced immediate, miraculous cures for what were lifelong health conditions.

Slowly but surely over the past decade, the credibility of conventional wisdom's grain-based, high-carbohydrate, fat-phobic diet has been destroyed, and a refreshing new movement has gained momentum. For the most part, the fundamental principles of evolutionary health have become widely accepted and validated—at least among well educated and open-minded health enthusiasts and health professionals. Granted, we still have a long way to go to overhaul government dietary policy, change the minds of those who earn their living peddling carbohydrate dependency, or help the average Joe who allows the advertising messages of fast-food and processed-food conglomerates to dictate his food choices.

There will be a sobering battle royal in the years to come. In one corner we have billions of dollars of corporate marketing muscle, hanging on to their sugar, bread, and margarine revenue streams by an ever more frayed rope. In the other corner we have an informed and enlightened segment of the population, disgusted by the massive financial costs and lost productivity of a fat, sick, carbohydrate-addicted general population. Diabetes alone afflicts 30 million Americans, with 86 million more diagnosed as pre-diabetic, together costing the United States $322 billion annually.

Fortunately, the information age allows good news to travel quickly and with great impact, and so the evolutionary-based eating and lifestyle principles have developed a tremendous hard-core base and an ever-growing reach into mainstream society. Thought leaders are finally getting their due, after resolutely swimming against the current for years, even decades. Dr. Phil Maffetone, the original fat-burning endurance coach and author of *The Big Book of Endurance Training and Racing,* has been advocating fat-adapted endurance training since the 1970s. Now his training and dietary principles, including his important calculation of "MAF heart rate" (stands for Maximum Aerobic Function, but also an ode to his last name) have become endurance lexicon.

Dr. Dominic D'Agostino, a researcher and world record–setting strength athlete from the University of South Florida (ketonutrition.org), has been generating breakthrough research about druglike therapeutic benefits of ketone burning (through both nutritional ketosis and supplement use) for cognitive and neurological disorders, cancer protection, athletic performance, and special applications of the neuro-protective benefits applicable to Navy SEAL divers and NASA astronauts preparing for a LEO (low earth orbit) mission.

Dr. Peter Attia (eatingacademy.com) is a San Diego physician who applies a multi-faceted approach to fight obesity and diabetes on the front lines; he is a thought leader in longevity and peak athletic performance, and a notorious extreme self-experimenter whose carefully chronicled cycling experiments have proven the profound benefits of fat- and ketone-burning for endurance performance.

Dr. Cate Shanahan, a family-practice physician from Connecticut, author of the acclaimed *Deep Nutrition,* and Los Angeles Lakers nutrition director who specializes in medically supervised weight loss through evolutionary-based eating, is lauded for her passionate crusade against refined high polyunsaturated vegetable oils and sugar. Her results with everyday patients, as well as elite professional athletes, and her ability to operate in both the traditional medical world and the progressive evolutionary health world make her a respected thought leader to a broad audience.

Luis Villasenor, a Mexico City–based personal trainer, bodybuilder, and power lifter, has been ketogenic for 16 years and counting! He has competed at a high level in explosive sports and helped thousands of clients drop excess body fat, and get healthier and stronger using a whole foods approach and context-modified ketogenic diet protocols. His thriving community at ketogains.com offers a great blend of scientific commentary and user experience.

While keto may be the latest hot dietary topic, the ketogenic diet has been around for nearly 100 years. It was developed in 1924 by Dr. Russell Wilder at the Mayo Clinic, who discovered that drug-resistant seizures could be managed with amazing effectiveness when patients adhered to an extremely low carbohydrate and moderate-protein eating pattern. In recent years, the ketogenic eating strategy has come into mainstream prominence owing to the profound and wide-ranging health, peak performance, and disease protection benefits it offers.

Thanks to the survival-of-the-fittest circumstances of evolution, the *Homo sapiens* genetic "factory setting" is one of metabolic flexibility, but our current lifestyle and eating habits have made us carbohydrate dependent, and have brought epidemic health problems like obesity and Type 2 diabetes as natural consequences. When you go keto, you are returning to your genetic setting for optimal health and longevity and are unwinding years, maybe decades, of metabolic damage caused by grain-based, high-carbohydrate eating patterns.

CHAPTER 3

The Health, Performance, and Disease Protection Benefits of Keto

SINCE my awakening to the rationale and principles of ancestral-style eating around 15 years ago, it quickly became crystal clear to me that humans were not meant for a grain-based, high-carbohydrate diet. Even before the dawn of the large-scale primal/paleo/ancestral health movement over a decade ago, the Atkins diet generated outstanding weight-loss success when people ditched the carbs and emphasized fat to the extent of entering ketosis. Unfortunately, Atkins flopped in time, seemingly due to a combination of significant flaws in the programming, PR faux-pas, and the fickle nature of the diet industry. But Atkins not only faded, it was also thrown onto the trash heap, derided as downright dangerous by mainstream medical, nutrition, and health practitioners who were stuck in the flawed carbohydrate paradigm.

The demise of Atkins—and the accordant, too brief cameo for the concept of ketosis for fat loss—is a great sociological example of how cultural forces like conventional wisdom can throw the baby out with the bathwater. The rudimentary approach of the Atkins diet indeed deserved critique, because its myopic emphasis on macronutrient ratios often resulted in people neglecting nutritional quality in favor of merely sticking to the designated fat, protein, and carb ratios. Giving a green light to snacking on highly processed pork rinds laden with chemicals and toxic vegetable oils might rightfully be viewed as a PR disaster for any diet or weight-loss program. However, the foundational biochemistry of Atkins—reduce carb intake, lower insulin, shed excess body fat—was accurate. The thought leaders in the ancestral movement knew this, and were familiar with the metabolic process of ketosis, but the concept was forgotten like a buried treasure for years. Frankly, I'll admit keto was an afterthought in comparison to the compelling goal of battling the conventional wisdom to transition people away from a grain-based diet. In the original 2009 publication of my book *The Primal Blueprint,* I referred to ketosis very briefly—as something you use on occasion for rapid fat loss.

Upon reflection at today's morbid rates of obesity in the western world, rapid and guaranteed fat loss is reason alone to take a closer look at ketosis. Today, with more science validating the epigenetic signaling effects of ketosis, the anti-inflammatory effects rivaling prescription drugs, and the mind-blowing potential for athletes to become bonk-proof through keto, I believe keto is poised to become the default dietary strategy for any open-minded, forward-thinking health enthusiast. I don't necessarily mean you should stay permanently in ketosis (although for some people this might be the best choice), but engaging in distinct periods of nutritional ketosis and eating a keto-friendly diet overall is an excellent way to drop fat on demand, promote athletic peak performance, and lower your risk of disease. My good friend Dr. Doug McGuff, emergency room physician and author of *The Primal Prescription* and *Body by Science,* assured me that ancestral health principles will one day be embraced by all, but that it would likely take 20 years, owing to the slow-moving "beast" that is mainstream health and medicine. And to that, Doug adds, "Personally, I don't want to wait that long." How about you? Let's dive into the wide-ranging benefits of keto right now!

Keto and Fat Loss

Perhaps the most immediate and dramatic benefit of ketogenic eating is the opportunity for quick and efficient reduction of excess body fat and easy, long-term maintenance of your ideal body composition. Ketogenic eating stabilizes appetite hormones, upregulates the metabolic processes that prioritize fat burning, and delivers a high satiety factor owing to the high fat composition of keto-friendly meals and snacks. Ketogenic eating can make you an efficient fat-burning machine. When you are in full-blown keto, you enjoy complete dietary satisfaction, rarely feel hungry (even if you skip meals!), and never have to struggle, suffer, restrict calories, or force strenuous workouts in order to burn extra calories. Instead, you allow your genetic setting as a fat-burning beast to naturally calibrate you to a healthy body composition. You will be able to properly utilize tools like Intermittent Fasting, nutritional ketosis, and ketone supplements to drop excess body fat whenever you want, without a struggle or a second thought.

While it's a literal truth—the law of thermodynamics—that you must burn more calories than you store to lose excess body fat, the secret is not burning extra calories through exercise while painstakingly restricting dietary calories. It's been scientifically validated that calories burned during exercise lead to a corresponding increase in appetite and a decrease in general physical activity. These dynamics are especially true for the chronic exercise patterns that desperate dieters engage in. The secret to reducing excess body fat is in *hormone optimization*—being a fat- and ketone-burner instead of a carbohydrate- or sugar-burner. When you eat keto, you correct the wildly excessive insulin production that is endemic to the Standard American Diet, since fat becomes your readily available fuel source around the clock.

In contrast, a high insulin–producing eating pattern shuts off fat burning and forces you to rely on ingested calories as your primary energy source. It starts disastrously with breakfast, the "most important meal of the day . . . *to not screw up*," says Dr. Cate Shanahan. At your highfalutin corporate retreat at the Ritz-Carlton, your "Healthy Start" breakfast buffet features fresh berries, low-fat Greek yogurt, homemade granola, low-fat banana-nut bread with apple butter, raisin bran muffins, steel-cut Irish oatmeal (with brown sugar, raisins, and pecans), orange or cranberry juice, and coffee. If you are conscientious and serve yourself moderate portions, you'll still consume at least 100 grams of carbohydrates and possibly up to 200 grams—more than our ancestors might have consumed over several days. And you'll be out 36 bucks. Seriously.

You'll burn some of this energy off right away (generating inflammation and free radicals in the process), then prompt a flood of insulin into your bloodstream to store as fat (in the form of triglycerides) any excess glucose that you don't burn right away. When insulin removes glucose from your bloodstream in the hours after your Healthy Start, you will become lethargic and start to feel hungry for lunch. You'll have another high-carbohydrate binge (yes, binge; because low blood sugar triggers a fight-or-flight reaction that causes you to overeat and your hormones to more likely direct those extra calories into storage as fat—all to protect you from the perceived life-or-death matter of low blood sugar). When you repeat this high-carbohydrate, high insulin–producing eating pattern day after day for the rest of your life, you'll contribute to the statistic that the average American gains 1.5 pounds ($^2/_3$ kilo) of body fat (and loses a half pound ($^1/_3$ kilo) of muscle each year from the ages of 25 to 55. If you fast or eat a keto-aligned meal for breakfast, none of this story happens. Instead, you sail along burning the clean fuels of fat (either from a meal or from storage), ketones, and an optimally minimal amount of glucose.

General Health and Disease Protection

It feels awesome to finally reach and attain your ideal body composition through keto, but the most life-altering benefits come from the profound ability of ketones to influence gene expression and cellular function throughout the body. Of particular interest is how keto might help you avoid the increasingly prevalent cognitive diseases and cancers that are becoming ever more closely linked with diet.

Anti-Inflammatory

Dr. Steven Phinney and Dr. Jeff Volek, early researchers of fat-adapted endurance training over 30 years ago and the co-authors of *The Art and Science of Low Carbohydrate Living,* cite research suggesting that ketones deliver an anti-inflammatory effect more potent than prescription drugs. This anti-inflammatory effect can particularly benefit age-related chronic diseases, autoimmune conditions, and colon cancer. While acute inflammation is a desirable element of your physiologic response to stress such as exercise demands (your muscles pump up to lift a weight or sprint to the finish line), uncontrolled chronic, system-wide inflammation is a sign that your body is battling adverse lifestyle practices such as poor nutrition, overly stressful exercise patterns, or insufficient sleep. You could categorize every lifestyle practice or food you eat as either promoting undesirable inflammation or helping you control inflammation.

You have likely heard the lauded anti-inflammatory benefits of omega-3 fatty acids. Beta-hydroxybutyrate, one of the two ketone bodies that your body produces along with acetoacetate (they both break down into acetone, so technically there are three types of ketones), disrupts the assembly of inflammatory processes inside your cells. This is essentially nipping inflammation in the bud before it has a chance to cause havoc throughout your body. Ketones are especially beneficial to your brain, which is most vulnerable to the damaging effects of inflammation. Conditions of cognitive decline such as Alzheimer's, dementia, ADHD, and autism are all characterized by inflammation and poor oxygen delivery to the brain (details shortly).

Antioxidant and Immune Function

Ketone burning upregulates the production of internal antioxidant enzymes like catalase, glutathione, and superoxide dismutase (SOD). These enzymes have extremely potent and wide-ranging effects in the body. They help protect against inflammation and oxidative stress caused by intense exercise, eating bad foods, and simply breathing air and burning calories. Having a powerful internal antioxidant system will boost immunity, delay aging, and protect you from cancer, neurological decline, and other degenerative diseases. SOD is particularly effective in keeping your skin looking healthy and youthful; SOD binds directly to collagen, preserving its elasticity and protecting it from the free radical damage that causes skin to wrinkle and sag. High glutathione levels are highly predictive of longevity, because this substance protects cells from the degeneration that leads to assorted diseases, especially cognitive conditions.

Ketogenic eating improves immune function in assorted other ways, such as the aforementioned promotion of autophagy (the natural cellular repair and detoxification process) and optimization of mitochondrial function (resulting in less free radical production when you burn caloric energy). Immune function is also enhanced when you transition from carb dependent to fat adapted, because you minimize the emergency production of gluconeogenesis as a component of the fight-or-flight response—something that happens every time a carbohydrate-dependent, high insulin–producing eater runs low on glucose. When you trigger fight-or-flight every time you experience an energy dip and you don't immediately slam more carbs, you significantly compromise immune function and many other aspects of general health. The immune system does its best work during downtime, such as your deep sleep cycles. Skimp on downtime with stressful blood sugar roller-coaster eating patterns or other stressful lifestyle practices, and your immune system skimps on its job. In contrast, when you are fat- and keto-adapted, your body rarely has to worry about making emergency conversions of amino acids into glucose, and all the energy systems of your body are able to exist in homeostatic balance.

Brain Function

As Dr. Dom D'Agostino relates, "Ketones readily cross the blood brain barrier and become a highly efficient energy source for the brain. Ketones promote elevated neurotransmitter and enzyme function such that your capacity to fire brain neurons increases, and you preserve that capacity better through increased oxygen delivery, reduced inflammation, and fewer reactive oxygen species generated." Enthusiasts report improved mental clarity and less brain fatigue when adhering to long-term nutritional ketosis eating patterns.

While your brain works more efficiently burning ketones, it also enjoys an enhanced level of protection against the breakdown that is characteristic of today's epidemic diseases of cognitive decline—diseases that are being increasingly associated with poor dietary habits. Beta-hydroxybutyrate has been found to deliver an assortment of neuro-protective benefits: it modulates a cell membrane receptor called hca2 that regulates inflammation; it helps preserve the GABA-to-glutamate ratio, which preserves brain homeostasis; and it prevents the activation of the mitochondrial "death switch" that results in the death of brain cells. This programmed cell death is known as *apoptosis,* and it can be undesirable—as in this brain cell example—and desirable, in the case of snuffing out dysfunctional or cancerous cells. Beta-hydroxybutyrate also has an anti-seizure effect because it raises the threshold at which mitochondria become deranged by a lack of oxygen, which is the trigger for a seizure. This is why the ketogenic diet has been a marvelously effective metabolic therapy for drug-resistant seizures for nearly a century.

Remember that your brain, since it cannot burn fat, is entirely reliant upon dirty-burning glucose—unless you make the sincere effort to serve up ketones as a cleaner, healthier option. In fact, impaired glucose metabolism is a hallmark of impaired brain function. This is why keto is particularly and profoundly beneficial for brain function. Even if you could care less about the athletic performance or weight-loss benefits of keto, protecting your brain from disease risk could be reason alone to overhaul your dietary habits and beliefs about food. The devastating loss in quality of life from mild cognitive impairment (MCI), dementia, Alzheimer's, Parkinson's, autism, and ADHD is now being seen as routine and also random, but it doesn't have to be. By simply eating keto, you can think and perform better in real time, and can achieve a drug-like neuro-protective effect against disease patterns.

The next time you have a headache, instead of popping an Advil, try a generous dose of supplemental ketones. According to Dr. D'Agostino, the enhanced oxygen delivery effects may bring immediate relief. Ketones even pass through the placenta to help provide the carbon atom foundation for fetal brain development. Here's the bottom line from Dr. D'Agostino: "When you burn ketones in your brain, you have less carbon coming out of the gas pipe and more horsepower coming out of the engine."

Cancer Fighting and Protection

Being in ketosis helps suppress the growth of cancer cells in numerous ways, most notably by starving cancer cells of glucose. Cancer cells thrive and proliferate by consuming glucose at a greater rate than regular cells. This unique metabolic behavior of cancer cells is known as the *Warburg Effect*, something that was discovered over 100 years ago by scientist Otto Warburg. It has long been known that fasting, calorie restriction, and ketogenic eating are effective metabolic therapies to reduce the availability of glucose for certain cancer cells, and serve as worthwhile complements to traditional chemotherapy and radiation to fight cancer. Only recently have studies appeared to suggest that fasting/keto benefits accrue not only from glucose restriction but also from the production of ketones. For example, beta-hydroxybutyrate is known to be an epigenetic modulator—able to influence the way genes are expressed throughout the body—and can play a role in preventing the expression of cancer-promoting genes.

Furthermore, when you lower insulin production through ketogenic eating, you produce the optimally minimum levels of prominent growth factors such as insulin growth factor (IGF-1) and mammalian target of rapamycin (mTOR). Minimizing growth factor stimulation supports the healthy functioning, repair, and motility of cells throughout the body, and makes for efficient protein synthesis and gene transcription. In contrast, when IGF-1 and mTOR are chronically elevated owing to excess carb intake and excess protein intake, you unnecessarily accelerate routine cellular functions. This leads to systemic inflammation, glycation, oxidative damage, insulin resistance, and ultimately accelerated aging. When growth factors are chronically elevated, you are more likely to have unregulated cellular activity that causes cancer, and more likely to have that cancer grow and spread to other areas of the body at an accelerated rate. Carbo loading and high-protein smoothies seem to be the default strategy for building huge guns in the gym; but they are not so great when you want to live a long, healthy life, fight cancer, or not get cancer in the first place. Furthermore, keto may be even more effective for muscle building and power gains than the traditional "overfeeding" approach to bodybuilding.

> **Chronic elevation of growth factors (from high-carb and high-protein eating patterns) accelerates aging and increases cancer risk.**

Someone with cancer who transitioned from a standard high-carbohydrate diet to a strict nutritional ketosis eating pattern would create a fundamental shift in the metabolic environment to make it highly unfavorable for glucose-dependent cancer cells. As you know by now, ketones can be effectively (and even preferentially) used for fuel by the heart, brain, and skeletal muscle, but most cancer cells are unable to use ketones for fuel. This is because mitochondria are required for ketones to burn (that's why they burn so cleanly—ample oxygen is used), and most cancer cells have dysfunctional mitochondria. This is one reason why they are cancer cells! And that's why most must burn glucose and don't require oxygen.

Besides being unavailable as fuel to cancer cells, ketones offer assorted other anti-cancer benefits. Ketones inhibit glycolysis (glucose burning) in cancer cells, essentially starving them since they can't burn ketones, either. Ketones help minimize free radical production in the body, while cancer cells thrive in the presence of reactive oxygen species. Ketones boost antioxidant production in healthy cells surrounding cancerous tumors—something scientists believe may help prevent cancer cells from growing and spreading. Ketones have also been found to help mitigate the effects of traditional radiation and chemotherapy cancer treatments. These treatments stimulate free radical production in tumors, but damage surrounding healthy tissues in the process. Being in a ketone-burning state would likely protect healthy tissues from the radiation and chemo damage without compromising the intended effects of these aggressive treatments.

Unfortunately, human cancer patients have been slow to adopt fasting, calorie restriction, and ketogenic eating strategies to fight cancer despite the phenomenal results seen in animal studies. The suggestion to take an extreme dietary departure from conventional wisdom is difficult to embrace for a patient fighting a serious disease with radiation and chemo protocols recommended by physicians. It's one thing to cut carbs to try and drop a few extra pounds, and quite another to perhaps go against the advice of the oncology doctor (who may have no nutritional expertise or training, but may still be inclined to dispense dietary advice, usually in alignment with the highly questionable USDA dietary guidelines). The advent of exogenous ketone supplements may be a wonderful opportunity for ketone therapy to gain a foothold in traditional cancer treatments, particularly when used in conjunction with a ketogenic eating pattern.

Cellular and Metabolic Health

Beta-hydroxybutyrate is more than just a clean-burning source of energy, it is a signaling molecule that can regulate cellular processes and inflammatory processes throughout the body. Beta-hydroxybutyrate is powerful enough to be considered an epigenetic switch that can actually turn an assortment of genes on and off, just as happens with powerful prescription drugs. Beta-hydroxybutyrate causes a direct modification of Kreb's cycle function such that you generate cellular energy with fewer free radicals and better cellular oxygenation. As mentioned earlier, enhanced oxygen delivery to the brain is especially important. In fact, seizures are triggered when the brain reaches a breaking point owing to insufficient oxygen delivery.

> **Beta-hydroxybutyrate is powerful enough to be considered an epigenetic switch that causes a direct modification in Kreb's cycle function.**

The minimized oxidative stress is especially relevant in the cardiovascular system, because your heart and your delicate artery walls are highly sensitive to oxidative damage from burning dirty fuel and assorted other stressful influences in modern life (including chronic exercise). According to Dr. Peter Attia and other experts, the heart seems to prefer burning ketones to any other fuel. Dr. D'Agostino cites research that ketones improve the hydraulic efficiency of the heart, enabling it to generate more ATP from a given amount of oxygen than when burning the inferior fuel source that is glucose. The brain, which cannot burn fatty acids, will burn ketones just as well as glucose. Interestingly, in a state of complete starvation, your brain will derive around one-third of its energy from glucose and two-thirds from ketones.

This is a good time to expose the popular health goal of developing a "fast metabolism" as a perk of vigorous exercise, meal timing, or high-tech supplements as ill-advised. Accelerated metabolic function promotes dysfunction and disease via increased free radical production from your beloved fast metabolism. The bodybuilders who train like crazy and choke down massive quantities of protein in their six daily meals will indeed increase muscle mass, but their pursuit of big guns compromises their longevity. Overtraining, overfeeding and overstressing (pumping out stress hormones, prompting gluconeogenesis to fuel your hectic, high-stress daily lifestyle patterns) promote metabolic *inefficiency.*

While accelerated metabolic function is not desired, neither is diminished metabolic function whereby your cells' energy needs are not met sufficiently. This can happen with a high insulin–producing diet that inhibits fat burning and forces you to rely on frequent feedings of external calories. This gets you back to metabolic inefficiency, lifelong accumulation of excess body fat, and increased risk of cancer, heart disease, and the many other conditions driven by oxidation and inflammation.

Ketone burning is also especially beneficial to mitochondrial health. Dave Asprey, author of *Headstrong* and *The Bulletproof Diet,* cites research that 46 percent of people over age 40 have compromised mitochondrial function, as evidenced by poor oxygen consumption rates. Remember, glucose can be burned without using oxygen or mitochondria, so a carb-dependent eating pattern can cause mitochondria to atrophy as a consequence. Things get worse for your mitochondrial health if you don't exercise or move enough, or alternatively are engaged in chronic exercise patterns.

In contrast, fat and ketone burning engage mitochondria in a lively manner, as do fasting and endurance or high-intensity workouts. As a consequence of these desirable cellular stimulations, your cells develop more and higher-functioning mitochondria through a process known as *mitochondrial biogenesis.* As described previously, if you envision fat and ketone burning as a campfire, you are taking the time to build clean-burning, long-duration logs (mitochondria-engaged fat- and ketone-burning logs), instead of constantly throwing more sticks and newspaper into a makeshift fire, which represents a carbohydrate-dependent pattern where energy must come from frequent high-carb meals and snacks. While you think you might be able to get away with a kindling-style diet in your younger years, once you hit your 40s, it's time to mind your mitochondria with exercise, fasting, and keto eating patterns.

One way to assess your cellular oxygenation health is to get a tiny, portable pulse oximeter (online, cheap ones are $25; a good one like the Massimo Mighty Sat is $400) and test your blood oxygenation rate. You simply stick your finger into the unit and obtain an instant readout. Unlike measuring glucose or ketones, there's no blood involved! This is a popular practice with hospital patients and also among elite athletes tracking recovery. A blood oxygenation value of 97 percent or higher indicates that you have good oxygen consumption, and likely good mitochondrial function.

Emotional Stability

Being a carbohydrate addict has far-reaching implications beyond nutritional inferiority and metabolic rigidity. When you suck at burning fat and are dependent upon regular high-carb meals and snacks for energy, you express an addiction to the powerful drug that is carbohydrate. When you free yourself from that addiction by unlocking the power to manufacture and burn energy internally, thereby stabilizing mood, concentration, and energy levels without needing regular meals, your emotional stability is greatly enhanced. Owing to enhanced oxygenation and neuron firing, ketogenic eating has been shown to reduce anxiety symptoms by 30 percent.

Mitochondrial Biogenesis

While it is not as sexy a sound bite as "rapid efficient weight loss," mitochondrial biogenesis is one of the most life-changing benefits of keto. Mitochondria are the energy generators located inside each cell. The better they function, the healthier you are. Mitochondria protect against oxidative damage from burning calories, breathing air, and living a high-stress modern life. The more mitochondria you have and the better they function, essentially the longer and healthier you live.

Mitochondrial biogenesis literally means the making of new mitochondria. Cells respond to stresses, or demands, by becoming stronger and more energy efficient—whether making new mitochondria or improving the function of existing mitochondria. Some of the most effective mitochondria-generating cell stressors are endurance workouts, high-intensity strength or sprint workouts (which stimulate mitochondria on a different energy pathway than endurance, which is why it's good to do both types of workouts), fasting (starving cells forces them to become more efficient), or ketogenic eating (you minimize dirty-burning glucose and recruit more mitochondria to burn fat and ketones). When you combine frequent fasting, keto-aligned eating, and a sensible exercise program, you get your mitochondria in top shape and enjoy maximum protective benefits against the oxidative damage caused by exercise and other forms of stress in modern life.

Enhanced Athletic Performance

If you're not an athlete, you might want to become one when you learn of the mind-blowing performance benefits offered by keto. Having been an endurance athlete for a full half-century, I can tell you that we have never seen any dietary strategy or magic pill that has anywhere near the potential of keto to elevate performance and speed recovery. The fact that ketones are now available in supplement form is even more interesting. We've already discussed how ketones are a high-octane fuel source that helps both muscles and brain operate more effectively, and generate much less inflammation and oxidative stress than glucose burning. This is a big deal to your general health and disease protection when you are working at your desk or sleeping, but when your central nervous system has better oxygen delivery and makes more bioenergetic compounds—brain firing on more cylinders—this has profound implications for peak physical performance.

For endurance athletes, the ability to burn fat efficiently as intensity increases is the essence of how to improve performance, and it's the main distinguishing feature of the winner from the slower athletes on the racecourse. For strength/power athletes, the anti-inflammatory, protein-sparing properties of keto allow you to work harder and recover faster, with less overall stress, inflammation, and risk of muscle breakdown.

When your brain gets more oxygen and neurons fire with more efficiency, your workouts seem easier, and this manifests as a literal truth per the *Central Governor Theory*. This theory has been popularized by Dr. Timothy Noakes, prominent South African exercise physiologist and author of the epic *Lore of Running*. Noakes has made headlines in recent years for renouncing much of his life's work in exercise physiology relating to the carbohydrate paradigm and becoming an enthusiastic convert to low-carb and keto principles. The consternation in the academic community was such that Noakes was put on trial in his native South Africa for his brazen rejection of conventional wisdom!

The Central Governor Theory asserts that the brain, not the muscles, is the ultimate limiter of peak physical performance. The theory suggests that your muscles are not really exhausted on that final rep or final mile before the finish line; it's your brain concluding that your muscles are cooked in order to protect yourself from injury and perhaps the unpleasant sensation of extreme energy depletion. This directly opposes the more superficial, simplified, and quite likely inaccurate "peripheral theory"—that the muscles themselves limit your performance—which has prevailed in exercise physiology forever. The idea of having a central governor might explain how we can sometimes achieve the impossible when duly inspired, or when in a state of extreme fight-or-flight stimulation.

Physiology lab data confirm that when you bonk (the sudden and severe decline of performance caused by glycogen depletion) during a long workout, there is actually still sufficient residual glycogen stored in the muscles to allow you to keep going. The bonk is your brain deciding to shut down operations in order to protect you from literally running out of energy—which is virtually impossible because when glycogen is gone you will tap into your abundant fat stores and ketone production to keep going. This is what Speedgolf world champion Robert Hogan did in his incredible tale of "violently rewiring appetite and metabolic hormones" (as described by Dr. Cate Shanahan) through a sequence of extreme depletion 17-mile training runs done without fluid or calories. (We'll discuss this in detail in Chapter 10.)

While muscle soreness, stiffness, and pain of strenuous, depleting workouts are real, as is the goofy feeling that happens when you run low on blood sugar, your brain can choose to override these signals if supremely motivated, shocked, or frightened. You can confirm the validity of the Central Governor Theory if you imagine someone putting a gun to your head on what you think is your last rep and demanding that you complete five more reps, or requiring you to run five more miles beyond a marathon finish line that your brain (and sore, stiff muscles) perceives to be your absolute limit of performance on that day. Amazingly, your brain will summon the motivation and inspiration to direct your muscles to comply!

Realize that just because your central governor can dig deep to summon a superhuman performance doesn't mean it's a good idea to do so. The Central Governor Theory is a concept to marvel at and occasionally tap into by accident (getting lost hiking in the mountains and somehow making it back to safety) or on purpose (giving it your all in a peak performance competition), but it's a much better idea to get into great shape so your body can deliver sensible peak performance efforts and recovery quickly. If you go to the well too often or too severely, the repercussions will be severe. As I relate in my book *Primal Endurance,* I can reference a single fateful track workout (16 x 800 meters in 2:24–2:28 for you runner geeks out there) that was so exhausting that I immediately fell ill for two weeks, and believe that I never had the same sharpness or competitive intensity afterward for the rest of my running career.

> **A brain on keto makes workouts seem easier, which becomes a literal truth because the brain is the ultimate governor of peak performance.**

When you are trying to perform an explosive movement like clear a high jump bar, hoist a heavy deadlift bar, or do one more rep or box jump when your muscles are fatigued, you must activate more motor units in existing muscle fibers and/or build more muscle over time to get the job done. When you go keto, it's easier for your highly oxygenated brain to activate more motor units to perform explosive efforts. Furthermore, you can sprint harder and longer before running low on oxygen. The brain perceives lack of oxygen as a life-or-death threat (remember, seizures occur when the brain reaches its oxygen threshold), prompting you to breathe harder and harder until ultimately you have to slow down. Better oxygen delivery leads to better performance, all other variables being equal. This is possibly another area where a pre-workout ketone supplement can provide a competitive edge. For endurance athletes, it's even easier to realize how much of the challenge is in your head. Staying mentally sharp, motivated, and oxygenated helps you go long and stay strong, regardless of the condition of your muscles.

In contrast, inflammatory glucose metabolism will lead to the familiar sensation of compromised/foggy brain function when you are doing multiple reps of explosive efforts, or trying to sustain your desired pace during a long endurance session. A brain that hasn't learned how to burn ketones gets groggy when blood sugar drops. Similarly, when you miss lunch and get the afternoon blues, or feel "fried" after a long, stressful day demanding peak cognitive function, part of this is fallout from burning dirty fuel. This fried sensation is a literal truth because when sodium-potassium pumps that optimize the chemical and electrical gradients your neurotransmitters rely on become depleted, your electrical circuits really are fried. At these times, you are obligated to refresh the pumps and reset the circuits through sleep, meditation, or any other winding-down behavior that minimizes demand and circuit activity.

This leads to the question: How much of your fatigue/performance limitation is a natural consequence of the energy expenditure, and how much can be attributed to the burning of dirty fuel? It's impossible to quantify, but very important to consider if you are interested in achieving your athletic potential and minimizing the damage to your body in the process. Even among the most highly trained athletes in power or endurance, it's commonplace to start workouts or competitions feeling fresh and energized, then struggle in the latter stages to the point of exhaustion. Post-session debriefings are rife with commentary about cramped muscles, blood sugar crashes, and involuntary zoning out—undesirable disengagement from peak performance focus—during the event.

It's time to pay close attention to the pioneers in the world of ketogenic athletic performance, and the incredible potential they are unlocking by delivering the most efficient fuel to their brains and muscles—nurturing their central governors in the process. Dr. Attia chronicles in detail at eatingacademy.com (read "my personal journey") how he significantly improved his cycling wattage output (the most accurate measure of power—translating to increased speed on the road) at anaerobic threshold heart rate when adhering to a ketogenic diet. His substrate utilization (mixture of fuels burned) at his anaerobic threshold (a strenuous "race pace" that a fit athlete can sustain for around one hour) went from 100 percent glucose at anaerobic threshold before dietary modification to 70 percent fat and 30 percent glucose while ketogenic.

This means that when keto adapted, he could continue—and at a faster pace!—for much more time before running out of glucose.

Sami Inkinen, a Silicon Valley entrepreneur and world champion amateur tri-athlete at the 70.3-mile half-iron distance, was able to extend his theoretical "time to bonk" at low-intensity bicycle pedaling wattage from 5.6 hours to *87 hours* after transitioning from a traditional higher carb eating pattern to a fat- and keto-adapted eating pattern. This time-to-bonk calculation was an estimate of when his body would run dry of glucose if he were to continue to exercise. Outside the realm of athletic performance, virtually everything you do with your brain or your body can become easier when you are burning fat and ketones as your preferred fuel instead of glucose.

"Bonk-Proof" Endurance

Becoming fat- and keto-adapted may represent the greatest breakthrough in the history of diet and exercise physiology for endurance performance. Unlike virtually any other type of athlete, carboydrate-dependent endurance athletes must deal with the potentially disastrous effects of glycogen depletion—something that happens after about two hours of sustained vigorous exercise. The essence of success in endurance sports is an athlete's ability, relative to the competition, to burn fat and preserve glycogen as effort escalates. The difference between the elite two-hour marathoner and a three-hour or four-hour runner is that the winner can click off sub–five-minute miles for 26 consecutive miles without blowing through glycogen stores, accumulating lactate waste products in the muscles, or running out of oxygen and having to slow down or stop—as would a mere mortal trying to perform at the elite level.

Since we were firmly entrenched in the carbohydrate paradigm for decades and unable to break out of the bubble, our obsession has been to stuff as much glycogen as possible into our liver and muscles before and after every workout (especially the quintessential endurance tradition of carbo-loading before important competitions), stretch the glycogen supply out as long as possible over the course of workouts and races (this happens when you get fitter through hard training), and succeed in the delicate art of assimilating additional carbohydrate fuel during workouts.

This challenge, as contemplated by the endurance community for the past several decades, spawned the multi-billion-dollar sports nutrition industry—energy bars, drinks, and gels became must-have tools of the trade. And it's never really worked. A study published in the journal *Medicine & Science in Sports & Exercise* reported that *31 percent* of Ironman triathlon competitors—a group of the most devoted, diligently trained, and well-prepared enthusiasts in the world—still experienced serious gastrointestinal distress during their event! It's no stretch to proclaim that *all* long and ultra-distance endurance athletes experience at least mild digestive issues in attempting the impossible task of processing sugary calories while blood has been shunted away from digestive organs and into the extremities to keep them moving along the road.

Here we are, some three decades since the invention of the PowerBar, over four decades since the first Hawaii Ironman event or the Western States 100-mile endurance run, and a huge percentage of highly trained participants are still bombing out because of GI issues rather than just the pure physical challenge of completing the course. Heavily advertised, cutting-edge designer sports nutrition products cannot overcome the reality that humans are not meant to assimilate calories during prolonged strenuous exercise, and that glucose is an extremely fragile and tenuous fuel source. What's more, how about the negative health aspects of eating a high-carbohydrate diet in general—something that's especially relevant for endurance athletes because they consume quantities far in excess of the average moderately active person.

Finally, we are busting out of the bubble and realizing that we can wean ourselves off glucose dependency through dietary modification away from carb dependency and toward fat- and keto-adaptation. In doing so, it's clear that we access an entirely new dimension of endurance performance potential. Or to put it more bluntly, doesn't it seem easier to improve your time to bonk from 5 hours to 87 hours by cutting carbs and adding fat in your diet, than it is by training 17 times longer and harder? The idea that a fat-adapted eating pattern is advantageous to endurance athletes is finally gaining mainstream acceptance, but pioneers like Doctors Phinney and Volek, and Dr. Maffetone have been advancing this theory quietly for over 30 years. The Phinney/Volek findings from the early 80s, although conducted and chronicled under exacting laboratory and academic protocols, were so counter to the paradigm that the scientific and athletic communities essentially ignored them until just recently.

Doesn't it seem easier to improve your "time to bonk" through dietary modification than by training 17 times longer and harder?

It's likely that the sports nutrition marketing dollars promoting carb dependency (and research dollars validating alignment with the carb-dependency premise) were a strong contributing factor in the suppression of these revolutionary ideas. In fairness, the pillars of conventional wisdom like the Gatorade Sports Science Institute were staffed with competent professionals doing meticulous research, but everything was happening inside a carbohydrate paradigm bubble. Science validates the idea that an athlete following a high-carbohydrate, high insulin–producing diet indeed needs a steady supply of glucose energy to sustain exercise output (especially as intensity level increases)—that's because he cannot access fat stores quickly or efficiently enough to sustain output levels beyond pedestrian (mostly fat-burning) intensities.

As Dr. Cate Shanahan explains (visit DrCate.com, or the "FatBurn Factory" You-Tube channel for more information), the reason the fat is inaccessible is the hyper-insulinemia caused by high-carbohydrate meals and snacks. In optimal metabolic circumstances, when you need to access and burn stored energy, a group of adrenaline-like hormones kick into gear and upregulate the activity of hormone-sensitive lipase (HSL). HSL unlocks triglycerides from storage, breaks down these three fatty acid molecules into free fatty acids, and releases them into the bloodstream for use as energy. Excess insulin inhibits this activity, instead stimulating the activity of lipoprotein lipase—LPL, which causes cells to pull energy from the bloodstream and into storage.

Dr. Cate calls this phenomenon in high-carb athletes *catecholamine resistance,* which is a precursor to becoming insulin resistant. Yes, those miles on the road help them fare better than a sedentary high-carb eater, but the picture of the carb-dependent endurance athlete is not pretty—and excess body fat is often visible in the picture. Your body will burn whatever ingested sugars you throw into the furnace, will burn through stored muscle and liver glycogen quickly, and then will commence gluconeogenesis to get more sugar from lean muscle tissue. Meanwhile, fat remains in storage as you struggle along with low brain and muscular energy during the final stages of your two-hour run or five-hour bike ride.

The masses never considered low-carb eating to access fat stores and instead subscribed to this program: carbo-load like crazy before long workouts or races; drain your sugary drinks and slam down a sugary gel every time your watch beeps on 15-minute intervals during your workout, and refeed on carbohydrates with reckless abandon immediately after workouts during the all-important "window of opportunity" when your muscles are most receptive to glycogen reloading. Like Professor Noakes, I am embarrassed to admit that I made a living in the sports nutrition/supplementation industry telling this story to athletes and providing them with the sugary products they needed to stay on the program. I was even lauded for developing one of the first products to deliver concentrated long-chain carbohydrate molecules into a powdered form, enabling the delivery of a massive amount of carb calories (as in 900!) in a single water bottle. The product was called Carbo Concentrate. Ouch.

In 2013, Dr. Volek and his colleagues conducted a landmark experiment with two distinct groups of highly trained endurance runners. Known as the FASTER Study (Fat Adapted Substrate oxidation in Trained Elite Runners), the experiment matched runners of similar ability from a group that ate in a traditional high-carbohydrate (60 percent), lower fat (25 percent) pattern, with runners who were fat- and keto-adapted for a significant time period before the study (averaging 70 percent fat, 20 percent protein, 12 percent carbs). Perhaps the greatest revelation to the scientific and athletic community from the results was the shockingly high rate of fat oxidation among the low-carb, high-fat athletes during a comfortably paced treadmill run lasting three hours. It was previously believed that the maximum potential for fat oxidation in a highly trained endurance athlete was around one gram of fat per minute (burning 540 calories per hour).

The study revealed that fat- and keto-adapted athletes were able to metabolize much more fat than the previously believed human limit. In fact, the low-carb group's *average* was 1.5 grams per minute, with the best individual reading at 1.8 grams/minute (burning 972 fat calories per hour!). What's more, the low-carb group burned fat at more than double the average rate of the high-carb dietary group, which averaged only 0.67 grams per minute and achieved peak fat oxidation at a higher percentage of maximum effort than the low-carbohydrate group.

In summary, low-carb endurance athletes easily access and burn more fat at all exercise intensities, unlike high-carbohydrate endurance athletes whose cellular energy is difficult to access. Fat- and keto-adapted low-carb athletes enjoy several important performance and recovery benefits. First, there is less reliance on external carbohydrate sources during exercise, resulting in less risk of digestive distress or bonking. Second, fat burning generates less inflammation and fewer reactive oxygen species than glucose burning. While this insight is important in general, it's especially important during exercise, because you elevate above resting metabolic function by a factor of 10 (jogging), 20 (tempo run/5k race), or 30 (full sprint). These values are known as Metabolic Equivalent of Task (MET)—so a sprint workout generates a score of 30 MET.

Finally, fat adaptation results in less glycogen depletion after workouts, so you don't require a massive high-carb recovery feeding the way a carb-dependent athlete does. When you gorge on a big meal after a workout, you increase oxidative stress to the gastrointestinal system, potentially delaying recovery and increasing the overall stress impact of the workout and the eating binge. Remember that the liver is the processing and distribution center for all the nutrients absorbed by the small intestine, including not only glycogen but also fatty acids, amino acids, and assorted vitamins, minerals, and micronutrients. The liver is also an important first line of defense to detoxify the bloodstream from alcohol and other toxins. If you overwhelm it with glucose processing from frequent carb slams, you can compromise your ability to recover from exercise and all other forms of stress.

Increased Strength and Explosive Power

Early into the popularity of keto, it was seen as the exclusive domain of endurance athletes, who could gain the obvious advantage of becoming largely independent of glucose needs during sustained efforts. Athletic endeavors that require lots of strength and power are *glycolytic*—the intensity is extremely high and the duration fairly short. It was even asserted by many that you would lose high-end power if you ate keto. This early speculation has now been refuted by respected science, and even the most explosive athletes can benefit from the protein-sparing, anti-inflammatory, neuro-enhancing effects of keto.

Ketone burning allows you to fire brain neurons at greater capacity and activate more motor units to get your desired work accomplished. Strength athletes know that motor recruitment is the essence of getting stronger—your brain calling more muscle fibers into play and messaging the nervous system to elicit maximum performance from each individual fiber. Sprinting or lifting the heavy bar feels easier because your brain works better, so the actions literally are easier. Another important benefit of keto for power/strength athletes is the likelihood that this type of dietary pattern will result in the reduction of excess body fat (if desired; some pure power athletes like to preserve bulk), which translates into a significant improvement in explosive performance with all other variables being equal. Like Brad and me, you'll go from being barely able to touch the rim to thunderous dunking—simply due to reduction of excess fat.

> **Ketogenic power/strength athletes will likely reduce excess body fat, delivering a significant improvement in explosive performance.**

When you are ketogenic, you can perform explosive efforts and not break down as much after as you would as a sugar-burner; that's because you generate less inflammation with clean-burning fat and ketones versus dirty-burning glucose. And because you don't need to burn as much glucose at rest when you're keto, you'll have plenty of stored muscle glycogen to power a high-intensity workout—even if it extends up to an hour.

When you are in a fasted or ketogenic state, you enjoy increased muscle protein synthesis due to an elevation of factors known as *myogens* in your bloodstream (an elevation that is directly attributed to the presence of the ketone acetoacetate). This makes sense from an evolutionary perspective. If you're starving and you score a feast, your body would want to use those calories to maximum efficiency. While the science is so new that we must be wary of sounding definitive, it appears that keto may actually be anabolic—not only as a convenient fuel source that spares muscle breakdown but also owing to the epigenetic effect: ketones switching on the genes that build or preserve muscle tissue.

Jacob Wilson, Ph.D., a skeletal muscle physiologist and director of the Applied Science and Performance Institute in Tampa, Florida, has published research that is particularly interesting because the subjects were hard-training athletes. As with the work of Phinney and Volek, using fit specimens is especially critical in the keto world because regular folks who are metabolically inflexible might deliver adverse results as a result of a shorter study period than the time it takes for them to become fat- and keto-adapted. Wilson's athletes increased blood levels of branched-chain amino acids while adhering to a ketogenic diet, and it seems that being in ketosis may also lower the threshold to stimulate protein synthesis in comparison to being in carbohydrate dependency.

Faster Recovery

If you're still worried about whether you can replenish glycogen and recover from workouts when consuming so few dietary carbs, understand that when you become fat-adapted, your fat oxidation rate is improved not only at the low intensities measured in the FASTER Study but also at levels all the way up to the anaerobic threshold. The stationary bike experiments performed by Dr. Peter Attia, and chronicled in detail at eatingacademy.com, are a great testament to this. Even if you are doing a strength workout, Crossfit class, or sprint session where you are delivering repeated near-maximum intensity efforts, a significant portion of these sessions is always devoted to low-intensity cardio warm-up and preparatory movements (burning mostly fat, because there is ample oxygen available) before you get into the juicy high-glycolytic, anaerobic stuff. In contrast, even a very fit person who is a sugar-burner starts draining his glycogen tank during the easy cardio warm-ups, and by the time a big-time effort is over, he'll be craving a sugar bomb to stave off the shakes.

Even for a keto endurance athlete doing long or ultra-distance workouts, glycogen can be spared as a consequence of optimized fat and ketone burning. Elite ultra-runner Zach Bitter, the USA national 100k champion and part of the low-carb athlete group in the FASTER Study, reported that he was able to complete a 8.5-hour overnight 38-mile endurance run through the river canyons of the Sierra Nevada mountains, pacing a teammate along the final segment of the Western States 100-miler, while consuming only water and liquid amino acids.

In addition to sparing glycogen during workouts, it's easy to restock depleted glycogen (however you deplete it—endurance or intensity—it doesn't matter) when you're fat- and keto-adapted. Even if you just eat a small keto-aligned meal or even decide to fast for a while after workouts to accelerate weight loss and keto progress, your body still finds a way to restock efficiently. First, you'll direct any carbs you do ingest right to your muscles because, as Dr. Cate says, "when the glycogen suitcases are open (muscles depleted), they take first priority." Furthermore, because your brain is burning ketones, it won't hog that ingested glucose.

Second, you will call upon gluconeogenesis on an on-demand basis to make just the glucose necessary to restock the muscles and no more. This is a huge contrast with the fight-or-flight abuse of gluconeogenesis experienced by the sugar-burner, who will strip down lean muscle mass to keep the crappy campfire going all day long. When you're keto, your mild, on-demand gluconeogenesis can come from ingested protein, or perhaps even from lean muscle mass now and then, but everything happens on a casual level instead of being the emergency fight-or-flight circumstances experienced by the sugar-burner.

Third, Dr. Cate speculates that during exercise, fat-adapted athletes might be able to reassemble unused glucose into its previous form of stored glycogen—because they are burning mostly fat and don't end up needing much glucose. While this is speculation at the very cutting edge of the new fat-adapted paradigm of exercise physiology, the FASTER Study confirmed that something interesting is happening inside the bodies of fat-adapted athletes. Both the high-carb and low-carb athletes significantly depleted their glycogen stores after the three-hour treadmill workout, but the low-carb athletes were able to restock glycogen even more efficiently than the high-carb athletes, despite consuming extremely minimal post-exercise carbohydrate!

> **Low-carb athletes were able to restock glycogen more efficiently than high-carb athletes, despite consuming extremely minimal post-exercise carbohydrate!**

Amazingly, glycogen reloading through post-exercise carbohydrate consumption is not the end-all athletes have perceived it to be for so long. In contrast, a carb-dependent athlete also burns mostly fat at rest in general, but in the hours after a high-glycolytic workout, glucose burning predominates over fat burning, as referenced often by Dr. Phil Maffetone. This is why carb-dependent athletes who exercise vigorously can't lose fat; they just end up burning more glucose in the hours after workouts, which stimulates an appetite for more carbohydrates.

The assortment of health, disease-protection, and peak-performance benefits from keto almost seem too good to be true. With modern society focused on technology and pharmaceutical breakthroughs to solve the illness of SAD eating and hectic, high-stress daily living, the idea that a metabolic therapy (a diet-based health intervention) could trump the most powerful drugs—or better yet, prevent disease conditions from taking hold in the first place—is nothing short of mind-blowing. In this context, we must create a big-picture definition for "keto" such that it conveys the metabolic state of low-carbohydrate intake (burning cleaner, less oxidative, less inflammatory fuel in fat), moderate protein intake (avoiding excess stimulation of cancer-causing growth factors IGF-1 and mTOR), and high-fat intake, which promotes optimally low levels of insulin production.

> **Dr. Peter Attia speculates that the insulin-lowering effects of a ketogenic diet could possibly be even more beneficial to health than the actual burning of ketones.**

Recalling Dr. Peter Attia's emphasis on optimizing insulin as the ultimate longevity marker, he further speculates that perhaps half of keto's vaunted neuro-protective benefits could be attributed to low insulin, and furthermore that lowering insulin could possibly be more important to health than producing ketones. The importance of this speculation will become clear in Chapter 11, when we summarize the undisputed critical assumptions about keto, and discuss options for long-term eating strategies. While some may be more adaptable to, and benefit further from, nutritional ketosis than others, a devoted effort to complete the journey outlined in the book—a 21-Day Metabolism Reset, a period of fine-tuning with fasting, and then going keto for a minimum of six weeks—is a highly recommended bucket-list objective for all of us. After all, of all the diets and strategies that we have been bombarded with over our lifetimes, it's more likely that something resembling keto was the default factory setting for our pre-civilized ancestors, and thus still of maximum health benefit to modern people.

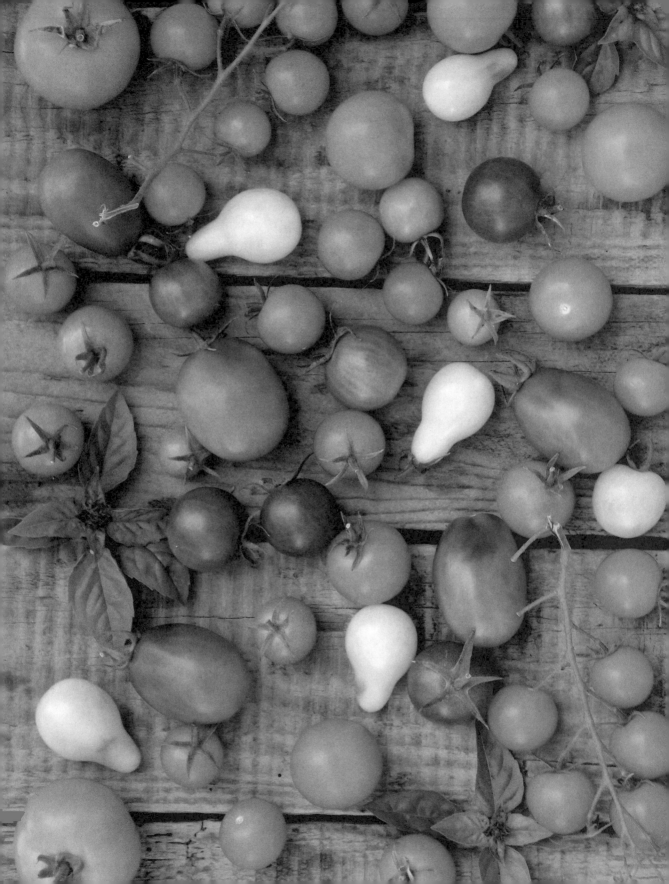

The 21-Day Metabolism Reset

CHAPTER 4

The 21-Day Metabolism Reset Overview

NOW that you've digested some extensive introductory material to (I hope) convince you of the benefits of ditching carbohydrate dependency, becoming fat- and keto-adapted, and doing everything right from the get-go, let's take a look at where you are headed on this journey. First, as the book cover promises, you are going to reset your metabolism in 21 days—downregulating your sugar-burning genes and upregulating your fat-burning genes in preparation for your initial foray into the wonderful world of keto.

The twenty-first day represents an important milestone in the effort to reprogram your genes, and it is also believed by many behavior experts to represent a sufficient length of time to establish and ingrain new habits. However, please don't misconstrue the message to think that this 21-Day Metabolism Reset is a miracle, a standalone cure for living happily ever after. We must steer clear of the quick-fix mentality that is the defining characteristic of the diet and fitness industry and instead envision the Reset as exactly that: a chance to reset your dial back to zero so you can give yourself a fighting chance at becoming fat- and keto-adapted for life. Before we begin, though, let's make the important commitment to go all out for the first 21 days. A firm commitment will go a long way toward lowering your insulin levels and optimizing your appetite and hormones, all key to helping you succeed.

> **The 21-Day Metabolism Reset is exactly that: a chance to reset your dial back to zero so you can give yourself a fighting chance at becoming fat- and keto-adapted for life.**

First things first; resetting that dial to zero means zero tolerance for any sugars, grains, or refined vegetable oils for 21 days. That's because during this period you will literally be detoxing from the addictive properties of sugar and wheat. To make your journey toward ketogenic eating easier, here's what you *don't* want to do during your 21-Day Reset: don't let carbs leak into the picture here and there to the extent that you still produce a significant amount of insulin, you lock fat away in storage, and you stimulate an appetite for more carbohydrates.

Instead, your 21-Day Reset will feature delicious meals emphasizing natural fats with a high satiety factor. This ensures that you will never go hungry, nor have to summon the very fragile attribute of willpower to stay aligned. No amount of will-power can stand up to the force of dysregulated appetite hormones and hungry opioid receptors in your brain. Hormone optimization (i.e., optimally minimal insulin production) and metabolic flexibility have to occur naturally, as a consequence of making diet, exercise, sleep, and stress-management choices that promote optimal gene expression.

> **Stress equals sugar cravings equals fat storage. Relax, enjoy life, and burn fat and ketones.**

In addition to your diet, there are three other areas you must dial in during the 21-Day Reset: exercise, sleep, and stress management. Any shortcomings in these areas will most certainly sabotage your success, even when you nail the dietary objectives.

For exercise, your primary objective is to increase all forms of general, everyday movement. This goes for everyone, even if you're already a big-time gym freak or high-mileage endurance machine. Even a devoted pattern of daily workouts is not sufficient to promote fat adaptation if you engage in prolonged sedentary periods, such as commuting, working in an office, and/or enjoying digital entertainment in your leisure time. If you aren't getting out for cardio exercise or gym visits at all, embarking on even just a moderate exercise program will greatly support your progress toward metabolic efficiency.

On the other hand, if you're a devoted fitness enthusiast, you must ensure that you steer clear of chronic exercise patterns, which will compromise your progress toward fat adaptation, as well as your ability to adhere to a restriction on dietary carbohydrates. Optimizing sleep is also critical to success in reprogramming your genes away from carb dependency and toward fat- and keto-adaptation. If you instead introduce artificial light and digital stimulation after dark, this promotes sugar cravings, dysregulates the appetite and fat-storage hormones, and actualizes the nasty quip that staying up late makes you fat, period. Finally, the hectic pace of modern life promotes chronic stimulation of the fight-or-flight response, which compromises fat metabolism and sucks you back into carbohydrate dependency, actualizing another quip: "stress equals sugar cravings equals fat storage." We'll cover assorted ways to counter rat-race dynamics with rest, recovery, and cultivation of a relaxed, intuitive process-oriented mindset toward your diet, exercise, and lifestyle goals.

Everything in Moderation, Including Moderation

People often raise an eyebrow when I add a packet of sugar to my coffee, reach across the table to grab a few french fries, knock back a shot of tequila, or even grab a slice of bread and dip it in oil and vinegar at a fine restaurant. I absorb the obligatory quip about my shocking lack of perfection as a health personality—quips that are often followed by a rationalization along the lines of "Well, if Mark's having some bread or fries, I guess we all can."

You can indeed do whatever you want in my presence, and I'll still be friends with you (or still be your husband, dad, boss, or business partner). Remember that I'm a guy trying to enjoy my life to the fullest, which means not stressing about food. Yes, it's possible for the same guy to be frequently poking his finger to record ketone and glucose levels, eating fewer grams of carbs in a *week* than I used to for dinner back in my marathon days (seriously), and express a sincere overall commitment to health and fitness; but also on occasion I say WTF (stands for, uh, "Welcome to Facebook," as my teenage friend Maria explains) and hit some bread, cheesecake, crème brûlée, or whatever other delicacy is offered at the right time, in the right place.

I'm definitely flexible about this diet stuff, but I don't want you to get the wrong idea. It's worth mentioning that I've spent nearly 15 years limiting my average daily carb intake to under 150 grams. I estimate that, for the last five years, I've averaged 50 to 70 grams per day. The fat- and keto-adapted foundation that I've worked diligently to build gives me more leeway than someone trying to recover from metabolic damage and carbohydrate dependency. Even if you aren't in dire straits, dietary indulgences and rationalizations can be a slippery slope for many people, owing to not only the physiological consequences of stimulating the glucose-insulin-hunger roller coaster but also the assorted background noise—psycho-emotional behavior patterns that play out both consciously and subconsciously.

I favor a bold and mindful approach to lifestyle transformation whereby you take full responsibility for your decisions and understand the repercussions of your choices. We are faced with a dizzying assortment of health-compromising temptations and distractions. If you outsource your fate to your medication regimen, you may end up in a world of regret and suffering. Even if you step up and make a decent effort on behalf of your health, but adopt the popular motto of "Hey, everything in moderation," you are likely to end in a moderate state of health. I don't know about you, but I prefer exceptional to moderate. I like Mark Twain's take on the motto: "Everything in moderation, *including* moderation."

What's more, we mustn't forget how pathetic our averages are these days. As popular American comedian and late-night talk show host Jay Leno reminds us, "Today there are more overweight people in America than average-weight people. So overweight people are now average. Which means you've met your

New Year's resolution." I'll take it a step further and second-guess the frequently lauded modern longevity statistics in developed nations. Great, Americans are now expected to survive to a "record high" of around 80 (albeit frequently connected to machines and forgetting our family members' faces), and that's certainly better than the U.S. life expectancy of around 50 from a century ago. However, organs wear out from natural use after around 120 years; that's a pretty disturbing gap between life expectancy and lifespan potential.

Rather than engage in heavy-handed dogma and heated right-and-wrong debate about eating, I prefer to think of everything as a series of choices. The choice to aggressively eliminate refined sugar, grains, and bad oils from your diet for 21 days might be one of the most life-altering choices you ever make. Do it right the first time, and you'll open up a whole new world of health. Once you experience even a hint of the benefits of being fat- and keto-adapted, you'll never go back to the annoyances and suffering associated with carbohydrate-dependency eating patterns.

21-Day Metabolism Reset, Action Items

The Reset is going to take commitment and discipline, but it must not and will not ever entail struggling or suffering. You are going to do things the right way such that the success you have reprogramming your genes and resetting your metabolism to prefer fat for fuel can be leveraged to make things easier the further you travel down this road. There are hundreds of thousands of people who have turned to ancestral eating principles after a lifetime of health struggles and excess body fat, and they have experienced rapid and stunning success. Now it's your turn; here's how we're going to get there: You'll focus your energy each week on specific action items. In week 1, the focus is on diet. Week 2 is on exercise, lifestyle, and stress management. The final week is when you put everything together to complete the Reset. Following is an overview of each week so you'll know what to expect. The objectives will be detailed in the ensuing chapters, so for now just let it all sink in.

Week 1—Out with the Old and in with the New

Your 21-day journey starts off with a bang, as you are going to ruthlessly purge your pantry and fridge (and office desk drawer . . .) of all sugars, grains, and refined vegetable oils. Unfortunately, these nutrient-devoid, inflammatory, and high insulin–stimulating foods constitute an estimated two-thirds of the calories in the Standard American Diet, and they cause nothing but trouble. This purge must be undertaken with great discipline, and is a mandatory first step toward going keto. While ditching your lifelong go-to staples might be a bit of a shock, you will immediately fill the void in your cupboards—and perhaps your psyche—by restocking with high-satiety, high-fat, nutrient-dense, primal/paleo/evolutionary-approved foods.

In Chapter 6, I detail which items to eliminate in numerous food categories (e.g., beverages, dairy products, fats and oils, and many more), and provide suggested replacements when appropriate. In Chapter 7, I present the rationale and benefits for primal-style eating, and cover the role of each macronutrient in your diet. You'll get a nice, big-picture understanding of the transition from the carbohydrate dependency caused by the SAD diet to the wide-ranging benefits of eating a nutrient-dense, whole-foods diet that promotes fat adaptation, and lays the foundation for going keto in the final section of the book. You'll get a quick summary of primal-style breakfast, lunch, dinner, and snacking patterns, along with a step-by-step meal plan to take you through the entire 21-Day Metabolism Reset.

Ditching your lifelong staple foods for an ancestral-style eating pattern can be a stressful transition, so the key is to surround yourself with delicious primal-approved foods and enjoy them liberally so you never struggle with or suffer from hunger or energy-level swings. Many low-carb enthusiasts make the mistake of diligently cutting carbs but harboring a latent aversion to high-fat foods, a relic of decades of conventional wisdom erroneously convincing us that fat makes you fat and clogs your arteries. If you cut carbs, you'll want to add more healthy fats to your diet to ensure that you stay satisfied and don't backslide into carb binges caused by hunger. This is easily achievable when you eat to your full satisfaction with nutrient-dense, high-fat meals and snacks. Eating food that is truly nourishing instead of just intensely tasty but nutrient devoid means your appetite and metabolic hormones are stabilized and you won't have to worry about crazy cravings.

Week 2—Dial in Exercise, Sleep, and Stress Management

With your dietary changes humming along nicely after the hard work in week 1, you will turn your attention to supportive lifestyle practices in week 2. In Chapter 6, I detail three areas to focus on: exercise, sleep, and stress management. Your objectives for exercise will be multi-faceted. Of foremost importance is to find ways to move more in your everyday life—taking leisurely walks in the morning or evening, taking the stairs instead of elevators, taking frequent breaks from prolonged sedentary periods at work, and finding time—even brief opportunities—for practices like yoga/stretching, calisthenics/mobility work, and even foam rolling.

Your next objective is to complete a respectable number of comfortably paced cardio workouts at aerobic heart rates, helping your body to become expert at burning fat not just during workouts but around the clock. Next, you'll focus on how to properly integrate brief, high-intensity strength training and sprinting—activities that will turbo-charge the fat reduction and accelerate your progress toward fat- and keto-adaption. You'll also learn the critical importance of avoiding chronic exercise patterns, whereby the frequent and prolonged overstimulation of fight-or-flight stress hormones can sabotage your efforts toward becoming fat-adapted and drive you back to carb dependency and burnout.

With sleep, the most urgent to-do item is to minimize artificial light and digital stimulation after dark, the combination of which is a disastrous affront to our hard-wired genetic expectation to align sleep and wake cycles with the rising and setting of the sun. Creating a mellow, dark, relaxing evening routine will help recalibrate your hormones to become more aligned with your natural circadian rhythm, which entails waking up around sunrise full of energy, and slowing down and eventually getting sleepy soon after it gets dark. This is important not just to ensure optimal sleep but also to transition out of the all too common evening sugar cravings and fat-storage hormonal patterns.

Finally, you'll turn your attention to stress management, honing your ability to chill in the face of overwhelming pressure to go, go, go in our hyperconnected, hyperspeed modern life. You'll be inspired to nurture meaningful live social connections, deemphasizing excessive use of technology and social media in the process. You'll learn how to use technology to make your life easier and less stressful instead of falling victim to the destructive effects of being hyperconnected. You'll build other healthy habits, such as walking for relaxation and problem solving, finding more ways to have fun and keep your motivations pure with your lifestyle transformation goals, keeping a gratitude journal, and carving out time for just *you*—enjoying hobbies or simply decompressing with some precious moments in nature.

Week 3—Completing the Reset

The objectives of weeks 1 and 2 are extremely ambitious, requiring plenty of your time, energy, and focus. So, in the third week of your 21-Day Metabolism Reset, you get to catch your breath and settle into a routine whereby you enjoy and appreciate your food choices, workout patterns, sleeping routines, and stress-management practices. This is a chance to take a closer look at any lingering needs to improve areas, whether it's been blasting your eyeballs with screen light late in the evening or still adding a couple-few-several pumps of peach sweetener to your iced tea.

By the time the 21 days are up, you'll want to have your operation super-tight, because when you reach the final section in the book, there is no turning back! As soon as you complete your Reset, you'll jump right into some fine-tuning exercises that will ensure your readiness for your initial six-week nutritional ketosis effort. This includes some extended morning fasts, as well as *The Keto Reset Diet* Midterm Exam. If you pass with 75 percent, you're ready to enter nutritional ketosis. If you aren't quite there yet, you'll spend a little more time in "week 3 mode" during which you can refine your behavior patterns to be more closely aligned with the diet, exercise, sleep, and stress-management objectives outlined in the 21-Day Reset.

If you are inexperienced in any of the areas of the Reset, such as monitoring your heart rate during cardiovascular exercise, or you haven't the faintest clue what 50 grams of carbs or 75 grams of protein look like, you may want to start doing some measuring in week 3. While I prefer to emphasize big-picture behavior change right out of the gate, and not get bogged down in details, it can be greatly illuminating to start measuring the most important parameters on your journey to keto.

Perhaps the most important things to measure are your heart rate during cardiovascular workouts and your daily carb and protein grams. Briefly, best results with cardio come when you exercise at or below your *maximum aerobic heart rate*. This is the point where you are burning mostly fat and minimal glucose, quantified by Dr. Phil

Maffetone's calculation of "180 minus your age" in heartbeats per minute during exercise. We'll cover this topic in more detail in Chapter 7.

For your daily carb intake, you'll want to remain under 150 grams of carbs per day during the Reset, and drop down to 50 or less when you go keto. For protein, your average daily intake should average around 0.7 grams per pound of lean body mass at all times. We'll cover this in more detail in Chapter 9 with the "Keto Kalculations" and "Journaling and Online Macronutrient Calculators" sections. If you jump over there now, you'll obtain some basic guidance on writing down everything you eat for a couple days, or ideally a whole week, and entering the results into an online food calculator to see where you stand and where to make necessary adjustments. While most consider it a pain to do something so tedious as record every calorie they ingest, it does bring more mindfulness to your eating, and food journaling can trigger red flags like nothing else. That said, if you are staying properly focused on the big picture (ditching bad stuff and emphasizing nutrient-dense, high-fat foods, exercising sensibly, and getting a proper handle on sleep and stress), you are going to emerge after 21 days with some awesome momentum to move you into the next phase of your keto journey. For now, let's hit Chapters 5, 6, and 7 hard, with total focus on and commitment to ditching carb dependency; you'll never go back, as you merge into the fast lane on the road toward fat- and keto-adaptation.

CHAPTER 5

Ditch Toxic Foods and Replace with Nutrient-Dense Foods

AS mentioned in Chapter 4, the 21-Day Metabolism Reset is not a miracle cure, but rather an opportunity to reset your metabolism and give you a fighting chance at fat adaptation. When you are ready to begin, make sure things in life are good for you, stress is moderate, and you have the time and energy to devote to meeting a health challenge. If you are considering a reset during a month of extensive business travel or with your little one battling an ear infection, hold off until your general life circumstances settle down.

Choosing a convenient time is especially important because you are going to hit the ground running: on the very first day you will grab a trashcan and commence the purge of pantry and fridge of all forms of sugar, sweets, sweetened beverages, white grains and whole grains, refined high polyunsaturated vegetable oils, and any form of processed, packaged, or frozen foods containing any semblance of these "big three" bad guys.

Sugars and grains are devoid of nutritional value, and they are the catalyst for the wildly excessive insulin production that many experts agree is the preeminent public health problem facing modern society. Refined vegetable oils share top billing with refined carbohydrates because they have sustained significant free radical damage during their high-temperature processing, and they are further damaged by exposure to heat, light, and oxygen, as when you heat these unstable oils during cooking. When you ingest these toxic agents, they are integrated into the membranes of healthy fat cells and cause dysfunction in healthy fat metabolism. When you are working hard to lose weight but notice a few stubborn pounds that won't go away, it could be that you are hanging on to dysfunctional fat cells that have been poisoned by certain vegetable oils that are known to be toxic.

Since the ingestion of these toxic oils causes an immediate disturbance to healthy cellular function at the DNA level, Dr. Cate Shanahan asserts that "consuming these oils is literally no different from eating radiation." Unfortunately, these calorically dense oils constitute a massive portion of the Standard American Diet. Noted author and alternative healer Dr. Andrew Weil suggests that soybean oil alone accounts for 20 percent of SAD calories. Dr. Cate cites an estimate that 40 percent of all restaurant calories—whether in fast food or from fine restaurants—come from vegetable oils (since most meals are cooked in gobs of oil—ask your waiter to use butter instead!).

Grains, sugars, and bad oils promote oxidation, inflammation, fat storage, dysfunctional fat metabolism, increased risk of cancer and heart disease, and accelerated aging. A complete elimination of these heavily processed, high insulin–stimulating foods is the only way to downregulate your inflammatory genes and sugar-burning genes, and open up the pipeline between your fabulous fat stores waiting to be called into service and the energy needs of your brain and muscles.

If you can't go all out on the first day, the first step, we can part ways right now and still be friends. However, your home environment has to be optimal to give yourself a fighting chance for overall adherence, because there are more temptations and detours in the big, bad outside world. Don't worry if you find yourself a little shell-shocked when you look into your empty pantry. You will be headed to the store to stock up instead on the primal/paleo/ancestral foods before the garbage truck even arrives to haul away your discards. That's important: don't make the mistake of ditching the refined carbs and oils and then sitting around without excellent snack or meal options, suffering from deprivation obsession. Your transition from oatmeal to omelet must be smooth and effortless!

Food Categories: Purging and Replacing

While the instructions to ditch refined sugars, grains, and vegetable oils are simple and clear, many enthusiasts have trouble recognizing the various forms and permutations of these offending foods, especially those that extend beyond the obvious characters and creep into even the finest restaurants and high-end grocery stores. Take the time to review these categories and product types to be sure you are breaking all ties with the bad guys. For each food category, replacement options are provided so you can get back into the swing of things quickly.

Alcohol

ELIMINATE: Alcohol calories have zero nutritional value and compromise body fat reduction goals. Known as "first to burn" calories (in the form of ethanol), these are immediately burned through because they are toxic in the bloodstream. This puts the burning of all other calories on hold, indirectly leading to fat storage (gotta store the glucose somewhere when you are burning off the booze) and even sugar cravings (since you don't have any other energy sources in the bloodstream after you burn through the alcohol).

REPLACEMENTS: If you insist on consuming alcohol during your 21-Day Reset or your efforts to go keto, it's best to consume it straight up. If you consume a mixed drink or have pizza with your beer, the carbs will get stored as fat. Red wines designated as "clean," "dry," or "additive-free" (yes, there are paleo-approved wines out there; google "dry farm wines" to learn more) or hard liquors like tequila are the least offensive forms of alcohol, while beer might be the most objectionable because it also contains carbs (they don't call it a "beer belly" for nothing!).

Beverages

ELIMINATE: You'll save enough money each year for a Hawaii vacation when you ditch designer coffees (typically laden with high-carb flavorings, syrups, creamers; regular coffee with real heavy cream is fine). Also toss out the following:

- Soft drinks and sodas: Obviously, these belong in the trash bin.

- "Energy" and sports/performance drinks like Red Bull, Gatorade, Vitamin Water, in both bottled and powdered forms (read the labels and notice the high carbohydrate counts)

- Bottled, fresh-squeezed, and refrigerated juices (fruit juices, exotics like acai and pomegranate, Naked Juice and Odwalla concoctions, Ocean Spray fruit preparations, and even fresh-squeezed antioxidant preparations from the trendy juice bar)

- Blended smoothies like Jamba Juice or homemade creations with fruit and fruit juice; sweetened alternative milks (almond, rice, soy, coconut, etc.; unsweetened varieties are fine)

- Sweetened teas like Snapple, Arizona, and premium brands from high-end markets (unsweetened is okay)

- Powdered drink mixes (chai-flavored, coffee-flavored, or hot chocolate preparations; besides lots of sugar, they often also contain bad oils)

- All diet sodas, zero calorie drinks, and other artificially sweetened concoctions (artificial sweeteners prompt sugar cravings)

- Most kombucha and similar fermented probiotic drinks (some are very low calorie, check labels)

- Sweetened cocktails (daiquiri, margarita, eggnog)

Sweetened beverages are the worst offenders because they give you a concentrated dose of carbohydrates without filling you up. Because they are not filling but still give you a wild ride on the blood sugar–insulin roller coaster, you will tend to consume more carbs and more total calories because of your fondness for sweetened drinks. If you're addicted to your daily Starbucks run, realize how much of the habit pattern is just ritual: getting out of the office and into your car, driving down to 56th & H, saying hi to the staff, and taking your crappy Frappy treasure back to your desk is a great way to break up a lazy afternoon of stillness. Perhaps you can maintain your comforting ritual, but swap out the caramel and nonfat milk sugar bomb concoction for a venti-size ice green tea (okay, 1 to 2 pumps of peach sweetener is fine . . . till it's time to go keto!).

REPLACEMENTS: Water is the drink of champions and should be the foundation of your liquid consumption. If you have an affinity for soda, you can prepare a concoction of two-thirds carbonated water, one-third kombucha, and generous squeezes of lime and lemon. Absolutely delicious! Coffee with cream and even a bit of sugar is an acceptable beverage, as are all herbal teas, caffeinated teas, or unsweetened teas available at most coffeehouses. Kombucha, the fermented and carbonated tea drink that has exploded in popularity in recent times, offers a nice dose of probiotics and other health benefits. Shop carefully for a product that has minimal carbohydrate content. Certain flavors contain only moderate amounts of carbs (5–20 grams/20–80 calories in a 16-ounce bottle—totally fine when you are cutting it with water as described), while others can go up above 40 grams/160 calories in a 16-ounce bottle—that's not much different from soda or fruit juice! You can also have fun making your own at home from a starter live culture known as a SCOBY.

Baking Ingredients

ELIMINATE: Toss all those ancient bags of powders (flours, starches, and powdered sweeteners like fructose or dextrose), and syrups like Karo, maple syrup, molasses, and even honey.

REPLACEMENTS: Almond meal and coconut flour serve as acceptable substitutes for wheat flour, and many primal/paleo cookbooks utilize these to help you welcome pancakes back into your world if you can't stand life without them. Stevia is an acceptable sweetener to use occasionally in small amounts.

Condiments/Cooking Items

ELIMINATE: Almost all condiments, mayonnaise, and salad dressings contain objectionable sweetening agents (both natural and artificial) and highly refined vegetable oils (details shortly). Jams, jellies, ketchup, and the like are significant hidden sources of sugar.

Toss everything in this category except cooking/flavoring/barbecue sauces. You can use these flavoring agents even if they have sugar or bad oils, because the amounts are trivial.

REPLACEMENTS: Healthy grocers and Internet resources now offer mayonnaise and salad dressings formed with a base of avocado oil (disclaimer: my company Primal Kitchen makes products in these categories. Disclaimer #2: They are absolutely delicious!). Products made with extra-virgin olive oil are also acceptable. Examine labels—even celebrity-branded salad dressings with "olive oil" in the title contain more refined high polyunsaturated vegetable oil than olive oil.

Dairy Products

ELIMINATE: Discard nonfat or low-fat milk, processed cheese and cheesy spreads, ice cream and other frozen treats and fruity yogurts. Any dairy product characterized as nonfat or low-fat is just a sugar bomb. Furthermore, many health-conscious consumers are concerned about potential allergenic, autoimmune, and growth factor stimulating effects of lactose (carbohydrate) and casein (protein) present in dairy. High-fat or fermented dairy products have little or none of these agents.

REPLACEMENTS: The best choices for dairy are raw, fermented, unpasteurized, unsweetened, and of the highest possible fat content: butter, aged cheese, cottage cheese, cream cheese, half and half, heavy cream, kefir, plain yogurt (full-fat), and whole milk (preferably raw).

Fats and Oils

ELIMINATE: High polyunsaturated vegetable and seed oils (canola, corn, soybean, sunflower, safflower, etc.) have been subjected to destructive high-temperature processing methods, along with the inclusion of chemical solvents. Significant oxidative damage has occurred during the processing of most of these oils, and things worsen significantly when the oils are exposed to light, oxygen, or heated for cooking purposes. These agents inflict cellular damage at the DNA level immediately upon ingestion. Dr. Shanahan cites one study with young, healthy subjects showing that eating a single order of french fries causes an immediate disturbance in healthy arterial function (stiffer, less able to dilate effectively) that can last for up to 24 hours! While vegetable oils don't stimulate insulin, they contribute to insulin resistance by creating oxidative stress in the liver.

Immediately discard all products made with these oils, including bottled oils (canola, cottonseed, corn, soybean, safflower, sunflower), buttery spreads and sprays (Smart Balance, Promise), and all products containing these oils (read labels—they're everywhere, including the aforementioned condiments and much of the packaged and frozen snacks at the supermarket). Of course, avoid the junky snacks and treats containing partially hydrogenated trans fats. When dining out, insist your meal is cooked in a temperature-stable fat such as saturated animal fats (butter, ghee, lard), olive oil, or avocado oil, or go elsewhere. It's a safe strategy to entirely avoid the lowbrow mainstream fast-food offerings, where you are sure to get heavy doses of free radicals from their assembly line offerings.

REPLACEMENTS: When an oil is made from a high-fat plant such as avocado, coconut, or olive, it's acceptable. Minimal processing is necessary and you are consuming a product that is close to its natural state. Until further notice, stick with avocado and extra-virgin olive oil for eating. For cooking, avocado, coconut, and macadamia nut oils are temperature-stable plant-based oils. Dark-roasted sesame oil is also acceptable for low-temperature cooking as in stir-fries. You can also cook with saturated animal fats like butter or lard. Even recycled bacon grease is vastly healthier than organic canola oil for cooking, believe it or not!

Fast Food

ELIMINATE: The popular global chains are mostly serving up sugars, grains, toxic vegetable oil, and inferior quality, heavily processed meats from feedlot animals. You can find less offensive offerings on their menus these days, but I typically view travel as a great opportunity to skip a meal or two and enjoy the benefits of Intermittent Fasting.

REPLACEMENTS: Numerous local restaurants and even national chains have a sincere commitment to sourcing the healthiest ingredients and preparing fresh, nutritious food for on-the-go consumers. For example, the fresh-Mex chain Chipotle has a "Food With Integrity" mission, and sources natural, local, planet-friendly meat and produce. Most popular chains either have alternative menu items or are happy to adapt to grain-free alternatives of the typical burger or sandwich offering.

Grains and Derivative Products

ELIMINATE: Grains come in many forms and clever disguises. Make sure you do a thorough purge of:

- Cereals, corn, pasta, rice, and wheat; bread and flour products (baguettes, crackers, croissants, Danishes, donuts, graham crackers, muffins, pizza, pretzels, rolls, saltine crackers, swirls, tortillas, Triscuits, Wheat Thins)

- Breakfast foods (Cream of Wheat, dried cereal, French toast, granola, grits, oatmeal, pancakes, waffles)

- Chips (corn, potato, tortilla)

- Cooking grains (amaranth, barley, bulgur, couscous, millet, rye)

- Puffed snacks (Cheetos, Goldfish, Pirates Booty, popcorn, rice cakes)

Told ya you were gonna make room in your pantry! Understand that corn is a grain, not a vegetable. Corn and its derivative products (such as the particularly offensive high fructose corn syrup, or HFCS) are ubiquitous in the modern diet—used to sweeten all manner of beverages and processed foods.

REPLACEMENTS: For meal staples like pasta, rice, corn, or bread, either skip them and enjoy the best part of the dish (meatballs and sauce, hold the spaghetti) or try fun replacements, like swapping out tortillas for lettuce leaves. For recipes, substitute coconut flour or almond meal for wheat flour. Swap out your grain-based snacks for high-fat alternatives such as nuts, seeds and their derivative butters, 85 to 90% dark chocolate, sardines, hard-boiled eggs, or fresh berries.

Legumes

ELIMINATE: Alfalfa, beans, peanuts, peanut butter, peas, lentils, soybeans, and tofu. Legumes are far less objectionable than grains because they offer some good nutritional benefits and have lower levels of harmful anti-nutrients. However, they deliver a significant dose of carbohydrates, and should be put on the sidelines during the 21-Day Reset, any time you are trying to reduce excess body fat, and especially when going keto.

REPLACEMENTS: Over the long-term, if you are at or near your ideal body composition, and have little or no concern about the leaky gut sensitivities that some experience when consuming legumes, you can enjoy your vegetables dipped in hummus, natural peanut butter in your smoothies or on your dark chocolate, and other legume favorites in moderation. Legumes are a reliable source of resistant starch to boot, something that's of particular concern for low-carb enthusiasts to regularly integrate into their diet.

Processed Meats

ELIMINATE: Don't confuse the evolutionary health message as that of giving free reign to consume unhealthy, heavily processed foods—and this includes the meat category. Avoid packaged meat products processed with bad oils, sweeteners, and chemical additives, such as breakfast sausage patties, dinner roasts, frozen meals, and sliced lunch meats. Avoid smoked, cured, nitrate- or nitrite-treated meats such as bologna, ham, hot dogs, jerky, pepperoni, and salami. Mass-produced meat, fish, fowl, and eggs often contain hormones, pesticides, and antibiotics, and they deliver an inferior nutrient and fatty acid profile because these animals' diets are vastly inferior to the diets of naturally raised animals.

REPLACEMENTS: Locally raised, pastured/grassfed animals are the best, followed by certified organic fare. If your local options are limited, utilize the Internet to have wild-caught Alaskan salmon or grassfed beef shipped right to your door.

Processed Snacks

ELIMINATE: Energy bars; fruit bars and rolls; granola bars; protein bars; frozen breakfast, dinner, and dessert products; and packaged, grain/sugar-laden snack products. If it's in a box, package, or wrapper, think twice! Take a closer look and see the typically excessive amount of carbohydrates—in addition to chemical additives and refined vegetable oils—that constitute many popular and even seemingly healthy snack and energy foods.

REPLACEMENTS: There are precious few options for healthy, low-carb packaged snacks. Many of the esteemed nutritious energy bar products such as LäraBar (made with raw fruit and nuts only) deliver an excessive carbohydrate count if you are trying to become fat-adapted. Strange as it may sound, an 85–90 percent cacao dark chocolate bar is a more favorable option than virtually any natural energy bar.

Sweets

ELIMINATE: Brownies, candy, candy bars, cake, caramel, chocolate syrup, cookies, do-nuts, ice cream, milk chocolate, milk chocolate chips, and pie. Also eliminate sugar/sweeteners (agave, artificial sweeteners, brown sugar, cane sugar, evaporated cane juice, HFCS, honey, molasses, powdered sugar, raw sugar, table sugar), sugar/chocolate coated nuts and trails mixes, ice pops and other frozen desserts, syrups, and other packaged/processed sweets and treats.

Consuming sweets generates a glucose spike and insulin flood with zero nutritional benefits. The glucose-insulin roller coaster eating pattern promotes inflammation, oxidative damage, and a suppression of immune function (glucose competes with vitamin C at cell receptor sites).

REPLACEMENTS: Giving up sweets for 21 days may seem daunting, but once you clear your system of excess glucose, you will see cravings minimize, crashes moderate, and health improve noticeably. You will soon become habituated to the rich and satisfying taste of 85 to 90 percent dark chocolate and forget what you are missing in the sweets department.

> **For the purposes of insulin moderation and fat reduction, a 200-calorie bowl of brown rice is no better than a 200-calorie bag of Skittles.**

But . . . What About Healthy Whole Grains?

Decades of conventional wisdom have led us to believe that whole grains should form the foundation of a healthy diet. The official U.S. government recommendation is "6–11 servings a day" from the bread, cereal, rice, and pasta food group, which occupies the base level of the familiar food pyramid. (Google "Primal Blueprint Food Pyramid" to find a version that honors our hunter-gatherer genetic hardwiring: no grains in sight!) While everyone is in agreement that refined "white" grains have no nutritional value, ancestral health experts argue that the recommended daily servings are 6 to 11 too many, even if you emphasize the vaunted whole grains.

Most forms of carbohydrates you consume are converted into glucose soon after ingestion in order to be burned. Complex carbs might burn a little slower due to their starchy composition and fiber content, but for the purposes of fat reduction, a 200-calorie bowl of brown rice is no different than a 200-calorie bag of Skittles. Sure, the Skittles cause a quicker glucose spike and insulin surge than would rice, but you still have to produce a similar total amount of insulin over time to deal with 200 calories of carbs in either form. The brown rice might have a tad more nutrition, but it pales in comparison to nutrient-rich foods like meat, eggs, nuts, or vegetables. Furthermore, as mentioned in Chapter 2, whole grains contain higher levels of anti-nutrients like gluten that compromise digestive and immune health.

Hungry for Quick Results?
Have Patience, Not Hunger

While the book's opening material detailed the longevity benefits of fasting, nutritional ketosis, and caloric efficiency, don't worry about this fun stuff at the outset of your journey. To ensure your success in eliminating these high insulin–producing foods, you can feel free to eat primal/paleo/ancestral foods as much and as often as you like. You are trading your morning oatmeal and O.J. for a delicious omelet, and your afternoon energy bar for a handful or two of macadamia nuts. You are doing whatever it takes to leave carbohydrate dependency in the rearview mirror once and for all, including obtaining total dietary satisfaction from high-fat foods. If at any time during the 21-Day Reset you feel hungry or deprived, or start obsessing about your old insulin-stimulating go-to treats, a handful of macadamia nuts could become your ultimate fail-safe go-to snack to obtain immediate and lasting satisfaction. I know mac nuts always do the trick for me. Other quick, easy go-to snack options include 85% dark chocolate smothered in almond butter, a couple spoonfuls of guacamole, a couple bunches of asparagus wrapped in bacon, or any of the enticing offerings in the "Bombs, Balls, and Bites" section of the recipe chapter.

Once you become fat- and keto-adapted, your energy dips and cravings will vanish, because your brain and body will have a steady supply of fat and ketones at all times in the event your food consumption is inconsistent. And when that time comes, you may be inclined on certain days to trade the omelet for an extended fast into your lunchtime salad, or start your day with a high-fat coffee or ketone supplement and consume nothing else until the afternoon. As a guy who loves to eat, this seems like one of the most beautiful benefits of keto—that the defining purpose of food in your life becomes that of gustatory pleasure instead of fuel for a gas tank that's constantly teetering on the verge of empty.

For now, we'll jump immediately into emphasizing wholesome, high-fat, high-satiety ancestral foods—the topic of the next chapter. Take out the garbage, and then it's time to go shopping.

CHAPTER 6

The Keys to High-Fat, Low-Carb, Primal-Style Eating

WITH unhealthy refined carbs and fats removed from your diet, they will be immediately replaced with more nutrient-dense, high-satiety primal/paleo/ancestral-style foods. A variety of fresh, colorful vegetables will be the centerpiece of your diet and occupy the majority of space on your plate. This is an important point to lead with, because casual critics often dismiss keto as unhealthy, based on an assumed restriction of high-antioxidant, nutrient-dense vegetables and fruits.

Yes, most of your calories will come from healthy fats during your 21-Day Metabolism Reset, but you will also enjoy a variety of nutrient-dense carbo-hydrates, such as vegetables and fruits. Vegetables are indeed composed almost entirely of carbohydrate, but they are high in fiber and water content, so even large portions of them deliver minimal carbohydrate calories in comparison to those heavily processed, concentrated sources of carbs like bread, cereal, sweetened beverages, energy bars, and sugary treats. Consuming a variety of colorful vegetables also plays an important role in supporting a healthy intestinal microbiome.

Mounting research suggests that our intestinal microbiome has a profound influence on digestive and immune function, inflammation control, mood stability and cognitive function (e.g., 90 percent of the "feel good" neurotransmitter serotonin is produced in the gut), insulin sensitivity and fat metabolism, improved thyroid function, improved sleep, and much more. Studies suggest that the gut microbiome presides over 6,500 different detoxification and metabolic functions. The ultimate goal is for healthy gut bacteria to preside over the ever-present harmful bacteria, because illness results when harmful bacteria predominate. It's especially important to eat your vegetables when going keto, because carbohydrate restriction automatically reduces your intake of certain other gut-healthy high-carbohydrate foods.

To facilitate and sustain nutritional ketosis (after you finish the 21-Day Reset), you must adhere to the hard limit of 50 grams of gross carbohydrate intake per day. Besides ditching all grains, sugars, and sweetened liquids, you will likely need to avoid all fruits, and also want to limit your intake of vegetables that grow in the ground (sweet potatoes or yams, rutabaga, beets, carrots, turnips, etc.). While these tubers are certainly nutritious foods that may have a deserved place in your long-term eating patterns, they are more starchy (delivering a more dense carbohydrate load per serving) than the above-ground groups like leafy greens and cruciferous vegetables (broccoli, Brussels sprouts, cabbage, cauliflower).

While fruit is also highly nutritious, today's year-round availability of extra-sweet, overly cultivated fruits is a far cry from our typical ancestral pattern of consuming wild, highly fibrous, less sugary fruits only during their narrow ripening seasons. Another concern about fruit when it comes to reducing excess body fat: Fructose, the prominent source of carbohydrate calories in fruit, must be processed in the liver before it can be burned for energy. The liver is also where excess carb calories are converted into fat, so fruit is known as the most lipogenic (fat-forming) form of carbohydrate. Because fructose goes straight to the liver, it's also great for restocking liver and muscle glycogen. Hence, if you're a devoted fitness enthusiast and maintaining ideal body composition, you can be more liberal with your fruit intake—it's going right into those glycogen suitcases. In summary, fruit has many nutritional and glycogen replenishing benefits, but it's off the table when you are going keto (okay, a handful of fresh berries now and then is fine, especially if you are active), and probably smart to avoid or strictly minimize when you are trying to drop fat. Otherwise, enjoy locally grown fruits during their ripening seasons, especially berries. Avoid big doses of winter fruits transported from distant locations, and never take concentrated doses of fruit in smoothies or juices. Don't stress too much about fruit consumption during your 21-Day Reset, but definitely don't go out of your way to eat it either. When in doubt, reference the ancestral consumption patterns and keep it real.

During your 21-Day Reset, your abundant vegetable intake and selective fruit intake will be complemented by nutrient-dense primal/paleo/ancestral-style foods such as meat, fish, fowl, and eggs; high-fat plant foods like olives, avocados, coconut, and their oils; nuts, seeds, and their derivative butters; and responsible consumption of high-fat dairy products and high-cacao percentage dark chocolate. After you learn about the ancestral eating philosophy and the ideal role of fat, protein, and carbohydrate in an ancestral eating pattern—and in a keto eating pattern—I'll present an at-a-glance summary of what ancestral meal and snack patterns look like, followed by a step-by-step 21-Day Metabolism Reset meal plan. You can follow the plan to the letter if you want to go on autopilot during your Reset, or you can peruse the suggestions to get inspiration for a delicious and easy way to adhere to the recommended eating patterns during your journey.

As I said earlier, your main goals are to kick your carb dependency and increase your fat intake so you remain satisfied and don't struggle. Don't worry about getting your carbs down to 50 grams per day until it's time to go keto. If you are diligently restricting refined grains and sugars, you will surely default into the more relaxed limit of 150 grams of average daily carb intake per day that frames the Primal Blueprint philosophy, and that's fantastic for right now.

Don't worry about dropping excess body fat during this reset period, either. Slimming down will happen effortlessly, and fat accumulation will cease to be a concern for the rest of your life when you build the right metabolic machinery. However, it's critical that you proceed through the steps presented in this book with precision and patience, never struggle or suffer, never backslide, and never rush anything. That's why you will do the fine-tuning and take and pass the midterm exam before you go keto.

A New Eating Philosophy

We've been conditioned to think that skipping meals, especially breakfast, is a disaster, but this concept is a relic from the carbohydrate-dependency paradigm. Indeed, if you are hyper-insulinemic and unable to burn body fat well, skipping a meal will make you tired, cranky, and likely to binge when you do eat something. Attempting a calorie-restrictive crash diet, a detox cleanse, or a programmed fast will simply cause more fight-or-flight stimulation, as you break down your body's lean muscle tissue to fuel your day with glucose. If you exist in carb dependency and attempt to crash-diet frequently, you will create metabolic damage that can make fat adaptation extremely difficult—even when you do things correctly.

Unfortunately, this story is extremely common, as well-meaning diet enthusiasts continue to fight the battle of the bulge with the wrong metabolic machinery. As you embark on the 21-Day Metabolism Reset, and eventually enter nutritional ketosis, you are accessing an entirely new paradigm of fat adaptation—one that carries completely different rules and realities than the carbohydrate dependency paradigm. In your new world, skipping meals, *especially* breakfast, earns you a gold star on the road to becoming fat-adapted and eventually keto-adapted.

> **If you exist in carb dependency and attempt to crash-diet frequently, you will create metabolic damage that can make fat adaptation extremely difficult.**

Again, your 21-Day Reset is only the first step in going keto, so don't be overly ambitious with fasting or calorie restriction until you have built more momentum. Just focus on making the right food choices, but at the same time realize that if you're not hungry, you don't have to eat. As you build your metabolic machinery, you can pay more attention to your hunger and satiety signals than you ever have before. You'll hone a deep-seated confidence that your world is not going to end if you push away your plate while there's still food on it, rush out of the house without preparing a ritzy unhealthy start breakfast, or work through lunch with a handful of almonds instead of the usual Tuesday all-you-can-eat Chinese buffet special. In the fat-burning-beast paradigm, regular meals are overrated, period. Hunger sensations, instead of being a telltale sign of fight-or-flight kicking into gear, are something that can help enhance your enjoyment and appreciation of food. And fat is your favorite thing to burn instead of something you hate.

For your first week of the reset, be sure you completely ditch the big-three offenders, eat as much nutritious low-carb, high-fat (LCHF) food as you want, be open to skipping or delaying meals if you aren't hungry, stop eating when you've reach a satisfaction point (instead of the usual feeling of "full"), and embrace an intuitive approach instead of the usual regimented approach. The great nation of Sweden has adopted the acronym LCHF as a mantra to transform the national consciousness and public policy about healthy eating. In America, I don't think we're close to toppling the food conglomerates and their manipulative advertising, nor the dated and special interest–tainted public policy any time soon—but you are free to try LCHF and see how it works for you.

While it's best that you focus on the big picture during the first three weeks—ditching processed junk and emphasizing ancestral foods—the following sections detail the evolved roles of fat, protein, and carbohydrate in an ancestral-style eating pattern, and the refinements required when you go keto.

Fat

The secret to becoming fat- and keto-adapted is to make natural fats the centerpiece of your diet and the vast majority of your calories (even though vegetables will still occupy the bulk of your plate). Hence, it's essential that you reject any lingering fat phobias that you harbor as a result of flawed cultural programming from dated, inaccurate science. Read Gary Taubes's books such as *Good Calories, Bad Calories; Why We Get Fat;* or *The Case Against Sugar* for exceptionally well-researched and referenced presentations about how ridiculously flawed and manipulative the scientific foundation for a grain-based diet is.

> **Eating fat won't make you fat. It will help regulate your appetite and satiety hormones so you need less food to achieve total dietary satisfaction.**

We've hit this point already from many directions, but it's essential to realize that eating fat won't make you fat. Rather, eating healthy sources of fat will help you better burn stored body fat (because fat doesn't stimulate insulin), stabilize your appetite and energy levels, provide high levels of satiety and satisfaction (because fat tastes good!), and help regulate the prominent appetite-stimulating hormone *ghrelin* and your prominent satiety/fat-storage hormone *leptin*. The end result is you require fewer calories to achieve total dietary satisfaction, can skip meals easily without adverse effects, and accordingly have stored fat (and ketones, too) easily accessible for energy. Under these circumstances, you can use tools like Intermittent Fasting or ketogenic periods to easily reduce any excess body fat, any time you want.

Enjoy Locally Grown Meals, *Really* Local

Escaping carb dependency and becoming fat-adapted is the only fail-safe way to manage your body composition over the long term. If you minimize insulin production, it's nearly impossible to add excess body fat. If you don't minimize insulin production, though, you will steadily pack on extra fat over the years. The severity of your fat accumulation depends on your unique familial genetics—the luck of the draw. Even if you come from skinny lineage, bad stuff happens inside when you are carb-dependent; becoming fat-adapted is the only true way to steer clear of the metabolic syndrome disease epidemic.

Now that you appreciate the urgency of escaping carb dependency and fully embracing your free pass to consume natural fats as your go-to food choice, let's talk straight about dropping excess body fat. If you go hog wild on bacon and other fats—obtaining all your energy needs from ingested calories—there won't be any stimulus to mobilize and burn your stored fat. Again, you won't gain fat on a high-fat diet; unlike with carbs, you'll be too satiated to overeat! But if you want to lose excess body fat, you must realize that you can get your next meal from your plate or, alternatively, from your butt and thighs. The elegance of being fat-adapted/metabolically efficient is that you won't know the difference; you'll breeze along on your busy morning whether you have had a big omelet or just some green tea with lemon.

If you are not fat-adapted, none of this works. Your carb-dependent hormonal situation (namely, the dysregulation of ghrelin, leptin, and other hunger/metabolic/satiety hormones) will stimulate hunger, and even cause you to overeat in response to any attempted caloric restriction. Remember, as a carbohydrate addict, you are lousy at burning stored energy like fat and ketones, and you are hugely dependent upon regular carb feedings to sustain your energy and ward off intense hunger. This is a much bigger problem than being fat-adapted and overdoing the macadamia nut snacks and morning bacon and eggs such that fat loss is stalled. If this is the case, just start eating more locally grown meals from the butt/thigh café; that is, ramp up your Intermittent Fasting, eat only when you're actually hungry, eat to satisfaction instead of to fullness, and move around as much as possible during the day. If you have a good fitness base and become fat-adapted, you can accelerate your progress by conducting long-duration aerobic workouts or brief high-intensity sessions.

Protein

Since the concept of a high-protein diet has been touted for years as something ultra-healthy and befitting a truly devoted fitness enthusiast, let's set the record straight: A high-protein diet (one routinely and significantly exceeding your baseline needs) is really a high-carbohydrate, fat-storage diet (details shortly). Your objective for protein intake is simple: consume the minimum necessary to preserve (or build, if desired) lean muscle mass and the healthy functioning of your organs. Mounting research suggests that we may require significantly less dietary protein than has been widely recommended by experts on either side of the low-carb versus low-fat debate. Furthermore, it's undisputed that there are an assortment of significant adverse effects to consuming more protein than you need to support basic metabolic function and preserve lean muscle mass.

When you're metabolically efficient, you can get your next meal from your plate or, alternatively, from your butt and thighs.

The widely agreed upon guideline has been to consume an average of 0.5 grams per pound (1.1 grams/kilo) of bodyweight per day as a baseline, then increase intake according to activity level. For the moderately active, that's 0.7 grams per pound (1.5 grams/kilo), and for devoted exercisers/high-calorie-burners, it is 1 gram per pound (2.2 grams per kilo). Some advocate even more than the gram-per-pound formula, particularly for special populations like bodybuilders and team sport athletes looking to add or maintain substantial amounts of muscle mass.

Dr. Ron Rosedale, author of *The Rosedale Diet,* asserts that 0.5 grams per pound of *lean body mass* is plenty for everyone, even hard-training athletes. Luis Villasenor, the keto bodybuilder and trainer, suggests that serious athletes as well as the elderly (who may be more resistant to mTOR signaling) need at least 0.7 grams per pound of lean mass, and possibly more at times. For comparison, a 200-pound athlete with 15 percent body fat following conventional recommendations would consume 200 grams of protein per day, or 800 calories. With the updated recommendation of 0.7 grams per pound of lean mass (200 pounds @ 15 percent fat means 170 pounds of lean mass), the recommended average daily consumption would be 119 grams (170 × 0.7), or 476 calories. If you are habitually overconsuming protein, optimizing your intake could increase longevity and reduce the risk of cancer and other disease patterns.

As was mentioned earlier about excess carb consumption, excess protein consumption also promotes accelerated cell division and the excessive stimulation of growth factors like IGF-1 and mTOR. Overfed cells influenced by excessive growth factors divide faster, are more likely to turn cancerous, and promote glycation, oxidative damage, and systemic inflammation. A handy chart to help you ballpark the protein contribution of common high-protein foods is provided in Chapter 9. When it comes to keto, it should also be noted that excess protein is insulinogenic (causes insulin to rise), so consuming lots of protein will shut off ketosis just like when you eat lots of carbs.

After your basic metabolic and lean tissue maintenance needs are met from dietary protein, any excess amino acids are sent from the small intestine to the liver to get processed. Since your body can't store protein as it can carbs and fat, your liver works hard to either convert the excess protein into glucose via gluconeogenesis (only if you need glucose) or commence a chemical process called *deamination* to clear the bloodstream of excess amino acids. Deamination results in a toxic buildup of ammonia and nitrogen, which must then be converted into urea and excreted by the kidneys. If you are slamming protein to the tune of your total bodyweight in grams per pound every day, as do many fitness enthusiasts, you definitely won't have to worry about going catabolic and losing muscle mass, but you might want to worry about increased risk of cancer, obesity, diabetes, insulin resistance, osteoporosis, kidney dysfunction, and accelerated aging.

> **Excess protein consumption promotes accelerated cell division and excessive stimulation of growth factors.**

Because you don't need to call upon gluconeogenesis excessively when you are fat- and keto-adapted, you may be particularly suited to thrive on moderate dietary protein consumption when you go keto. Experts like Doctors Attia, D'Agostino, Phinney and Volek, and Luis Villasenor assert that optimal intake varies among individuals, but the consensus recommendation is 0.5 grams per pound of lean mass as a baseline, up to 0.7 grams per pound of lean mass if you are active, and potentially up to 1 gram per pound of lean mass for extreme subjects such as an ectomorph doing heavy athletic training, an active, growing teen who is not overweight, a pregnant or lactating mother, or an active elderly person. Consequently, we have to appreciate the critical distinction between the optimal keto strategy of high fat, moderate protein, and ultra-low carb, in contrast with a shaky keto approach of medium-ish fat, medium-ish protein, and low-but-not-ultra-low carb intake. It's easy to blur these lines when you're a novice, or you don't take the time to calculate accurate macronutrient intake with an online calculator, or you are a bit cavalier or absentminded about your meal and snacking habits, or if you have embedded in your psyche an irrational affinity for protein thanks to the dated bro-science that pervades the fitness community.

If you are stressing about trying to pinpoint your protein intake, realize that your body is really good at dealing with occasional insufficiencies, as well as excesses. If you fall short now and then (e.g., fasting), your body will engage in protein-sparing efforts such as the aforementioned autophagy to get you back to even par. If you get into a routine of underconsumption, you won't feel so hot—you'll be sluggish and notice your muscle mass decreasing. Considering that your baseline requirements are minimal, this might only happen if you are chronically overtraining, following a severe calorie-restricted crash diet, have a serious chronic illness like celiac disease or a severe leaky gut that prevents you from absorbing nutrients, or go on a hunger strike to protest the bro-science in the fitness community.

On the flip side, if you overconsume protein now and then, you'll excrete it or make a little extra glucose—no big deal. A bigger concern for low-carb/keto enthusiasts is dutifully restricting carbs and bad oils, but being overly ambitious about protein intake and/or reluctant (both consciously and subconsciously) to make nutritious natural fats a dietary centerpiece. When going for lean meats instead of fatty meats, hitting the high-protein smoothies every day, or doing truly silly stuff like consuming egg whites instead of the entire egg, you risk overstimulating the undesirable growth factors. Interestingly, protein stimulates both insulin and insulin's counterregulatory hormone, glucagon (which mobilizes energy from storage to burn). For this reason, protein doesn't promote fat storage as directly as do carbohydrates (which stimulate just insulin, while suppressing glucagon).

Knowing that carb intake is restricted to a maximum of 50 grams/200 calories per day, and that even top-end protein consumption for most people will only be 300 to 600 calories a day, it follows that when you do the Reset, and even more so when you go keto, the vast majority of your calories will come from nutritious natural fats.

Carbohydrate

I've mentioned many times the hard limit of 50 grams of carbohydrate intake per day to facilitate ketosis. This is a widely accepted general guideline, but it's time to drill a little deeper in an effort to optimize your carbohydrate intake. First, there is good support for the idea that carb intake to facilitate ketosis should be lower if you are minimally active, perhaps down around 20 grams per day. If you are extremely active, you can likely consume significantly more than 50 grams per day and still be in the keto club. A Tour de France cyclist pedaling through the mountains for five hours a day can probably consume 200 grams of carbs per day (that's still way less than the 600 grams a traditional high-carb pro rider might consume) and still be in ketosis.

This athlete's hall pass (I know, reminds me of high school, too . . .) is a consequence of dietary carbohydrates going directly to refuel glycogen stores that have been depleted through exercise. Because there are no excess carbs in the bloodstream needing to be cleared, there is minimal production of insulin and therefore no disruption of ketosis. Only when glycogen storage tanks in the liver (around 100 grams) and muscles (400–500 grams) become full will dietary carbs be converted into triglycerides and stored as fat. Doctors Attia, D'Agostino, and Shanahan concur with the idea that the timing of carbohydrate intake can affect your keto efforts, and also your general health, immune function, and fat-burning capabilities. Whether you're trying to stay in nutritional ketosis or just maximize the benefits of a low-carb lifestyle, the trick is to consume carbs in a manner that doesn't disturb homeostasis, immune function, or optimal hormone balance. If you consume too many carbs at one sitting, you'll not only quickly shut off the ketone burning but you will also stimulate that objectionable insulin response and the consequent chain of events that disturb homeostasis.

What's more, it's been shown that a sugar binge can suppress immune function for hours afterward, because glucose competes with and crowds out vitamin C on cellular-entry pathways. If you consume an appreciable amount of carbs and then go sit on your butt in the office for eight hours, this is going to promote dysregulation of appetite, energy level, and mood, and promote insulin resistance and fat storage. This is why Dr. Cate urges people to not screw up breakfast with a carb bolus. Conversely, if you consume a larger than usual carbohydrate meal the night before a challenging workout, these carbs will likely be put to good use during your session. Similarly, if you enjoy some of your favorite nutritious carbs in the aftermath of a challenging workout, those go directly toward restocking muscle glycogen, and will be far less likely to stimulate excess insulin or disturb hormone balance.

Your best carb intake strategy is to not overconsume at any single meal—and of course in general, too! You don't need to be tightly wound here and eat one Brussels sprout per hour instead of a bowl of them at dinner, but it's great to start tightening up your carb intake in preparation for going keto. This should not be a big issue, because when your metabolic machinery is burning stored energy well, you'll become less likely to stuff your face. This common habit has been attributed to subconscious fears of running out of energy before your next meal. This is understandable, because it is in fact what happens when you are a sugar-burner. When you reset your metabolism and your appetite is always stabilized, you'll enjoy just the right amount of food to give you maximum satisfaction, rather than eat to the point of that silly post-meal discomfort we are all so familiar with.

You may have heard of the concept of *net carbs,* whereby the amount of fiber contained in a certain food is factored into a calculation with the gross carbohydrate volume to produce a lower net carb number. The thinking here is that the fiber minimizes the glycemic response, and hence a soda with 50 grams of gross carbs has a more deleterious impact than a fibrous bowl of fruit with 50 grams of gross carbs but a net carb value of only 30. This is relevant on many levels, especially when spacing carbs out in small doses to try and not disturb ketone production. However, I'd rather you err on the safe side with your carbohydrate intake patterns, and track your gross carbohydrate intake. Besides, this is what the online macronutrient calculators generate, so record-keeping is less laborious than having to factor out fiber to derive net carb figures. Note an important exception per Villasenor's Ketogains program: Avocados and greens and other nonstarchy veggies have such high fiber and nutrient density that you can essentially ignore them when you are tracking to stay under 50 gross carbs per day (i.e., their net carb values are extremely low).

Primal/Paleo/Ancestral Eating
at a Glance

The delicious recipes in this book, the 21-Day Metabolism Reset meal plan at the end of this chapter, and a 21-Day keto meal plan that's at the end of Chapter 9 are all low carb and grain free. I hope you take the time to prepare some interesting selections. For now, you may want to build some momentum by establishing a routine of simple, repeatable go-to meals. Here are a few ideas:

Breakfast

EGGS: Prepared any style, perhaps with some bacon. Try a bowl of chopped hard-boiled eggs, chopped bacon, walnuts, and sun-dried tomatoes, drizzled with avocado or olive oil.

OMELET: Enjoy ingredients like pan-fried chopped veggies, bacon, cheese, and perhaps topped with avocado and/or salsa.

HIGH-FAT COFFEE OR TEA: Enjoy your warm morning beverage with a tablespoon of melted butter, coconut oil, or MCT oil. This will give you calories to burn until your first proper meal, and potentially be less difficult than a complete fast.

MACRONUTRIENT BALANCED SMOOTHIE: Base with unsweetened coconut or almond milk, add ice cubes, whey protein powder, a generous pile of fresh kale or spinach, and perhaps a tablespoon of coconut oil or MCT oil. This is a great way to get a concentrated dose of greens.

Lunch

SALAD: My midday Bigass Salad (page 259) is the centerpiece and greatest joy in my overall eating strategy—especially beneficial in delivering nutritious carbs and resistant starch when I'm keto. Enjoy leafy greens, assorted colorful veggies, nuts, and a protein source like chicken, fish, steak, or turkey. Coat generously with a healthy oil like extra-virgin olive, avocado, or a dressing made from these bases.

Dinner

MEAT AND VEGETABLES: This suggestion obviously covers 1,001 possible combinations. Dive into the recipe ideas in this book and the many other primal/paleo/ancestral-style cookbooks available.

Snacks

BERRIES: Locally grown, in-season.

COCONUT PRODUCTS: The high-fat king of the plant kingdom, providing an excellent source of hard-to-find medium-chain triglyceride fats. MCTs provide assorted anti-inflammatory and immune-boosting properties. Add thick flakes to a homemade trail mix of nuts and dark chocolate. Refrigerate full-fat coconut milk and enjoy out of the can like pudding. If you can find the delicacy of coconut butter, a spoonful will change your life!

DARK CHOCOLATE: 85% cacao is a delicious high-fat, relatively low-carb treat. Once you habituate to the less sweet, more bitter taste, you'll never go back to the sugary milk chocolate.

FISH: Oily, cold-water fish have the best omega-3 profile and are inexpensive, convenient snacks. Pack some herring, mackerel, sardines, or tuna wherever you go.

HARD-BOILED EGGS: Put some salt, garlic spice, and olive or avocado oil in a baggie, roll the egg around in the mixture, and enjoy.

NUTS AND SEEDS: Enjoy a handful any time you have the inkling for a snack—a great protection against backsliding to the high-carb energy bar days.

NUT BUTTER: Take a straight-shot spoonful or smother on celery or dark chocolate. Choose almond, cashew, tahini, or other nut butter instead of peanut butter if you have allergies.

OLIVES: A great source of monounsaturated fatty acids.

21-Day Metabolism Reset Meal Plan

The Reset will help you align with ancestral eating patterns and get into a rhythm of eating delicious meals and snacks that are completely free of grains, sugars, and refined vegetable oils. We are not going to worry about restricting carbs down to keto levels yet, as it's important to build momentum toward fat- and keto-adaptation without unnecessary struggle. Of course, by ditching SAD foods and eating ancestral-style foods, your carb intake will naturally land at around 150 grams per day. If you are coming to your Reset off a deep immersion in SAD eating, you may experience a brief period of "low-carb flu," characterized by symptoms such as low energy, headaches, and brain fog. This is your body literally detoxing from carb addiction and working hard to transition to a fat-adapted eating pattern. Your brain, used to a fresh supply of glucose every few hours for years, hasn't yet built the metabolic machinery to burn ketones. With each passing day of ancestral-aligned eating, your fat-burning genes will upregulate and you will have more energy, focus, and appetite stability than ever before.

The 21-day sequence is thoughtfully designed to give great variety and satisfaction while adhering to the defined food and macronutrient guidelines. You can follow it exactly, but there is nothing wrong with moving the meals around or even repeating your favorite dinner three nights in a row. Besides the following meals, there are fantastic recipes in Chapter 12, and more low-carb and keto-friendly ideas online and in bookstores. Check out the recipe section at marksdailyapple.com/recipes to start.

During your 21-Day Reset, you don't need to worry about restricting calories; it's best to focus on eliminating harmful modern foods and eating patterns. Eat as much as you need to feel satisfied and to have sufficient energy for your workouts. After you complete the Reset and the six-week nutritional ketosis experience, you can then target fat reduction with tremendous momentum and virtually guaranteed results.

You will notice that I did not include any treats or desserts in the meal plan. This is because I think it is important to avoid sweets, even primal- and keto-friendly versions, during the transition phase as much as possible. If you are craving something sweet, start with a few squares of extra-dark chocolate and see if that does the trick. If over the long term you want to enjoy some creative low-carb treats, check out the desserts section of Chapter 12.

Tips for Success

‣ Don't worry about getting fancy in the kitchen unless you enjoy that sort of thing. Primal and keto eating can be as simple as an omelet and a couple Bigass Salads (page 259) every day, if you want.

‣ Double or even triple the recipes to have prepared food on hand. In particular, make large batches of protein staples like grilled chicken or shredded pork or beef. Make big pans of roasted vegetables. Hard-boil 6 to 12 eggs to have ready for salad prep.

‣ Keep the fridge stocked with raw veggies and fruit. I find it helpful to wash them as soon as I bring them home from the market (except that fresh berries should not be washed until you are ready to eat them). Some veggies like carrots, bell peppers, radishes, and cucumbers can be sliced ahead of time. Keep washed mixed greens on hand so that you can always throw together a quick salad.

‣ Stock your pantry, car, gym bag, and work desk with a few healthy snacks like macadamia or other nuts, high-quality jerkys, or, weather permitting, 85% dark chocolate.

- Embrace leftovers. Remember, almost any leftover can be turned into an omelet or stir-fry the next day for a whole new meal. Chop meat and veggies into bite-size pieces and sauté in avocado oil, bacon fat, or butter. Add some garlic powder or taco seasoning, pesto or Pea-NOT Sauce (page 219), or salsa and cheese for a whole new dish.

- Add healthy fats to every meal: heavy cream in your scrambled eggs, extra-virgin olive oil on your lunch salad, Primal Kitchen Mayo on your burger, and so on.

- If you are following the meal plan, look ahead a day or two to see if there are things you can do in advance. Especially if you will be taking lunch to work, you will likely want to prep lunches the night before so you can easily assemble or reheat them the next day.

Primal- and Keto-Approved Snacks

- Nuts and trail mix. Ideally make your own with raw or dry-roasted nuts, seeds, unsweetened coconut flakes, dark chocolate pieces (85% cacao or higher) or cacao nibs, unsweetened dried fruit (optional, use sparingly when keto), and a dash of Himalayan sea salt.
- Half an avocado with salt and lime juice.
- Hard-boiled egg.
- Primal Kitchen protein bars, or other bars made with only primal-approved ingredients.
    Recipe suggestion: marksdailyapple.com/primal-fuel-bars/
    Recipe suggestion: https://philmaffetone.com/phils-bars-revisited/
- Olives.
- Raw or roasted veggie sticks with dip (see the "Sauces, Dressings, and Dips" recipes), such as Primal Kitchen Ranch Dressing, guacamole, or aioli.
- Bone broth (see page 216).
- High-Fat Coffee (page 210; decaf if after morning).
- In-season berries or frozen organic berries with heavy cream or full-fat coconut milk.
- Organic apple or celery sticks with almond butter.
- Pork rinds/chicharrones (check ingredients—should only contain pork rind and seasoning like salt, pepper, etc.).
- Fat bombs (see the "Bombs, Balls, and Bites" recipes in Chapter 12).

DAY 1

Breakfast	Lunch
Primal Omelet (page 196)	Go-to Green Smoothie (page 212)
Coffee or tea with heavy cream	

Dinner	
Hamburger (6 ounces meat with 2 tablespoons Primal Kitchen Mayo, wrapped in lettuce leaves)	½ medium avocado, sliced
	Sliced tomato (approximately ½ cup)
	Dill pickle spears

DAY 2

Breakfast	Lunch
2 eggs, fried in 2 tablespoons butter	Bigass Salad (page 259)
Chicken sausage (2 small links)	
Fresh berries	
Coffee or tea with heavy cream	

Dinner	
The Best Grilled Chicken (page 237), with pesto (store-bought or homemade, pages 223 or 262)	Grilled asparagus spears (+1 teaspoon avocado oil, per serving)

DAY 3

Breakfast	Lunch
Primal n'oatmeal (see marksdailyapple.com/primal-noatmeal/)	Bigass Salad (page 259), with leftover grilled chicken
Coffee or tea with heavy cream	

Dinner	
Chili (see marksdailyapple.com/sweet-potato-chili-fries/)	Green beans sautéed with butter and garlic

DAY 4

Breakfast	Lunch
Greek Yogurt Crunch Bowl (page 201)	Baked sweet potato topped with:
1 cup fresh berries	*½ cup leftover chili*
Coffee or tea with heavy cream	*2 tablespoons shredded cheese*
	1½ tablespoons sour cream
	1 tablespoon chopped green onions

Dinner	
Creamy Gorgonzola "Mac" and Cheese (page 268)	Side green salad (¼ Bigass Salad, page 259) with 1–2 tablespoons Perfect Vinaigrette (page 221)

DAY 5

Breakfast	Lunch
Primal Omelet (page 196)	Go-to Green Smoothie (page 212)
Coffee or tea with heavy cream	

Dinner	
Slow-Baked Salmon with Dill Aioli (page 242)	Spinach Salad with Warm Bacon Vinaigrette (page 260)

DAY 6

Breakfast	Lunch
Coconut Flour Macadamia Pancakes (page 198), made with 1 cup blueberries	Collard Green–Turkey Club Wraps (page 243)
3 slices of bacon	1 small apple
Coffee or tea with heavy cream	2 tablespoons almond butter

Dinner	
Beef stew (see marksdailyapple.com/beef-stew-and-chicken-soup-in-35-minutes-or-less/)	Cauliflower Rice (page 266; make extra for tomorrow's dinner, too!)

DAY 7

Breakfast	Lunch
Egg Muffins in Ham Cups (page 204)	Leftover beef stew
Coffee or tea with heavy cream	

Dinner	
Thai Soup with Shrimp (page 252)	Veggie Sushi with Cauliflower Rice (page 264)

DAY 8

Breakfast	Lunch
Go-to Green Smoothie (page 212)	Cheesy Chicken and Ham (or turkey) Roll-ups (page 244)
	Raw veggies with 2 tablespoons Primal Kitchen Ranch Dressing to dip
	Mandarin orange

Dinner	
White chicken chili (see marksdailyapple.com/white-chicken-chili/)	Note: Also make Chai Chia Breakfast Pudding (page 205) for tomorrow morning
Sautéed zucchini and yellow squash	

DAY 9

Breakfast	Lunch
Chai Chia Breakfast Pudding (see day 8)	Leftover white chicken chili
Coffee or tea with heavy cream	

Dinner	
Slow Cooker Carnitas (page 229)	Sautéed Cabbage with Bacon (page 263)

DAY 10

Breakfast	Lunch
Primal Omelet (page 196)	Leftover carnitas in (raw) cabbage cups
Coffee or tea with heavy cream	¼ cup guacamole
	¼ cup salsa

Dinner	
Pan-Fried Cod with Dill Caper Sauce (page 254)	Side green salad (¼ Bigass Salad, page 259) with 1–2 tablespoons Perfect Vinaigrette (page 221)
Perfect Roasted Brussels Sprouts (page 271)	

DAY 11

Breakfast	Lunch
Turmeric Scrambled Eggs (page 206)	Ginger Beet Smoothie (page 213)
1 cup cubed cantaloupe	¼ cup almonds
Coffee or tea with heavy cream	2 squares dark chocolate

Dinner

Turmeric and kale soup (see marksdailyapple
.com/turmeric-kale-soup-with-ground-lamb/)

Roasted baby carrots with cumin

DAY 12

Breakfast

Brad's "Ketoatmeal" (page 203) topped with
½ cup fresh berries and ¼ cup shredded
coconut

Coffee or tea with heavy cream

Lunch

Leftover kale soup

½ baked sweet potato with 1 tablespoon butter
and cinnamon

Side green salad (¼ Bigass Salad, page 259)
with 1–2 tablespoons Perfect Vinaigrette
(page 221)

Dinner

Macadamia-Crusted Mahi-Mahi with Browned
Butter (page 256)

Steamed broccoli with ¼ cup finely grated
Parmesan cheese

DAY 13

Breakfast

Katie's Keto Granola (page 207), with ¾ cup
full-fat coconut milk and ¼ cup fresh berries

Coffee or tea with heavy cream

Lunch

Antipasto plate:

  3 ounces salami and/or prosciutto

  1 ounce cheese, sliced or cubed

  ½ cup roasted red pepper (store-bought,
    in olive oil)

  ½ cup olives

  ¼ cup artichoke hearts (store-bought, in water)

  ¼ cup Marcona almonds

  1 small pear or apple, thinly sliced

Dinner

Sausage and Kale (page 240)

DAY 14

Breakfast

3 eggs, scrambled with 1 cup Sausage and Kale
left over from last night's dinner

Coffee or tea with heavy cream

Lunch

BLT wrap in collard greens, with Primal Kitchen
Mayo

½ baked sweet potato

Dinner

Chicken Kabobs (page 238)

Butternut squash roasted with avocado oil, salt,
and pepper

DAY 15

Breakfast	Lunch

Brad's "Ketoatmeal" (page 203), topped with:
   ½ banana, diced *(the greener, the better)*
   1 tablespoon cacao nibs
   1 tablespoon almond butter
 	
Coffee or tea with heavy cream
	Bigass Salad (page 259), with leftover chicken and veggies

Dinner	
Zucchini Noodles (2 cups; see page 262)	Marinara sauce (homemade or store-bought with no added sugar), with 1 cup ground beef, turkey, or chicken; and ¼ cup shredded Parmesan cheese added

DAY 16

Breakfast	Lunch
2 hard-boiled eggs 1 cup diced cantaloupe 1 ounce prosciutto Coffee or tea with heavy cream	Crunchy Tuna Salad (page 245) in collard green wrap (see page 243) Small green apple

Dinner	
Slow cooker Korean beef, with kimchi (see page 248)	Steamed broccoli with 1 tablespoon butter (make a big batch!)

DAY 17

Breakfast	Lunch
2 eggs, scrambled 2 slices bacon Turnip Hash Browns (page 200) Coffee or tea with heavy cream	Baked sweet potato with leftover Korean beef, topped with 2 tablespoons sour cream Leftover steamed broccoli

Dinner	
Baked chicken breast with pesto Cauliflower Rice (page 266)	Steamed green beans with butter

DAY 18

Breakfast

Go-to Green Smoothie (page 212)

Lunch

Collard green wrap (see page 243) with 2 slices of ham, 1 piece of provolone cheese, and 2 tablespoons Primal Kitchen Mayo

Small green apple

2 tablespoons almond butter

Dinner

Shrimp sautéed in butter with garlic

Massaged Kale Salad with Goat Cheese (page 269)

1 cup roasted beets

DAY 19

Breakfast

High-Fat Coffee (page 210) or Chicken Bone Broth (page 216), then delay until hungry

2 eggs, scrambled with 1 cup spinach and ¼ cup feta cheese (*if eating breakfast*)

Lunch

Bigass Salad (page 259) with leftover shrimp (or canned tuna)

Dinner

Grilled chicken thighs (brine and marinate; see page 237, but do not cut into pieces before grilling)

Cheesy Broccoli and Cauliflower Casserole (page 271)

DAY 20

Breakfast

High-Fat Coffee (page 210) or Chicken Bone Broth (page 216), then delay until hungry

Greek Yogurt Crunch Bowl (*if eating breakfast*)

Lunch

Smoked Salmon Spread (page 227)
   1 small cucumber, sliced
   3 small radishes, sliced

Dinner

Flank steak, 6–8 ounces, topped with:
   1 cup mushrooms sautéed in avocado oil
   ¼ cup blue cheese crumbles
   Steamed broccoli with 1 tablespoon butter

DAY 21

Breakfast

High-Fat Coffee (page 210) or Chicken Bone Broth (page 216), then delay until hungry

Go-to Green Smoothie (*if eating breakfast*)

Lunch

Cheesy Ham Roll-ups (page 244)

Celery sticks

2 tablespoons almond butter

Dinner

Seared Ahi with Herb + Lime Dressing (page 233)

½ avocado

Side green salad (¼ Bigass Salad, page 259) with 1–2 tablespoons Perfect Vinaigrette (page 221)

CHAPTER 7

Live a Keto-Friendly Lifestyle

AFTER the hard work of your dietary transition in the first week of the Reset, it is now time to make sure your exercise, sleep, and stress-management behaviors support your progress toward fat adaptation instead of compromising it. Of foremost importance is to avoid the assorted forms of chronic stressors that are endemic to hectic modern life. The main offenders are overly stressful exercise patterns, insufficient sleep, and a type-A, hyperconnected mindset. All these stressors overstimulate the fight-or-flight sympathetic nervous system—something that strongly promotes sugar cravings and fat storage.

Even if you are diligent with your diet, other chronic stressors trigger sugar burning with a significance similar to your slamming a slushy at the convenience store. In this chapter, we cover the big-ticket items—the deal breakers for all the diet guidelines in the book if you screw them up. First is exercise, whereby you'll conduct an optimal balance of frequent everyday movement, structured cardio workouts at aerobic heart rates, and brief, intense strength and sprint sessions. Most important of all, you must make absolutely sure you avoid chronic patterns that promote carbohydrate dependency. Next is sleep, for which it's critical to minimize artificial light and digital stimulation after dark. Our innocent use of screens at night causes an extreme dysregulation of your appetite and fat-storage hormones. Finally, we cover stress management, where the objective is to slow down and tone down your type-A tendencies, which promote sugar burning and fat storage. Consequently, when you are transitioning out of carb dependency and into low-carb patterns, or transitioning from low-carb to keto, the best results will come when life is good in general.

> **Stress drives cortisol drives sugar cravings drives insulin drives fat storage!**

Exercise: Move, Lift, and Sprint!

My Primal Blueprint exercise philosophy entails a blend of moving frequently, lifting heavy things, and sprinting once in a while. This honors the lifestyle behaviors of our ancestors and promotes optimal gene expression. Moving frequently (blending formal cardio sessions with increased everyday movement) makes you a good fat-burner around the clock. Lifting heavy things—a regular routine of brief, high-intensity resistance/strength training exercises—enhances organ function, supports mobility and functionality, and prevents injury and breakdown of joints and connective tissue. Sprinting once in a while (ideally, it's running for weight-bearing benefits, but no-impact options are fine, too) delivers a pulse of anti-aging adaptive hormones, actualizing the natural law to "use it or lose it."

Unfortunately, hectic modern life is causing us to really mess things up on the exercise front. Many fail to obtain a bare minimum of basic movement, cardiovascular workouts, or any form of intensity or resistance exercise. Once we hit the big 4-0 or thereabouts, we sit on the sidelines, welcome in disease risk factors, and experience a dramatically accelerated decline into feeble old age. Even devoted fitness enthusiasts who do their hour-long daily workouts package that with so much downtime commuting, working at a desk, and indulging in screen entertainment during leisure hours that they cannot escape the disease risk factors associated with sedentary lifestyle patterns. This is a scientifically validated phenomenon known as the "active couch potato syndrome."

Many ambitious fitness enthusiasts drift into chronic patterns—workouts that are a bit too difficult, last too long, and are conducted too frequently with insufficient rest in between. If you are part of the endurance running or triathlon scene, or the Crossfit scene, or you have your personal trainer set to autopay on your online banking, this story might hit home. A type-A approach to fitness definitely gets you out from under the covers and into your workout, but over time your fervent discipline and resilience can end up compromising your health. I am painfully familiar with these dynamics due to my background as an elite marathoner and Ironman triathlete. My heavy training regimen (I ran 100 miles per week for a decade) made me a picture of fitness on the outside, but destroyed my health on the inside.

> **Chronic exercise is stressful and depleting. Consequently, your brain will crave and prompt you to consume additional carbohydrates.**

Let's acknowledge that your keto journey is mostly about diet: that's what will remove the excess body fat and deliver the wide-ranging health and metabolic benefits. Sensible exercise habits will support and even accelerate your progress, but we mostly want to be sure they don't compromise your progress. Chronic exercise is stressful and depleting. Consequently, your brain will crave and prompt you to consume additional carbohydrates. This drives excess insulin production, which drives excess fat storage and hormonal dysregulation. It's time to reel in your type-A patterns, slow down your cardio pace, take more leisurely walks and flights of stairs, and then occasionally hit it hard with short-duration workouts. Believe it or not, this evolutionary-tested approach is more effective, less stressful, and less time-consuming than the traditional chronic, time-consuming "consistency is key" approach to exercise.

Move Frequently

Your active lifestyle and regular cardio workouts promote a strong cardiovascular and metabolic system. You can efficiently process oxygen and fuel with your robust network of mitochondria, making you an excellent fat-burner around the clock. This is the true secret to lifelong weight management. As discussed in Chapter 2 with regard to the compensation theory, increased general movement and avoiding stillness is arguably more important to health and weight loss than being a high-calorie-burning gym rat or road warrior.

Walking is the obvious foundational element here. Get your dog out every day, or twice a day, as any faithful companion deserves. Take phone calls or in-person meetings while strolling through the office complex courtyard or pacing in your office, instead of sitting at your desk. Swear off elevators and enjoy all the stairs life has to offer. Save on door dings by parking in the farthest spot from the building and walking it in. Realize that this movement objective also includes deliberate practices like yoga, Pilates, and tai chi; flexibility and mobility exercises, from formal stretching regimens to impromptu squats or quad stretches you can do at your desk or while watching TV; and self-care techniques such as foam rolling and the like.

Remember, this is not about burning calories in the name of weight loss, it's simply about moving. The accordant wide-ranging health benefits include optimized fat metabolism around the clock, increased range of motion in joints, improved insulin sensitivity, improved overall cardiovascular health (not just workout fitness, but improved function of the circulatory system throughout your body), and enhanced oxygen delivery to your brain, improving cognitive performance.

Aerobic Workouts

In tandem with your movement efforts, strive to accumulate a minimum of two hours of structured cardiovascular workouts (fitness walking, jogging, cycling, swimming, cardio machines, and so forth) each week. It's critical that you remain at or below your *maximum aerobic heart rate* for the duration of these sessions. Maximum aerobic heart rate correlates with the point of your maximum fat oxidation (burning the most fat calories) per minute. At this heart rate, you obtain maximum fat-burning benefits. When you exceed your maximum aerobic heart rate, peak fat oxidation drops and you trigger a spike in glucose burning. This greatly compromises the intended benefits of the workout and pushes you back in the direction of carbohydrate dependency, because the workouts are a bit too stressful and depleting to support fat-adaptation. If you feel a tiny bit punky and craving something sweet after a routine cardio workout, you are assuredly exercising at too high a heart rate, cementing your status as a sugar-burner accordingly. When you combine increased general movement with cardio workouts that are truly aerobic and emphasize fat burning, you improve your ability to burn fat both during exercise and at rest, and you can recover quickly because the workout is minimally stressful.

> **Maximum aerobic heart rate = maximum fat oxidation per minute. Exceeding the aerobic maximum can result in more glucose burning, more stress hormones, and slower recovery.**

Your maximum aerobic heart rate can be calculated using Dr. Phil Maffetone's highly respected formula of "180 minus your age" in beats per minute. For example, a 30-year-old exerciser would have a maximum aerobic heart rate of 150 (180 minus 30). If you are not healthy and fit right now, you'll want to subtract five beats from your calculation. Super-fit, successful endurance athletes can add five beats to their calculation. Beware: this heart rate limit arrives for most of us at a perceived exertion that is surprisingly easy. Even though it's no trouble to speed up your heart rate by the tune of 5, 10, or even 20 more beats per minute without feeling any significant strain, the metabolic effect of the workout changes and you drift into what exercise scientists call the *black hole*—a pace that's below the red-line anaerobic threshold at which you can really feel strain, but is too difficult to be an effective fat-burning session.

When you enter the black hole, burning less fat and more glucose, you end the workouts feeling a bit tired, depleted, and hungry for quick-energy carbohydrates. You have also generated more oxidation and inflammation, elevated the production of stress hormones, and increased the fatigue and acidic damage in the muscles. What's more, kicking into glucose burning during the workout shapes your metabolic pattern for many hours afterward—up to 72 hours, according to Dr. Maffetone. That's plenty of time to throw down your next black hole workout and keep the glucose-burning campfire going 24/7. After your lively morning Spin class (and high-carbohydrate post-workout snack or meal), you'll burn sugar instead of fat. Meanwhile, your cubicle neighbor who slept later, walked her dog, and had bacon and eggs for breakfast will be burning fat. She'll be better off in many health categories, likely including more success at dropping excess body fat.

> **Slow down, burn fat, go keto. Speed up, burn sugar, fail keto, store fat.**

Conventional wisdom has conditioned the fitness community to believe that going faster, working harder, and burning more calories is the path to weight loss, but this logic has been unequivocally refuted, both anecdotally and scientifically. I realize that it can be really tough to discipline yourself to slow down and smell the roses, especially in group workout settings when you are encouraged to keep pace with others who may be more fit. That's why it's essential that you monitor your heart rate carefully for the duration of your cardio workouts. You can get a quality unit with a chest strap that transmits data wirelessly to a digital wristwatch for less than fifty dollars—Polar F1 is a reliable no-frills model. If you don't have a heart-rate monitor, you can use a watch with a second hand to count your pulse for 10 seconds and multiply by 6, or use a nose-breathing test with which you attempt to breathe with your mouth closed during your workout. If you can't breathe comfortably with your mouth closed, you are most likely above your maximum aerobic heart rate.

As discussed with the admonition to use tremendous discipline in ditching sugars, grains, and vegetable oils, you must apply the same rigor in regulating your cardio sessions to proceed at or below your maximum aerobic heart rate at all times. Even a couple of careless minutes at a glucose-burning heart rate can compromise the desired fat-burning benefits of the workout. Once glucose burning kicks in, it's difficult to shut it down and return to a predominantly fat-burning state. For this reason, it's essential to warm up gradually at the beginning of your workouts. If you progress too quickly from a rested state into even just a routine aerobic pace, you will burn glucose initially while your body's fat-burning engines are still warming up. Remember the campfire analogy given earlier—the big logs take a while to get started. Even for the fittest athletes, it's a great idea to walk (or do very slow movement of your chosen activity) for a few minutes at the beginning of a training session to ensure fat oxidation is optimized for the duration of the effort.

Lift Heavy Things

The objective here is simple: put your body under some type of resistance load regularly to promote overall health, broaden your fitness competency, and delay the aging process. Do whatever types of workouts are most appealing to you. Two workouts per week lasting as little as seven and no longer than 30 minutes is plenty to get you really fit and strong—really! Don't worry about the bro-science debates between free weights and machines or cords, tubes, sandbags, or just plain bodyweight. The main goal here is to achieve an adaptive hormonal response from a workout that is brief in duration and that challenges your muscles to perform functional, full-body, explosive movements. If you are short on ideas or experience in this area, search YouTube for "Mark Sisson—Primal Essential Movements." The PEMs—pushups, pullups, squats, and planks—are safe and simple to learn, and they give you a fantastic, full-body workout. If you are a novice, you'll find that each movement has a sequence of easier progression exercises to allow you to gradually progress toward performing the baseline movement. For example, doing chair pushups for a while helps you build the strength to perform traditional pushups on the ground.

Whatever type of resistance workout you choose, it should be performed at high intensity, be brief in duration, and be balanced with sufficient rest between challenging sessions. What you want to avoid are workouts that are too long in duration (and accordingly, not intense enough), and/or are conducted too frequently without sufficient rest. You want to finish even your most intense workouts feeling mildly and pleasantly fatigued rather than exhausted. To achieve the temporary spike in fight-or-flight hormones that stimulates the genetically optimal adaptive response (you adapt and become stronger from the workout stimulus, instead of breaking down from a chronic workout pattern), the workouts need never extend longer than 30 minutes. If your workout lasts too long, such as when you move through station after station at the gym until you finish feeling depleted and exhausted, you will overextend the fight-or-flight response and drift into a chronic carbohydrate-dependency pattern. Only conduct strength workouts when you feel fresh and motivated, then go hard and go home. If you're sore or sluggish, wait it out until you are chomping at the bit to get back at it.

Sprint Once in a While

I call sprinting the ultimate primal workout—the proper way to stimulate the fight-or-flight response that served our ancestors so well and became hardwired into our genes. While we commonly abuse the fight-or-flight response in hectic daily life and through carb/insulin roller-coaster eating patterns, we also fail to perform the occasional, brief, all-out efforts that deliver extremely potent metabolic, fitness, and anti-aging benefits. Sprinting stimulates lean muscle development or preservation; improves energy, alertness, and mood (by improving oxygen delivery and decreasing inflammation in the brain); increases your resilience to fatigue (both mental and physiological) when you exercise at lower intensity levels; stimulates the all-important mitochondrial biogenesis; strengthens muscles, joints, and connective tissue; and can be an extremely effective catalyst to help you break through fat-loss plateaus. "Nothing cuts you up like sprinting" is my favorite comment to the primal living enthusiasts I encounter who are frustrated with weight-loss plateaus despite diligent adherence to dietary guidelines.

The extreme metabolic stimulation of a sprint workout sends a powerful adaptive signal to your genes to reduce excess body fat.

After your sprint workout, adaptive hormones such as testosterone and human growth hormone circulate in the bloodstream, targeting specific organs to deliver an assortment of anti-aging benefits—enhanced libido (for both males and females) being a good example. Here's why nothing cuts you up like sprinting. The extreme stimulation of a 30 Metabolic Equivalent of Task (MET) sprint session sends a powerful adaptive signal to your genes to reduce any excess body fat, because the penalty for carrying extra body fat along while sprinting is so severe. This is also why weight-bearing sprinting is ideal for fat reduction (it also helps with bone density). However, if you aren't fit enough right now to perform high-impact running sprints, you'll get the same anti-aging hormone pulse with any sort of low- or no-impact all-out effort, such as uphill running or stair climbing, swimming, stationary cycling, elliptical, rowing machine, Versaclimber, or other cardio machines.

You may have seen news and magazine headlines touting sprinting as a "better" workout than cardio owing to its more pronounced metabolic benefits. However, it's important to understand the big picture: First, you must ditch carb dependency and get fat-adapted; otherwise, all fat-reduction bets are off—morning sprint leads to evening Ben & Jerry's (see "The Skinny on Impossible Dieting" below). When you are fat-adapted, a high-intensity sprint workout will elevate mitochondrial and metabolic function for up to 24 hours after the session. Even though you burn mostly glucose during the brief session, you'll burn more fat at rest for many hours afterward—*if* you are fat-adapted. If you are pondering the logically flawed question of "What's better between cardio and intensity?" understand that they are both essential elements of the big picture. Low-carb/keto eating patterns, combined with comfortably paced movement and strictly aerobic cardio sessions, make you good at burning fat around the clock. Intense strength training and sprinting turbo-charge your overall mitochondrial and metabolic function, as well as provide a direct stimulation to reduce excess body fat owing to the nature of the effort.

The Skinny on Impossible Dieting

The disastrously flawed foundational premise of the diet industry is that you can reduce excess body fat by disciplining yourself to restrict dietary calories, then burn off excess body fat during strenuous exercise. But when this challenge is undertaken in a carbohydrate-dependency state, you don't lose fat very well, if at all. Instead, you experience fatigue from insufficient calories, combined with chronic exercise patterns. Our primal genes perceive this combo to be a matter of life or death, and they respond with emergency production of glucose via gluconeogenesis. This temporarily alleviates your fatigue by providing a stable fuel source to your sugar-addicted brain and muscles (since they can't burn fat and you are restricting normal caloric intake), but you may lose lean muscle mass in the process. Ultimately, you end up burned out from chronic overstimulation of the fight-or-flight response and the fatiguing effects of suboptimal nutrition (a synthetic shake for breakfast and lunch, followed by a high-carb, nutrient-devoid dinner anyone?).

When you engage in a pattern of impossible dieting, you will likely find yourself always hungry, you will commonly overeat to the point of discomfort (a survival mechanism against the combo of starvation and chronic exercise), you will still feel less energetic overall (your body doesn't want to be energetic when you are starving and overexercising), and you will become more likely to store whatever calories you consume as fat (due to dysregulation of the prominent satiety/fat-storage hormone leptin). All this bad stuff happens because your genes don't want you to die of starvation, but you keep trying to starve (and exhaust) yourself, and you're ineffective at burning stored body fat.

Owing to sprinting's high degree of difficulty and profound hormonal and metabolic effects, occasional efforts will deliver the best results. Once every 7 to 10 days, and only when you are feeling fully rested and motivated to deliver a maximum effort, you can conduct a sprint workout honoring these precise guidelines:

RESPECT YOUR CURRENT ABILITY LEVEL: If you are worried about the weight-bearing risks of running sprints, choose no- or low-impact options such as swimming, stationary cycling, elliptical, or other cardio machines. Strive to work up to actual running sprints. Uphill sprints have less impact and are a great way to transition from low impact to no impact. Realize that "all out" doesn't mean to the point of collapse; all your efforts should be under control, with good technique preserved.

SPRINT WHEN YOU FEEL FRESH: Only attempt sprints when you feel high energy and motivation levels—never when feeling fatigued during daily life or when experiencing soreness or injury hot spots. Realize that sprints are a maximum challenge to your brain, as well as your body, and you need to be sharp in every way to deliver an effective workout. Top coaches assert that you should feel quick and springy during warm-up exercises in order to get a green light to continue with the hard efforts that await. If you feel flat, sluggish, or stiff during warm-ups, save your energy and try again another day.

THOROUGHLY WARM UP AND COOL DOWN: Warm-ups and cool-downs not only protect your muscles from injury and ease the stress impact of the workout but also prime your central nervous system for explosive action. Before your workout, do slow-paced cardio until you break a slight sweat, feel your joints lubricate, and you experience sharpened psychological focus. Spend at least 5 minutes doing a gentle warm-up. Proceed with dynamic stretches (moving through a range of motion, not static), preparatory technique drills, and brief maximum efforts (often called "wind sprints") before you commence the hard stuff—at least 10 minutes' worth, for a total warm-up of 15 minutes. After your final sprint, cool down with easy cardio for 5 to 10 minutes. Make sure you have stopped sweating and that your breathing rate is back to normal before you stop moving. Try to remain active and mobile for the remainder of the day to help speed recovery.

CONSISTENT QUALITY EFFORTS: Each sprint should be similar in both measured performance (e.g., time over a certain distance) and perceived effort level. If you have to dig deeper to deliver the same sprint time, deliver a significantly slower time with the same effort, or notice your form compromised or muscle tightness/pain arise owing to fatigue, it's time to stop the workout. This is a very important concept to grasp, and it may require you to transition away from the typical "no pain, no gain" thought process that pervades the cardio/endurance community in particular. Give a *controlled maximum effort* on each sprint, and end your workouts feeling pleasantly fatigued, but not exhausted. With sprinting, a little goes a long way. Don't even contemplate another session until you are completely recovered and chomping at the bit to deliver more maximum intensity efforts.

TAKE AMPLE RECOVERY INTERVALS: For the most difficult activity of running, 4 to 6 sprints of 15 to 20 seconds each is plenty. Take enough recovery—in the form of slow jogging (don't be stationary or sit or lie down!)—between your sprints so that your breathing returns to near normal, and you are mentally refreshed and focused to deliver another effort. Your recovery time may range from 30 seconds early in the workout to

60 seconds between your final efforts before turning on the jets again. Low- or no-impact sprints have less impact trauma and require more time to ramp up to reach maximum intensity, so you can try longer duration sprints of 20 to 30 seconds each, again taking complete recovery between the efforts.

Sleep: Create Dark, Mellow Evenings!

While we all understand the importance of good sleep and we pay plenty of lip service to the subject, the reality is that sleep is getting the shaft in high-tech modern life. While I offer an assortment of tips and techniques for optimizing your sleep in this section, the essence of the problem is this: *excess artificial light and digital stimulation after dark*. Our delicate circadian hormonal processes have been synchronized with the rising and setting of the sun for millions of years. When the sun sets, humans are hardwired to wind down, start to feel sleepy in a few hours, and gracefully transition to a fully restorative night of sleep. Many sleep experts believe we also may be hardwired for biphasic sleeping habits, such that a midday nap is the default human expectation for hormone optimization.

Today, instead of experiencing a mellow and graceful transition to sleepiness during the evening hours, our exposure to artificial light after sunset kicks off a chain reaction of adverse hormonal events. Artificial light and digital stimulation after dark suppress the release of melatonin, the hormone that makes us feel sleepy in the evening (a process known as dim light melatonin onset, or DLMO). In tandem, we experience a spike in the primary stress hormone cortisol. Initially, cortisol floods the bloodstream with glucose, giving us a "second wind" to stay awake and finish our emails or Netflix series binge. Thus, if you stress yourself in this manner every night, chronically elevated evening cortisol can bind with the appetite receptors in the brain and trigger you to consume high-calorie foods. Late nights also dysregulate ghrelin (spiking appetite) and leptin (promoting fat storage). Indeed, our digestive systems also have a circadian rhythm, and eating late at night can mess things up (details in the appendix), making it likely that you'll eat beyond feeling satisfied and store those calories as fat.

From a genetic perspective, your artificially lengthened days have tricked your genes into thinking it's summer all the time. During the long, bright days of summer, we became hardwired over 2.5 million years of evolution to consume extra carbs (i.e., ripe fruit) and to store those calories as fat—to prepare for the long winters of food scarcity. It may be hard to believe, but your innocent use of a computer, television, or smartphone has a profound effect in locking you into fat-storage patterns. When nights of digital stimulation and insufficient sleep are a fixture in your life, you can become insulin resistant, meaning you are more likely to store your midnight snacks as fat, and more likely to crave sugar because you do a poor job of accessing and burning internal energy stores. One study from the University of Chicago showed that just two weeks of sleep deprivation (subjects slept for four hours per night) resulted in a 50 percent increase in insulin resistance!

Excess artificial light and digital stimulation after dark makes you fat.

During a quality night's sleep, assorted other hormonal and metabolic processes work to help turbo-charge your immune system, build a healthy intestinal microbiome, manage oxidative stress, repair and rebuild muscle tissue, organize short- and long-term memories, replenish neurotransmitters like serotonin and dopamine, and refresh depleted brain neurons and synapses to help you awaken refreshed and cognitively sharp for the busy day ahead. You also normalize cortisol, ghrelin, and leptin—the metabolic troublemakers on the late show. When these influential hormones are optimized (by sleeping in alignment with your circadian rhythm, low-insulin eating patterns, and sensible instead of chronic exercise), your appetite will spike only when you're hungry, your brain will tell you to stop eating when you're satisfied, and you will be better at burning stored energy instead of accumulating it.

Your most urgent assignment on the sleep issue is to make a concerted effort to minimize the amount of artificial light and digital stimulation after dark. I realize that this may be cramping your style big-time, especially in the winter when there may be up to seven hours of darkness between sunset and your bedtime. On that note, realize that our bodies are hardwired to sleep much more during the short days and long nights of winter, while we can function better on less sleep during the longer days of summer. The farther away from the equator you live, the more disparity you might have between your summer and winter sleeping patterns.

Extending from your basic commitment to having darker evenings, you'll also want to strive for optimal sleep habits and sleeping environment. Make a strong effort to go to bed at the same time each evening, and to (hopefully) awaken naturally, near sunrise, without an alarm clock, feeling refreshed and energized. Following are more tips to get your sleep game in top shape:

BEHAVIOR: Author and business mogul Arianna Huffington has done a great job championing the need for sleep in her bestselling books *Thrive* and *The Sleep Revolution*, where she chronicles her recovery from burnout and her renewed devotion to sleep. Huffington urges us to create a relaxing evening ritual to prep mind and body for sleep—shutting off technology, taking a warm bath, changing into special pajamas. These are deliberate and patterned behaviors that help us unwind from the high-stress disposition we exhibit during our busy days. Forget the chatter about eating certain sleep-inducing foods—it's likely best to not eat anything in the final hours. Be sure to stay away from carbs, alcohol, caffeine, and tobacco. With your doctor's support, try to ditch prescription sleep medications, which knock you unconscious but interfere with true hormonal restoration.

ENVIRONMENT: After dark, get in circadian sync by minimizing your indoor light use. Use candles instead of lamps, read with a headlamp in bed, or don a pair of yellow or orange-tinted UV-protective sunglasses after dark. These lenses allow plenty of light in so you can see safely, but effectively block the harmful "blue light" spectrum emitted from regular lightbulbs and digital screens that disturbs melatonin. Consider switching out some of the white bulbs in your lamps for orange bulbs (often called insect bulbs, available at home supply stores). If you must use TV or computer screens, use them as early as possible in the evening, and keep them as dim as possible. Download a free software program called f.lux, which automatically softens the color temperature (similar to brightness, but not exactly the same) of your screen to lessen the intensity of the light emission when it gets dark.

Create a minimalist bedroom with no clutter—especially no television or work desk! Make it completely dark by covering or removing any light-emitting devices (even tiny stuff like LCD clocks or hallway night-lights; use a small flashlight if you have to get up) and using blackout curtains. Make the room as quiet as possible; use a noise-canceling device or smartphone app (try Rainmaker Pro for a great variety of rainfall) if there are disrupting noises from outside. Keep the temperature cool—60 to 68°F (16 to 20°C) is ideal. I sleep on a mattress cooling device called the Chili-Pad, which facilitates my maintaining a desirably low body temperature throughout the night.

NAPPING: At times when you fall short on optimal evening sleep, napping can be an extremely effective strategy to help you recalibrate quickly. Feeling foggy, fried, or sleepy during the day is a sign of "sleep pressure," indicating you fell short of optimal restoration the previous evening. A high-quality nap (find a dark, quiet, cool area away from the stimulation of your busy day) as short as 20 minutes can literally refresh a fried brain by rebalancing important chemicals responsible for efficient neuron firing. What's more, as you become fat- and keto-adapted, you may find that your afternoon blues are minimized to the extent that you don't need to nap as frequently.

TIMING: Strive to get to bed at the same time each evening. The critically important deep sleep cycles predominate early in your sleep cycle, so sleeping in after staying up late doesn't quite cut it—even if you bag a similar number of hours. In an ideal morning, you will awaken naturally, near sunrise, without the need for an alarm clock, and you will feel refreshed and energized. If this is not your current story, try to improve your evening habits so that it can become a reality shortly.

Rising before sunrise—something we romanticize as a sign of a true peak performer and/or ultra-disciplined exerciser—is another affront to our genetic expectations of a sunrise-triggered natural awakening. Our circadian rhythms respond to sunrise with a graceful reduction of melatonin in trade for an elevation of feel-good hormones such as serotonin, and also a desirable bump in cortisol. If you jump out of bed to a pre-dawn alarm, you'll spike cortisol in an undesirable manner, and you'll get into a similar pattern as described with chronically elevated evening cortisol.

Stress Management: Slow Down and Focus!

My apologies to the type-A brigade, but slowing down the pace of your life and relaxing more can make you leaner, more energetic, and ultimately fitter, stronger, happier, and healthier. As a lifelong entrepreneur responsible for my own destiny, I understand as well as anyone else the need for discipline and goal setting—staying focused and getting stuff done against the constant temptation to drift into the mind-numbing passive entertainment options of the digital age. To those who like to misinterpret or criticize my platform, know that primal living is not a recommendation to disavow your worldly possessions and regress to primitive times; rather, it is a suggestion to model the lifestyle behaviors of our ancestors and adapt them to the realities of high-tech modern life. You can do that with whatever revisions and compromises are necessary to ensure you enjoy the heck out of your comfortable modern existence.

While the disconnects between the SAD diet and our ancestral hunter-gatherer eating patterns are obvious, it requires a little more reflection to consider how our genetic expectations for the distinct stress and rest patterns of primal life conflict with the chronic stress that is the essence of modern life. Our ancestors certainly had some unspeakably tough times, but they generally lived—by modern comparison today—incredibly mellow everyday lives. The stresses they faced were typically brief, fight-or-flight occasions that—if they survived!—served to fine-tune their overall survival-of-the-fittest abilities. Today, we may be too far over in the fast lane to strive for an incredibly mellow life—even beach bums get stressed about credit card late-payment penalties. However, you can leverage technology to make life easier instead of more stressful, and you can apply the same exceptional prioritization skills that you use to get through law school, manage your sales team, or keep the kids on schedule, making health and balance your top priorities. In addition to moving more, exercising sensibly instead of chronically, making sleep a priority, and eating a low-carb, high-fat diet, here are some suggestions to help you minimize the stress of hectic daily life and nurture a healthy mind, body, and spirit:

CONNECT: Form and nurture positive, uplifting social connections. This is one of the most profound longevity markers known—right up there with healthy eating, exercise, and sleep. I'm talking about live, interpersonal connections, not digital connections! Unfortunately, the latter have compromised the former for the first time in human history. It might be helpful to envision your relationships as an *intimate circle* of family and close friends, and a larger *social circle* comprising co-workers, neighbors, workout partners, or friends from hobby, community, or religious groups. Most of your energy should be directed toward nurturing these circles, with only minimal energy toward maintaining superficial connections with larger groups of people via social media.

Depending on your personality and your preferences, your intimate circle might number between 6 and 12 people, while your social circle might include another 12 to 24 people. Your nuclear or extended family would predictably be in your intimate circle, but you can decide to include or exclude whomever you want, at any time. Anthropologist and evolutionary biologist Robin Dunbar characterizes an authentic and strong personal relationship by *an ability and willingness to do each other favors*. While you don't have to go around validating the thumbs-up status of your relationships on a daily basis, you can apply the spirit of this message to focus more on face time than on Facebook. As Dunbar reminds us, "A touch is worth a 1,000 words any day." Furthermore, envisioning these circles and who's in them helps you pay close attention to relationships that may have reached their expiration date or might benefit from a little more distance at times.

DIGITAL DISCIPLINE: Discipline your use of technology so that it makes your life easier and more efficient, but you never become a slave to it. While email is a lot easier than typing letters and licking stamps, and social media enables us to nurture distant relationships that might otherwise get diminished, the efficiency and accessibility of technology can compromise your health if you are unable to observe realistic boundaries. Of foremost importance is to ruthlessly filter out or strategically edit all information you are exposed to in the course of a day. Allow only high-priority communications from high-priority people into your figurative, and literal, inboxes. Be especially vigilant with mobile technology so as to not let it interfere with your appreciation of wherever you are, whomever you're with, and whatever you're doing right now. When you get a phone call or text buzz during your kid's soccer game or during afternoon tea with grandma, you are allowing intrusions into some of life's most precious and fleeting moments. If you disagree, check back with me in ten years when the soccer games and afternoon teas are gone forever. Remember *Way of the Peaceful Warrior* author Dan Millman's admonition that "there are no ordinary moments."

When it's time to engage with technology, be sure you focus on a single peak performance task at a time, instead of trying to multitask. Stanford University research reveals that attempts to multitask can compromise learning, memory, creativity, and focusing, and lead to increased mental fatigue. MIT research suggests that there is literally no such thing as multitasking, because your brain can process only one stream of information at a time. Hence, multitasking is actually a quick switching of focus back and forth between disparate tasks. You can pull this off when the stakes are low (e.g., stamping envelopes while talking on the phone), but diminished performance and increased stress are the results when the tasks are demanding, such as driving to GPS navigation while negotiating an important business deal. When you overload, both of your inputs have an increased potential to go south. Instead of multitasking, focus on your top priority over the course of the day and single-task through your list in a methodical manner. If you are a peak performer charged with creating original content, batch your emails and phone calls into specified time blocks, then go offline when it's time to be creative.

Even when you are successfully implementing the aforementioned strategies, it's essential to take frequent breaks from periods of peak cognitive focus. Take a quick 1- to 3-minute break for every 20 minutes of intense focus, particularly if you're at a desk job. Stand up, move your body, look at distant objects, or close your eyes and take a few deep breaths before returning to the hot seat. For every two hours of busy engagement, take a 10-minute break and engage in behaviors that counterbalance your work tasks. Get outdoors into sunlight and fresh air and move your body—a quick set of squats or planks is a great way to build fitness when you make fitness breaks a daily habit. You can also choose to go into a quiet, dark area and listen to guided meditation. Play a game of Ping-Pong or strum a few guitar chords, and you'll return to work refreshed and inspired.

> **Take a 10-minute break for every two hours of busy cognitive engagement—get outdoors into sunlight and fresh air and move your body!**

If you proclaim that you are too busy to engage in these productivity-boosting, stress-reducing behaviors, realize that if you *don't* disengage regularly, the breaks will be taken for you unwittingly. These breaks will come in the form of your taking twice as long to complete simple tasks versus when you are sharp, or zoning over to a succession of short-attention-span digital entertainments—YouTube videos, afternoon Facebook cameos—or lingering at the water cooler to jabber about sports or celebrity worship. Granted, any type of break can be restorative at some level, but purposeful breaks are much more supportive of peak performance. If you're going to hang out at the water cooler, make it be on your terms—be fully present and appreciative of your socializing opportunity, and make a graceful and polite exit when your intended duration is reached.

After a busy stressful day, we all deserve to unwind however we want, perhaps by indulging in a great selection of digital entertainment options. However, please consider prioritizing your sleep and then backing into digital entertainment with what time is still available. If you have time to enjoy a show or two, or three (one of my favorite technological innovations of all time—binge-watching!), then do so. If your consistently observed bedtime is approaching, though, wrap it up and take comfort knowing that your show will be there for you when you are ready (thanks again to technology making our lives better!). Here are some additional tips for relieving stress:

EXERCISE: Walking delivers the aforementioned metabolic benefits, and it is a great way to de-stress and even to get a fresh perspective for problem solving. Your favorite fitness pursuits are the ultimate way to blow off steam and counterbalance the long periods of inactivity in home and workplace. The social and convenience aspects of a fitness club are great, but be sure to include outdoor workouts to enjoy the additional benefits of fresh air, open space, and nature.

FUN: Never forget that this lifestyle transformation stuff is supposed to be fun. Instead of stressing about daily carb totals or looking like a social outcast at the next dessert club gathering, view your keto journey as an opportunity to try some interesting new foods, engage in spontaneous and intuitive fasting efforts, and perhaps serve as a role model for others interested in transformation. With fitness, consider that wearing high-tech biofeedback gadgets, keeping precise workout logs, and being consistent with your schedule are highly overrated. Instead, just get outside, connect with nature, and appreciate any form of physical challenge that appeals to you. Understand that your inclination to be hyperconnected is not a character flaw; it's a hardwired genetic attribute that keeps us vigilant for changes in our environment that can affect our safety. Yep, the dopamine burst we get from jumping to respond to a text message buzz today is akin to our ancestors' urgent reaction to a rustling in the bushes. Consequently, it's essential to be mindful of your programmed reactions to digital stimulation and disciplined about powering down. When you power down, you open yourself up to exciting new opportunities to take interactions with your partner, children, or friends to the next level of significance. Being healthy—ever super-fit and super-healthy—should never involve any suffering or deprivation, and can actually be fun!

GRATITUDE JOURNAL: My wife, Carrie, is a huge devotee of this habit, and her passion has inspired many others to adopt the practice. Pick a consistent time each day to spend a couple minutes jotting down things you are grateful for in your life. Following through with this simple and empowering exercise—perhaps before bed or first thing each morning—might quickly become a life-changing habit. Anything goes with gratitude journaling: you can be grateful for that awesome party last night, or your new car, or the warm weather, the health of your children, or the park in your neighborhood. Being able to stay true to this exercise and make consistent daily entries is a great counterbalance to the shared human tendency to complain. No kidding; psychologists assert that humans are hardwired to commiserate with each other. While this can be cathartic for the tribulations and unfairness of daily life, it can also be destructive to the extent that you get stuck telling your sob story, and listening to others' sob stories, like broken records.

PERSONAL TIME: It's essential to nurture healthy social connections, but it's also critically important to carve out time for just you. I'm not so much talking about holing up in bed with your iPad. This is more like unplugging from the civilized world entirely: no screens, no people—just getting out into nature and quieting your mind. Even if

I have only 5 minutes to spare, I enjoy going into my backyard and looking at the city view in the distance, or getting onto my slackline (balance-walking on a wide tightrope), becoming completely engrossed in quieting my mind and balancing my body. Making an occasional grand solo outing (from a two-hour hike to a two-week backpacking trip) can be deeply life affirming and relaxing in a manner entirely different from hiking with a partner or a social group.

PURE MOTIVATION: Cultivate a pure motivation for all of your lifestyle transformation goals. This entails your having a deep love and appreciation for the *process*—of healthy eating, sensible exercise, prioritizing sleep, and all the rest—and that you do not attach your happiness or self-esteem to the outcome. This admonition plays out graphically with goals related to body composition and fitness. Dieters who stress about the scale every day and experience disappointing results will often tailspin into self-destructive behaviors because their motivations are impure. Ditto for athletes who get discouraged and distracted when they lose to a superior performer.

Remember Johnny G's words in Chapter 1: that true success can only come when your endeavors are natural, enjoyable, and easy to maintain. While assorted sacrifices are necessary to achieve esteemed peak performance goals of all kinds, and we can't have fun all the time, it's valuable to frequently step back and ask yourself the big-picture question: Is this overall journey fun, fulfilling, and bringing more happiness to my life? If the answer is no, or even "Uh, maybe," that's not good enough. It's time to make some changes. Sometimes it's changing the mechanics, such as quitting the hyper-competitive cycling club and enjoying more leisurely solo rides. Other times a shift in mindset will do wonders, as in getting over yourself and allowing the fun and pure motivations to be rediscovered.

See You on the Other Side!

With your carbs-to-fat transition in full swing, and the supportive lifestyle behaviors in place, you are ready to take the next step toward going keto. Chapter 8 will assess your metabolic fitness and give you the final launch preparations before commencing your first formal effort at nutritional ketosis in Chapter 9.

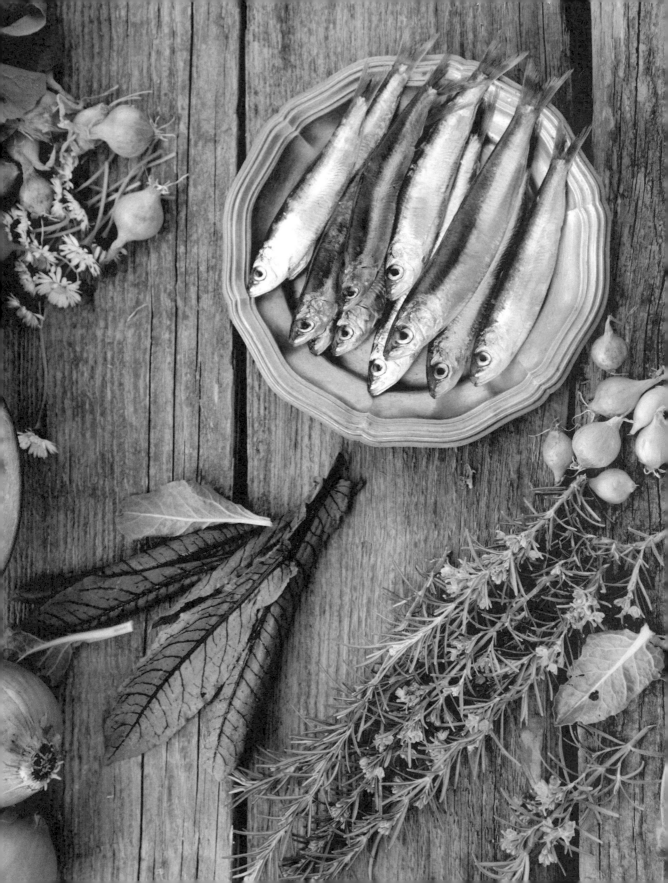

III

Going Keto

Are You Ready? Final Launch Preparations

THE successful completion of your 21-Day Metabolism Reset has upregulated your fat-burning genes and laid an excellent foundation for you to make your initial foray into nutritional ketosis. If you were locked into a significant carbohydrate-dependency pattern, it's likely that the hardest part of this journey is behind you, and the rest is all about testing, evaluating, and fine-tuning, as well as creating an optimal long-term eating strategy. To ensure your success in going keto, it's time to challenge the current limits of your metabolic flexibility and stimulate some further improvement. You will do this through fasting in the morning until you are truly hungry,

and perhaps (if you are really fit) using fasted workouts to accelerate your adaptation. Once you make some solid progress in this area and can hit some impressive milestones (e.g., feeling comfortable and energetic while fasting for 16 hours), you can confidently enter nutritional ketosis using the guidelines in the next chapter.

At the end of this chapter is a fun midterm exam you take to determine your readiness to enter nutritional ketosis. The questions were prepared in consultation with Dr. Cate Shanahan and serve as much more than just a midterm exam at Keto College. Owing to the individual variation in how we produce and utilize ketones, your subjective answers to these metabolic questions are likely more significant than the numbers you produce on a blood or breath ketone meter. For example, Doctors Shanahan, Attia, D'Agostino, and others have mentioned how some keto enthusiasts, particularly well-conditioned athletes, often post low blood ketone readings despite adherence to the dietary guidelines. Dr. Cate speculates as follows:

> It's possible that the athlete is producing a significant amount of ketones, but the tissues are sopping them up so quickly and efficiently that blood levels don't rise very high. It's an efficient gating system in an efficient metabolic specimen. While this phenomenon is not discussed often, it's known in science that our bodies regulate the production of *everything* to prevent the wasted efficiency of excess production. It seems that ketone production would be regulated in the same way.
>
> What's more, you might see higher numbers early into your keto-adaptation phase, because your muscles and brain are both starving for their usual fuel of glucose, and your body is trying hard to supply their energy needs via ketones. Later, as your muscles get more enzymes involved in the beta oxidation of fatty acids, ketones can be used preferentially by the brain, and lower levels will be found circulating in the blood when you take a reading.

The laboratory studies conducted by Doctors Phinney and Volek confirm this phenomenon: when blood ketone levels are high, the muscles are using more ketones. When blood levels are lower, a greater percentage of ketones is being used by the brain, and the muscles are efficiently burning mostly fatty acids. While I support taking frequent readings of both blood ketones and blood glucose to notice the effects of different meals, exercise, and sleep patterns, make sure you give proper weight to the assortment of commonsense subjective evaluations about whether your keto journey is working. The Precision Xtra meter mentioned in Chapter 1 can test both ketones and glucose. Don't worry; the glucose strips cost pennies, unlike the costly ketone strips. Also, check eBay for the same Precision-branded ketone strips at bargain prices.

Fasted Mornings

The simplest way to building your fitness for going keto is to delay your first meal of the day until WHEN—When Hunger Ensues Naturally. This simple, intuitive strategy will turbocharge your fat- and ketone-burning genes, enhance your insulin sensitivity, and set you up for easier adherence to a low-carb or keto eating pattern for the rest of the day. When you act in accordance with your hunger instead of pursuing a fixed schedule for fasting, you will free yourself from the pressure and anxiety that can often cause you to rebel when your willpower weakens or you lose interest in being so regimented. With the WHEN approach, you can allow progress to happen naturally, instead of forcing it. This is important because with metabolic fitness, as with physical fitness, progress often happens in a haphazard fashion. You may notice yourself making steady progress, getting stuck on a plateau despite devoted effort, then having a major breakthrough out of nowhere.

Furthermore, owing to the many stress variables of daily life, some days are better than others to stretch the limits of your metabolic fitness. For example, I'm extremely comfortable eating in a compressed time window during which I routinely fast for 18-hour periods with no trouble—even if I throw an intense workout or jet travel into the mix. However, on certain days, hunger grabs me in the morning hours, possibly due to some interesting triggers. For example, if I have a public-speaking event, my nervous energy sometimes manifests as hunger. I also notice on mornings when I do little or no exercise, I often get hungry sooner. This might seem counterintuitive, because in the carbohydrate paradigm, exercise drives glycogen depletion drives hunger. However, I suspect that exercise increases my fatty acid and ketone oxidation, and thereby allows me to power along for longer on internal energy sources than if I had not exercised. With the WHEN approach, you essentially take what your mind and body give you each day, do your best with your eating, exercise, sleep, and stress-management strategies, and allow progress to happen naturally.

If you are feeling some trepidation at the idea of routinely skipping an early morning meal, just focus on avoiding carbs at breakfast and enjoy a high-satiety omelet or other low- or no-carb preparation, if you desire. This will help you preserve the nice momentum you carry into each day from an overnight fast, but will also provide for your escalating energy needs in the morning. Over time, you will likely experience a reduced appetite for morning calories and can dabble in either fasting, consuming only a high-fat coffee or a ketone supplement, or just keeping the omelet in place as your go-to morning meal.

On the other hand, when you wake up and slam orange juice and cereal in short order, you spike insulin, shut off ketone production (even those who aren't keto-adapted still make a bit of ketones every morning, until the first bite of carbs arrives), lock fat into storage, and send a message to your genes that carbohydrates are going to be your go-to fuel source for the rest of your busy day. From this example, Shanahan says it's critical not only to regulate your total carbohydrate intake but also to strategize the timing of your carbohydrate intake to promote fat adaptation. As described, morning may be a bad time because you are primarily in fat-burning mode after resting for a long period, and you rudely interrupt the pattern with a high-carbohydrate breakfast. In contrast, when you ingest carbs after a prolonged fast or before or after an ambitious workout, they will be prioritized to refilling depleted glycogen stores, and hence not spike insulin adversely.

Similarly, in the evening after a busy day, ideally one in which you bagged many hours of fasting and enjoyed the accordant benefits, Shanahan theorizes that enjoying some nutritious carbs is not objectionable: "Prompting an insulin response under these circumstances can help assist with recovery from exercise, and may actually improve insulin sensitivity by keeping your cells adept and alert at responding to the signals of insulin trying to deliver nutrients to the cells," Shanahan explains.

At first, WHEN might arrive 30 minutes after you wake up. If so, take note of the time, relax and enjoy your meal, trust the process, and try again the next day. As the benefits and momentum created by your 21-Day Metabolism Reset strengthen over time, you will be able to skip or delay meals without experiencing the disturbing sensations of a sugar crash. This will take a bit of mindfulness to refrain from habitual morning calorie consumption when you aren't really hungry, but you should never extend to the point of suffering or diminished energy.

Many people in the low-carb, fat-adapted world advocate for the ingestion of fat calories in the morning, such as with a coffee containing butter, coconut oil, or MCT oil. Getting some fat calories into your system to burn might make it easier to extend into the afternoon hours before eating a proper meal. Since you aren't consuming any carbohydrate calories, a high-fat coffee or tea will not compromise your goals of becoming fat- and keto-adapted. Others argue against consuming high-fat coffee because the calorie load can be significant, but of minimal nutritional value in comparison to a breakfast of eggs and vegetables, for example. Like so many other elements of the *Keto Reset Diet* approach, your guiding principles will be personal experimentation and personal preference, while respecting the guidelines and restrictions of a fat- and keto-adapted eating strategy.

> **Fasting until WHEN—When Hunger Ensues Naturally—is the simplest way to fine-tune fat adaptation.**

For the fine-tuning goals of this chapter, I suggest you tackle the challenge cowboy style, and not consume any calories after your final evening meal or snack (try to wrap things up early—this facilitates good sleep, too) until WHEN the following morning. You can consume water, coffee, or tea, but don't enhance your beverage with anything more than a squeeze of lemon or heavy cream. I allow for another exception here, and that is a ketone supplement in the morning—something explained in detail in the next chapter.

After you awaken and launch into your busy day, you should expect normal concentration and energy levels as you get into your busy morning routine, with no hunger sensations and no strong desire to eat. At some point you will start thinking about food or experience true hunger sensations, such as a growling stomach. That's the time to enjoy a snack or a proper meal, ideally low in carbohydrate so you don't disrupt the momentum you have created from your fasting. Realize that this is not a forced fast, whereby you struggle to reach some predetermined time goal before you allow yourself to take a bite. You'll want to generate authentic results that reveal how long you can comfortably last before you feel like eating—even if it's not that long initially. Here are some benchmarks to consider as you progress toward going keto:

12 HOURS (E.G., 8 P.M.–8 A.M.): NEEDS TO IMPROVE. If you wake up and feel hungry, or experience energy lulls soon into your morning, reflect on the previous evening's meal or late-night snacks or desserts. If they were high-carbohydrate and insulin-stimulating, you may experience a spike in hunger hormones and compromised fat-burning ability the following morning. Ditto if your sleep was poor.

14 HOURS (8 P.M.–10 A.M.): GOOD. You've made a good effort to escape carb dependency, and are likely sleeping well and not binging on carbs the night before.

16 HOURS (8 P.M.–12 NOON): VERY GOOD. This is a routine lifestyle pattern for many ancestral living enthusiasts, often called *compressed eating window.* If you can do this once or twice a week, you are definitely ready to try nutritional ketosis.

Even if you exceed the carbohydrate threshold for keto with your chosen meal after 12, 14, or 16 hours, that doesn't negate the many hours of fasted-state benefits (autophagy, inflammation control, fat reduction, etc.) you'll enjoy each day. There are many ancestral living enthusiasts eating at the range of 50 to 150 grams of carbs per day in a compressed eating window and enjoying exceptional health. Of course, this assumes you're avoiding sugars, grains, and bad oils, and are not consuming excess protein.

If you are a devoted fitness enthusiast, you can fine-tune your fat adaptation and improve your metabolic fitness by conducting fasted workouts. This strategy is best contemplated when you have a strong fitness base already established. It's certainly not necessary to be a fitness enthusiast to succeed with keto, and in fact the morbidly obese population segment arguably stands to gain the most profound benefits from keto. However, if you're fit and want to quickly accelerate your fat- and keto-adaptation, you can dabble in fasted workouts before you enter nutritional ketosis, and explore the strategy deeper after you've completed your first nutritional ketosis stint. During your first keto effort, you may want to tone down your exercise efforts overall (and especially avoid chronic patterns!) to make sure the drop down to 50 grams of daily carbohydrates is not harder than it needs to be.

The entry-level effort for fasted workouts is to conduct a baseline fitness maintenance workout first thing in the morning—this assumes an approximately 12-hour fast. On either side of this baseline fitness maintenance standard you have recovery workouts (easier and shorter than maintenance workouts) and breakthrough workouts (workouts that are difficult or lengthy enough to stimulate an improvement from your current level of fitness). For example, a competent endurance cyclist might consider 1½ to 2½ hours at an aerobic pace to be a baseline ride. A breakthrough workout would be a century event (100-mile organized ride) or an hour-long time trial effort at anaerobic threshold heart rate. A recovery ride would be one hour or less on flat ground at aerobic heart rates well below the "180-age" aerobic maximum.

It's likely that you already do fasted baseline workouts as part of your normal routine, so you can up the ante a bit by either fasting for a significant period after the workout or escalating the duration or difficulty of the workout. Advanced strategies for fasted exercise are in Chapter 10.

The Keto Reset Diet Midterm Exam

The following subjective questions will help you assess your level of keto readiness. Dr. Cate Shanahan, whose medically supervised weight-loss practice integrates state-of-the-art metering equipment to measure rates and variables affecting fat oxidation in real time, nevertheless strongly advocates for the accuracy and relevance of subjective evaluators. For the following questions, give yourself an honest rating on a 1–10 scale, 1 being failure and 10 being outstanding compliance with the question. If your aggregate score is 75 percent or better (90 points out of 120 total points), you are ready to commence a period of nutritional ketosis—ideally for a minimum commitment of six weeks, per the recommendations of Dr. Dom D'Agostino.

If these characterizations are still a little out of your league and you score below 75 percent, there is no harm in exercising some patience, dabbling further in morning fasting and fasted workouts, and giving your genes and hormonal processes more time to transition from carbs to fat. With two to three additional good weeks under your belt, try the test again and see if you can deliver an authentic score of over 75. Because your keto commitment is significant, you want to be absolutely certain you are in top form before going for it.

While there is great interest in tracking blood glucose and ketone values to validate metabolic fitness, subjective markers are quite likely a more effective way to assess readiness and track progress. As discussed in detail in the next chapter, there is a lot of complexity, individual variance, and ambiguity when it comes to number tracking. Recall the paradox of highly trained athletes often delivering low blood ketone readings because they are making and using ketones with great efficiency. Take some time to provide honest and thoughtful answers to each question. With your passing grade, you then proceed to the section that follows to outline the particulars of your nutritional ketosis effort.

THE KETO RESET DIET MIDTERM EXAM

21-DAY METABOLISM RESET

Write your score for each of these questions on a 1–10 scale, 1 being failure and 10 being outstanding compliance.

_____ 1. Have you completely eliminated sugars and grains from your diet (including natural stuff like honey and agave), eating 150 grams of carbs per day or less?

_____ 2. Have you completely eliminated refined vegetable oils from your diet?

_____ 3. Are you in a comfortable routine of eating a variety of nutrient-dense foods in a macronutrient composition of very high fat, moderate protein, and very low carb intake?

_____ 4. Are you getting optimal cardiovascular exercise from both frequent everyday movement and structured aerobic workouts at 180-age heart rate?

_____ 5. Are you conducting regular brief, high-intensity workouts featuring full-body functional movements, and doing occasional maximum effort sprints?

_____ 6. Do you have excellent sleep habits, including minimizing artificial light and digital stimulation after dark; maintaining a simple, dark, quiet, cool, environment; following deliberate and relaxing bedtime rituals; and observing consistent bed and wake times?

_____ 7. Are you managing stress expertly, including increased daily movement and regular breaks from peak cognitive focus; disciplined use of technology, including powering down to enjoy the present moment; enjoying quality social time and personal time; expressing gratitude every day; and making sure you cultivate a pure motivation and have fun on the road to lifestyle transformation?

FASTING

_____ 1. Can you handle frequent 12- to 14-hour (overnight) fasting periods and occasionally extend to 16 hours (e.g., from 8 P.M. to 12 P.M. the following day), with stable energy and cognition?

_____ 2. Can you skip lunch, or just eat a small high-fat snack, and carry on productively until dinner?

ENERGY/METABOLISM

_____ 1. Are you completely free from crash-and-burn episodes characterized by strong sugar cravings, indulgences in high-carbohydrate sweets and treats, afternoon sleepiness, post-meal sleepiness, or early evening burnout when you collapse for a spell after you arrive home?

_____ 2. Do you rarely notice your mood or concentration levels adversely affected by food?

_____ 3. Do you rarely experience significant hunger, say twice a week or less?

Maximum possible points: 120

Passing score: 90 (75 percent)

_____ **YOUR SCORE**

_____ **YOUR PERCENTAGE** (your score divided by 120; e.g., 90 /120 = 75%)

CHAPTER 9

Go Keto!

IF you've completed an excellent 21-Day Reset and posted a 75 percent or better on your keto exam, I can assure you with great confidence that the hard part is definitely behind you now. With dietary fat or stored fat as your primary fuel choice, you have entered a fabulous new dimension of health, peak performance, and longevity potential. As long as you adhere to your baseline metabolic conditioning over the long term with ancestral-style eating patterns, you can largely avoid the struggling with and suffering from lifelong weight gain, elevated disease risk factors, and fatigue/illness/burnout patterns caused by carbohydrate dependency. Now it's time to bring more lofty health, body composition, and peak performance goals into the picture by going keto. Your nutritional ketosis effort will require significant discipline, focus, and restraint each day, but your appetite hormones will normalize to the extent that you will never struggle with hunger and deprivation in the familiar model of a calorie-restrictive diet.

If you require another 5, 10, or 20 pounds of body fat to drop to your personal ideal, a ketogenic eating phase will prepare you for success more certainly than anything else you have ever tried. Being fat-adapted can keep you at your ideal body composition indefinitely, even if your exercise volume fluctuates. The druglike anti-inflammatory effect of ketone burning might also help you improve stubborn inflammatory or autoimmune conditions. You can make some huge and rapid changes in your blood lipid panels to push you out of disease risk-factor categories. You can experience peak brain performance from improved oxygen delivery and neuron firing. Finally, you can pursue profound breakthroughs in fitness performance, both in endurance endeavors and in strength/power endeavors.

Note that all these lovely benefits are available only if you've really done your homework and are showing clear signs that you are fine-tuned and ready for nutritional ketosis. If you plunge deep into the extreme carb-restriction world from even mild residual carbohydrate dependency, or as a stress-head with hectic work habits, deficient sleep, and/or insufficient or chronic exercise patterns, you will most assuredly crash and burn. These ambitious but ill-prepared folks often find themselves tired, hungry, irritable, and giving up their keto effort after three weeks—if they even last that long. After they bomb out, many of them enter the fray on social media, rationalize excuses about their failed experiment, and plunge back into some level of mild to significant carbohydrate dependency. Let's make sure this won't be your fate! Relax, take a deep breath right now, and realize that there is no harm in spending two to three more weeks in Reset mode and retaking the midterm exam later. Remember, we are talking about honing a metabolic efficiency that lasts for the rest of your life.

Here's the lowdown on keto: Make a sincere commitment to go a minimum of six weeks observing a hard limit of 50 grams of gross carbohydrates per day (20 grams if you are inactive—and don't forget you can net-out nonstarchy veggies and avocados), coupled with a protein goal of around 0.7 grams per pound of lean mass per day. Owing to the fragility of the liver's ability to make ketones, the carb intake limit applies *every single* day. If you eat 100 grams of carbs one day, you'll shut off ketone production for a while (opinion varies on this—some experts suggest it can take several days to get back in the groove after a single carb binge!), even if you consume zero the next day to maintain a 50 average (although that's not a bad idea if you get derailed).

You have a little more flexibility with your protein intake limit, which can be averaged out over the course of a week or a month. Let's set a hard limit of never exceeding

1 gram per pound of lean mass on any single day, and a goal to average out at 0.7 grams per pound.

> **Observe a hard limit of 50 carbohydrate grams per day, coupled with a protein goal of 0.7 grams per pound of lean mass per day.**

It's going to be tough to maintain nutritional ketosis if you don't have accurate data on your macronutrient intake, so it's time to get familiar with journaling and online macronutrient calculators. It will also be helpful to gain a basic understanding of the carbohydrate, protein, and overall macronutrient values of keto-friendly foods so you can ballpark your 50 carb grams or your protein target on the go. In forthcoming sections of this chapter, you'll learn the macronutrient contributions of many keto-friendly foods, along with tables that isolate for carb values and for protein values.

With the tight parameters on carbs and protein, fat becomes the operative variable to avail total dietary satisfaction at all times, and also to manipulate in order to facilitate fat reduction any time you desire. Even with the stringent carb and protein guidelines, you can enjoy a rich and deeply satisfying diet featuring foods high in nutritious natural fats: meat, fish, fowl, and eggs; nuts, seeds and their derivative butters; high-fat plants like coconut products, avocados and avocado oil, olives and olive oil; high-fat dairy products like raw milk, cheese, cottage cheese, cream cheese, and heavy cream; and 85% or higher dark chocolate.

Out of the gate, understand that the first three weeks may be tough, especially if you've made rapid progress from carb dependency to an ancestral-style pattern whereby your carb intake is around 150 grams per day, and now you are trying to bump quickly down to 50 grams. Remember Dr. D'Agostino's observation that people who fail usually bail out at around three weeks, right when things are about to get easier! And furthermore, the six-week mark is when you will experience the transformational benefits in athletic performance, weight loss, mental clarity, or correction of disease risk factors.

Carefully Counting Carbohydrates

During your 21-Day Metabolism Reset, you likely lowered your carb intake from SAD levels to under 150 grams per day—derived from abundant vegetable intake; sensible fruit intake; nutrient-dense carbs like sweet potatoes, wild rice, and quinoa; incidental carbs from nuts, seeds, and their butters; high-fat dairy and 85% dark chocolate; and maybe a bit of leaking here and there with a corn tortilla or a sushi roll. If you are not a regular exerciser and want to go keto, many experts recommend you limit your carb intake to 20 grams per day. If you are working with the 50 number, realize that you certainly don't need to make a point to max out every day. Getting into NLS* mode to drop below 50 carb grams entails the following:

‣ **Absolutely zero grains, sugars, or sweetened beverages:** Sorry, Starbucks, the desired number of pumps for your exotic teas and coffees is zero when you are going keto.

‣ **Little or no fruit:** This is just a temporary measure to ensure you succeed with keto. Eventually, even when you stay keto for long periods, you can enjoy sensible intake of seasonal fruit, particularly the low-glycemic, high-antioxidant berries.

‣ **Little or no nutrient-dense, in-ground vegetables:** Root vegetables and tubers like sweet potatoe/yams, squash, rutabaga, carrots, and beets are more starchy and warrant temporary elimination or sincere moderation during your keto efforts. The same goes for the otherwise ancestral-approved wild rice and quinoa.

‣ **Selectivity with incidental carbs:** You can creep up and over 50 grams if you go hog wild on nuts, nut butters, 85% dark chocolate, plain yogurt, and coconut milk. Exercise a little moderation and selectivity. If you are inclined to indulge, emphasize the delicious snack and treat recipes in Chapter 12 that are predominant in fat and low in carbs.

CARB CHART: Here is a quick look at the carbohydrate levels in various keto-friendly foods. (Fitday.com was the resource for most of those measurements; you will find variation in the calculations depending on which macronutrient calculator you use.)

---

* NLS = Next Level Shit

Dairy and Other Proteins/Fats	Size	Carbs
Cheese, cheddar or colby	1 cup	3 grams
Cheese, feta	1 cup	6 grams
Coconut milk, full fat	1 cup	12 grams
Coconut flakes	½ cup	7 grams
Cottage cheese	½ cup	4 grams
Cream cheese	½ cup	5 grams
Dark chocolate, 85%	40 g—⅓ bar	13 grams
Eggs		Little to no carbs
Fats and oils		Little to no carbs
Meat, fish, fowl		Little to no carbs
Yogurt, Greek full-fat	⅔ cup	5 grams

Fruits	Size	Carbs
Avocado	⅓ medium	4 grams (net gross is 19)
Banana, Green	1 medium	5 grams
Banana, Yellow	1 medium	27 grams
Blackberries	½ cup	7 grams
Blueberries	½ cup	7 grams
Raspberries	½ cup	7 grams
Strawberries	½ cup	6 grams

Nuts, Seeds, and Their Derivative Butters	Size	Carbs
Almonds	½ cup	6 grams
Almond butter	2 tablespoons	6 grams
Cashew butter	2 tablespoons	9 grams
Macadamia nuts	½ cup	9 grams
Pecans	½ cup	7 grams
Pumpkin seeds	½ cup	7 grams
Sesame seeds	½ cup	9 grams
Sunflower seeds	½ cup	14 grams
Walnuts	½ cup	6 grams

Vegetables (cooked except when otherwise noted)	Size	Carbs
Broccoli florets	1 cup	7 grams
Brussels sprouts	1 cup	11 grams
Cabbage, green	1 cup	8 grams
Cabbage, red	1 cup	7 grams
Chard	1 cup	6 grams
Cucumber (raw)	1 cup	3 grams
Kale	1 cup	6 grams
Kohlrabi	1 cup	11 grams
Pepper, green	1 cup	4 grams
Pepper, red	1 cup	6 grams
Spinach	1 cup	7 grams
Tomatoes	1 cup	10 grams

Protein Primer

Here are some tips to ensure you don't exceed your recommended average daily protein intake of 0.7 grams per pound of lean mass:

DON'T OVERDO PROTEIN SUPPLEMENTS: High-protein meal replacement powders or isolated protein powders with whey, soy, egg, or vegetarian protein sources may someday be utilized as a nice addition to a macronutrient balanced smoothie (especially whey—the other sources are inferior), but they may unnecessarily bump up your protein levels during keto efforts if you go overboard.

EMPHASIZE HIGH-FAT ANIMAL FOODS: Respect our ancestral tradition of consuming animals nose-to-tail style. Choose ground beef with the highest fat content, not the lowest. Instead of ultra-lean chicken breast, cook an entire chicken, then make bone broth from the carcass. Don't do any deliberate high-protein modifications to foods or meals. Say no to egg whites only, extra-lean meats, or any recipe or concoction that overemphasizes protein (often by reducing fat content)—not only during keto but at all other times as well. These strategies make your macronutrient ratios much more keto-friendly, and they dramatically increase the overall nutritional value of your diet.

PERSONAL CALCULATION: Identify your personal protein target at 0.7 grams per pound of lean mass per day:

My total bodyweight: _____

My estimated (or known) body fat percentage: _____

Calculated fat weight (body fat percentage × bodyweight): _____

Calculated lean body mass (total bodyweight minus fat weight): _____

Average daily protein gram intake target (0.7 × lean mass): _____

Daily protein grams: _____ Daily protein calories (grams x 4): _____

Practically speaking, what does consuming 0.7 grams of protein per pound of lean mass look like? First, let's consider the upper and lower extremes of lean body mass. A lean, muscular male at 200 pounds and 10 percent body fat has 180 pounds of lean mass. His protein target is an average of 126 grams/504 calories per day. A petite female at 120 pounds with 25 percent body fat has 90 pounds of lean mass. Her protein target is an average of 63 grams/252 calories per day.

Most people fall somewhere inside these extremes, with target consumption between 60 and 120 grams. For this exercise, let's split the difference and target consumption at 90 grams per day. This hits close to home for a male weighing 180 pounds with 22 percent fat (98 gram/day target) or a female weighing 160 pounds with 27 percent body fat (82 gram/day target).

PROTEIN CHART: Here are some common high-protein foods and the approximate amount of protein grams a typical serving provides. (Fitday.com was the resource for most of those measurements; you will find variation in calculations depending on which macronutrient calculator you use.)

Nuts, Nut Butters, and Seeds	Size	Protein
Almonds	½ cup	15 grams
Almond butter	2 tablespoons	8 grams
Macadamia nuts	½ cup	10 grams
Sesame seeds	½ cup	11 grams
Sunflower seeds	½ cup	12 grams

Dairy and Other Proteins	Size	Protein
Cheese, Swiss	1 cup	35 grams
Cheese, cheddar	1 cup	32 grams
Cheese, colby	1 cup	31 grams
Cheese, feta	1 cup	21 grams
Cheese, gouda	1 cup	33 grams
Eggs	3	18 grams
Whey protein	1 scoop	25 grams
Yogurt (Greek)	⅔ cup	11 grams

Fish	Size	Protein
Salmon (baked)	4 ounces	29 grams
Sardines (water-packed)	1 tin	17 grams
Sardines (oil-packed)	1 tin	22 grams
Tilapia	4 ounces	30 grams
Tuna, fresh	4 ounces	28 grams
Tuna, canned	4 ounces	51 grams

Meats	Size	Protein
Beef, ground (80% lean)	8 ounces	57 grams
Beef, filet mignon	8 ounces	70 grams
Beef, sirloin	8 ounces	68 grams
Chicken (breast)	4 ounces	35 grams
Pork (chop, center loin)	1 chop (146 g)	41 grams
Pork (tenderloin)	4 ounces	32 grams

At a glance, it's apparent that it's quite easy to hit your 0.7 gram per pound of lean mass target, and that you might have to be vigilant to avoid overconsumption. What's more, when you realize how minimal your carb intake is when you ditch grains and sugars, it's apparent that most of your dietary calories will come from fat so as to maintain ideal body composition and avoid excessive growth-factor stimulation.

Keto Kalculations

Following are macronutrient values in the food categories of cheese and dairy, coconut products, dark chocolate, eggs, fruit, meats, nuts, seeds, and their derivative butters, oils, vegetables, and yogurt. Formulating your meals and snacks from these categories will help you stay keto-aligned, but even with these rich foods you have to be careful not to exceed recommended carbohydrate and protein guidelines over the course of a day. Notice the high carbohydrate values in even modest servings of fruits, and the high protein content of things like Greek yogurt, and most fish and meats.

Maintaining keto is clearly about getting most of your calories from fat. When strategizing my meals during keto phases, I like to make quick ballpark calculations to stay keto-friendly. If I'm making a keto calculation for an 85% dark chocolate bar with 13 grams of carbs, 20 grams of fat, and 4 grams of protein in a good serving, I'll quickly total up 52 calories of carbs and 16 calories of protein (knowing each has 4 calories per gram). With 20 grams of fat at 9 calories per gram, I get 180 fat calories. While 180 fat calories with 16 calories of protein and 52 calories of carbs is not quite boilerplate keto of 75 percent fat, 25 percent protein, and 10 percent carbs (it's actually 73 percent fat, 6 percent protein, and 21 percent carbs), it's close enough to eat! Now, if I had fish or hamburger with steamed vegetables for dinner before my chocolate, the macros would be starting to look out of balance, with insufficient fat. However, because fat is so calorically dense, it's easy to balance things out over the course of a day by simply drizzling an extra tablespoon of avocado oil on my lunchtime salad (14 grams of fat, zero carb, zero protein) or slathering my steamed vegetables at dinner in two tablespoons of butter (23 grams of fat, zero carb, zero protein).

Don't get too worked up over hitting your targets at every single meal, just use the information presented to get a good basic education in the macronutrient contributions of common primal/paleo/ancestral foods, and get into the rhythm of pairing sensible servings of foods that are mostly carb or protein with plenty of nutritious natural fats from clean animal sources or high-fat plants like avocado, coconut, and olive, and their oils. Note: Fitday.com was the reference for the following measurements.

Cheese and Dairy

	CARBS	FAT	PROTEIN	CALORIES
Butter, 2 tablespoons (30 g)	0 G	23 G	0 G	204
Cheddar cheese, 1 cup diced (132 g)	3 G	43 G	32 G	525
Colby cheese, 1 cup diced (132 g)	3 G	42 G	31 G	520
Cottage cheese, ½ cup (112 g)	4 G	3 G	12 G	88
Cream cheese, ½ cup (112 g)	5 G	40 G	7 G	397
Feta cheese, 1 cup crumbled (150 g)	6 G	32 G	21 G	396
Gouda cheese, 1 cup diced (132 g)	2 G	37 G	33 G	471
Yogurt, Greek (²/₃ cup, 150 g)	5 G	8 G	11 G	13

Coconut Products

	CARBS	FAT	PROTEIN	CALORIES
Coconut milk, 1 cup full-fat (240 ml)	6 G	45 G	0 G	420
Coconut flakes, ½ cup (28 g)	7 G	17 G	2 G	191
Coconut oil, 1 tablespoon (15 ml)	0 G	14 G	0 G	117
Dark Chocolate (85% Trader Joe's, 40 g)	13 G	20 G	4 G	250

Eggs

	CARBS	FAT	PROTEIN	CALORIES
Primal Omelet (page 259)	12 G	38 G	30 G	510
Scrambled, 2 large (100 g)	2 G	14 G	14 G	204

Fish

	CARBS	FAT	PROTEIN	CALORIES
Salmon, 4-ounce fillet, wild-caught (112 g)	0 G	9 G	29 G	206
Sardines, 1 tin (packed in water)	0 G	7 G	17 G	130
Sardines, 1 tin (packed in oil)	0 G	10.5 G	22.5 G	180
Tilapia, 4-ounce fillet (112 g)	0 G	3 G	30 G	145
Tuna, 4-ounce fresh fillet (112 g)	0 G	6 G	27 G	163
Tuna, 5-ounce can (140 g)	0 G	6 G	35 G	200

Fruits

	CARBS	FAT	PROTEIN	CALORIES
Avocado, 1/3 medium (50 g)	4 G	8 G	1 G	80
Banana, medium yellow (120 g)	27 G	0 G	1 G	105
Banana, medium green (120 g)	5 G	0 G	1 G	24
Blackberries, ½ cup (62 g)	7 G	0 G	1 G	31
Blueberries ½ cup (50 g)	8 G	1 G	2 G	42
Raspberries, ½ cup (62 g)	7 G	0 G	1 G	32
Strawberries, ½ cup sliced (100 g)	6 G	0 G	1 G	27

Meats

	CARBS	FAT	PROTEIN	CALORIES
Beef, ground (80% lean), 8 ounces (225 g)	0 G	37 G	57 G	137
Beef, filet mignon, 8 ounces (225 g)	0 G	20 G	70 G	462
Beef, sirloin steak, 8 ounces (225 g)	0 G	10 G	68 G	362
Chicken breast, boneless, skinless, 4 ounces (112 g)	0 G	5 G	35 G	196
Chicken thigh, boneless, skinless, 4 ounces (112 g)	0 G	7 G	31 G	196
Pork chop, center loin, 1 chop (146 g)	0 G	8 G	41 G	248
Pork tenderloin, 4 ounces (112 g)	0 G	6 G	32 G	192

Nuts, Seeds, and Their Derivative Butters

	CARBS	FAT	PROTEIN	CALORIES
Almonds, ½ cup (56 g)	14 G	37 G	15 G	422
Almond butter, 2 tablespoons (30 ml)	6 G	2 G	7 G	196
Cashews, ½ cup (56 g)	20 G	31 G	11 G	378
Cashew butter, 2 tablespoons (30 ml)	9 G	16 G	6 G	188
Macadamias, ½ cup (60 g)	9 G	51 G	5 G	481
Pecans, ½ cup (56 g)	7 G	36 G	5 G	342
Pumpkin seeds, ½ cup (59 g)	12 G	32 G	17 G	373
Sesame seeds, ½ cup (75 g)	17 G	31 G	11 G	363
Sunflower seeds, ½ cup (70 g)	14 G	38 G	12 G	415
Walnuts, ½ cup (60 g)	8 G	39 G	9 G	392

Oils

	CARBS	FAT	PROTEIN	CALORIES
Avocado oil, 1 tablespoon (15 g)	0 G	14 G	0 G	124
Coconut oil, 1 tablespoon (15 g)	0 G	14 G	0 G	116
Olive oil, 1 tablespoon (15 g)	0 G	14 G	0 G	119

Vegetables

	CARBS	FAT	PROTEIN	CALORIES
Broccoli florets, 1 cup cooked (156 g)	7 G	2 G	2 G	51
Brussels sprouts, 1 cup cooked (223 g)	11 G	4 G	4 G	81
Cabbage, green, 1 cup shredded raw (70 g)	5 G	0 G	1 G	22
Cabbage, green, 1 cup cooked (150 g)	8 G	3 G	2 G	60
Cabbage, red, 1 cup shredded raw (70 g)	7 G	0 G	1 G	28
Cabbage, red, 1 cup cooked (150 g)	10 G	3 G	2 G	69
Chard, 1 cup cooked (175 g)	6 G	3 G	3 G	50
Cucumber, 1 cup sliced raw (104 g)	3 G	0 G	1 G	14
Kale, 1 cup chopped raw (16 g)	6 G	1 G	3 G	33
Kale, 1 cup cooked (130 g)	7 G	3 G	3 G	62
Kohlrabi, 1 cup sliced raw (135 g)	8 G	0 G	2 G	36
Kohlrabi, 1 cup cooked (165 g)	11 G	0 G	3 G	48
Lettuce, 1 cup shredded (47 g)	2 G	0 G	1 G	8

	CARBS	FAT	PROTEIN	CALORIES
Pepper, green, 1 cup sliced (92 g)	4 G	0 G	1 G	18
Pepper, red, 1 cup sliced (92 g)	6 G	0 G	1 G	26
Spinach, 1 cup chopped leaves (30 g)	1 G	0 G	1 G	7
Spinach, 1 cup cooked (180 g)	7 G	3 G	5 G	67
Tomatoes, 1 cup sliced (176 g)	7 G	0 G	2 G	32
Tomatoes, 1 cup diced cooked (240 g)	10 G	0 G	2 G	41

Journaling and Online
Macronutrient Calculators

All this talk about macronutrient numbers means you are going to have to keep some records. First, you will write down everything you eat in the course of a day, carrying around a small notepad to be sure you don't forget anything. You must be mindful of every time you open your mouth, and make an effort to accurately measure, weigh, or make a good estimate of the amounts of food you consume. Definitely measure your foods, using a tablespoon and a measuring cup; you can even consider getting a food scale if you want to get enthusiastic about repeating the food journaling exercise frequently. You then input the data, a day at a time, into an online macronutrient calculator. The calculator generates a report, in both numerical and pie-chart form, to reveal your macronutrient percentages. A couple of the most popular websites for this are fitday.com and myfitnesspal.com. Creating an account is free and it is a great way to automatically archive your daily macronutrient reports.

You'll notice that common foods like eggs, bacon, salmon, broccoli, or 85% dark chocolate already exist in the database, so you just enter the amount you consume. For example, 1 cup of cooked broccoli has 55 calories—11 grams of carbs, 4 grams of protein, and 2 grams of fat. Four squares of Lindt's 90% cacao dark chocolate (an excellent choice, by the way) has 12 grams of carbs, 4 grams of protein, and 22 grams of fat. If you can't find your food in the list but have a Nutrition Facts label to refer to, you can make a custom entry to add to your daily intake list. For example, a tablespoon of Primal Kitchen Mayo (an excellent choice by th . . . whoops, I digress!) has 0 grams of carbs, 0 protein, and 12 grams of fat.

I'd love to see you keep the records for an entire week at the outset of your nutritional ketosis journey. The mere act of keeping these records brings greater mindfulness and accountability to your eating habits. Doing it for a week will give you great insight into your eating habits and an inkling of success you can expect if you stay the course (or, inversely, reveal where you need to right the ship in order to stay in keto ranges). In many cases, novice keto enthusiasts initially come in too high on both carbs and protein, despite devoted efforts. Sometimes this happens when a person overdoes even keto-approved foods and blows past 50 without even noticing, just like a speeding motorist. Common offenders are dark chocolate (4 squares—we're square; 14 squares—beware) and nuts, seeds, and nut butters. Honestly, it takes a little getting used to the sensation of not being hungry, to the extent that you have to catch yourself when you absentmindedly reach for yet another handful of nuts during a lull in your afternoon work schedule.

Keto-Friendly Environment

As was covered in detail in Chapter 7, going keto entails more than just nailing your macronutrients. I discussed previously how stress equals sugar in real life and how sleep insufficiency can also push you back toward carbohydrate dependency. Your eating environment must be pristine as well. Surround yourself with keto-approved groceries and snack foods; be completely clear of sugars, grains, and refined vegetable oils in your home. If you are going to a Monday night men's group or a Tuesday night bowling league where you can count on finding potential diversions away from keto, address the issue proactively: steel your resolve and/or bring your own snacks.

Another thing you can consider adding to your bag of tricks is ketone supplements. While these recent innovations are still being tested and validated, they seem to have some good potential to generate leverage to keep you on track with your keto goals. Granted, you're trying to achieve ketosis by nutritional means, so taking a supplement that will quickly throw you into ketosis by nondietary means seems like cheating. Alas, supplementing into a ketone-burning state may be particularly helpful in getting you through periods of struggle, such as an afternoon energy lull that might otherwise be met with a carbohydrate backslide or a high-calorie almond butter binge. You might also try the supplements first thing in the morning, as you attempt to extend your fast as long as possible. Before you consider using them as a crutch or hangover cure, realize that best results will come when the supplements are used within a framework of ketogenic eating. We'll discuss supplements further in the Appendix.

As far as following a daily routine, figure out whatever works best for your particulars. I've mentioned fasting in the morning, but if you are going to be working hard without access to food for many hours after you leave the house, it's perfectly acceptable to enjoy some bacon and eggs every morning. Perhaps you can fast during the workday and last until dinner, as an alternative to an extended morning fast. Definitely carry some keto-approved snacks with you, such as a baggie of macadamia nuts. Your central governor will thank you for providing that psychological comfort, whether you need it every day or not.

Evaluate your first week of macronutrient reports carefully for red flags. Of particular concern is staying out of that no-man's-land where you cut carbs down from around 150 grams per day to the 80 to 100 range—a significant belt-tightening, but not low enough to unlock your keto weaponry. While "low but not keto" might be a winning long-term strategy, it will stall your progress out of the gate.

Exercise During Keto—Avoid Chronic!

Even if you are doing a good job avoiding chronic exercise patterns—keeping cardio workouts in the aerobic zone and making your high-intensity workouts brief and infrequent, it's a good idea to back off from your overall energy expenditure during the initial keto effort if you are worried about your ability to comply. Remember, your muscles, heart, lungs, and brain have been ravenous at the glucose gas station for a long time, and they require an adjustment period to get used to the solar panels you just installed. I'm not suggesting sitting on your butt when you switch from oatmeal to eggs, for too much inactivity will make going keto more difficult than if you are generally active and energetic. Instead, just tone down your workout caloric output for the first few weeks, with particular attention to avoiding overdistance aerobic sessions, prolonged strength-training sessions, or anything that has the slightest whiff of being chronic. My best advice is simply to walk as much as you can during your keto efforts, and during daily life in general.

As detailed in Phinney and Volek's *The Art and Science of Low Carbohydrate Performance,* there are important nuances for fitness enthusiasts in the process of becoming fat- and keto-adapted. In the early stages of adaptation, your muscles and brain may compete for ketones as they wean off glucose. This may result in some unpleasant symptoms, such as energy lulls and periods of foggy brain when your muscles are winning the tug of war, or perhaps diminished workout performance on the other side of the rope. As you become more adapted, though, your muscles will burn fat with greater efficiency and have less need for ketones—allowing the brain to enjoy express delivery from the liver.

When you get to that esteemed level of possessing fat-adapted muscles and a keto-adapted brain, you receive the full effect of bonk-proof endurance, less oxidative stress, improved body composition, and faster recovery in comparison to your glucose-burning former self. Just be patient and don't overtax your muscles as they transition from mostly glucose to a blend of fat and ketones, and finally over to mostly fat. If you go long, go slower than usual; if you go hard, make the workout shorter than usual.

After six weeks of nutritional ketosis, your intense or prolonged workouts transition from potential liability to effective accelerator of your metabolic fitness. As you'll discover in the next chapter covering advanced strategies, you can pair fasting with exercise to quickly get back on track if you have a dietary departure or you want to drop a few quick pounds of fat that somehow snuck back into place. You'll also discover how you can launch yourself into ketosis any time with a single major depleting workout, and prime your appetite hormones and pleasure center in your brain away from carbs and toward fat.

The Keto Meal Plan

The foods you eat during keto won't actually differ much from the foods you ate during the 21-Day Metabolism Reset; you'll just make some tweaks to your meal patterns to keep the carbs under 50 grams and make sure your protein averages 0.7 grams per pound of lean mass per day. This means going from occasional trickles to zero with sweeteners like honey or sweetened beverages, temporarily cutting out fruit and starchy in-ground vegetables like sweet potatoes and squash, and watching out for excess consumption of nuts, seeds, and dark chocolate. To make sure you are hitting the ideal keto macronutrient percentages, you must also find deliberate ways to increase your fat intake, such as being more liberal with your healthy salad dressing or application of butter to your steamed vegetables, throwing avocado into whatever you're eating (including smoothies!), or trying out some of the "Bombs, Balls, and Bites" section of Chapter 12.

The Keto Meal Plan mixes in some different strategies and techniques, such as a range of morning options like fasting, green smoothies, delicious omelets, high-fat beverages, and more. See what works best for you, or throw caution to the wind and try the exact plan for the 21 days provided, then reassess what works the best for you over the long term. Note: All the meals in this section can be found in Chapter 12.

WEEK 1

DAY 1

Breakfast

Fast until lunch; black coffee or herbal tea is okay

Lunch

Baked Avocado (page 279), one of two ways

½ cup macadamias

2 squares dark chocolate

Dinner

Slow Cooker Carnitas (page 229)

Primal Coleslaw (page 261)

Steamed cauliflower, mashed with 1 tablespoon butter and 1 tablespoon sour cream

DAY 2

Breakfast

Ginger Beet Smoothie (page 213)

Lunch

Cuban Un-sandwich (page 231) with leftover carnitas

Sliced avocado

Dinner

The Best Grilled Chicken (page 237; make extra!)

Caesar Salad with Anchovies and Pancetta (page 276)

Parmesan Crisps (page 285)

DAY 3

Breakfast

Sausage, Kale, and Goat Cheese Frittata (page 202)

High-Fat Coffee (page 210), or coffee or tea with heavy cream

Lunch

Bigass Salad (page 259), with leftover grilled chicken

Dinner

Cashew Beef (page 253)

Cauliflower Rice (page 266)

Steamed broccoli, with 1 tablespoon butter

DAY 4

Breakfast

Fast until lunch

Lunch

Stuffed Tomato (page 236)

Side salad (¼ Bigass Salad, page 259), with 1–2 tablespoons Perfect Vinaigrette (page 221)

½ small green apple

2 tablespoons raw almond butter

Dinner

Turkey Fajita Salad with Chipotle Lime Dressing (page 241)

DAY 5

Breakfast

Greek Yogurt Crunch Bowl (page 201)

High-Fat Coffee (page 210), or coffee or tea with heavy cream

Lunch

Collard Green–Turkey Club Wrap (page 243)

Sweet Pepper Nacho Bites (page 289)

Dinner	
Grilled chicken thighs	Green Bean Casserole (page 272)

DAY 6

Breakfast	Lunch
Go-to Green Smoothie (page 212)	Leftover Green Bean Casserole
	½ avocado
	¼ cup almonds

Dinner	
One-Pan Shrimp and Asparagus (page 239)	Side green salad (¼ Bigass Salad, page 259), with 1–2 tablespoons Perfect Vinaigrette (page 221)

DAY 7

Breakfast	Lunch
Turmeric Scrambled Eggs (page 206)	Smoked Salmon Spread (page 227)
Leftover asparagus with 1 tablespoon butter	1 small cucumber, sliced
High-Fat Coffee (page 210), or coffee or tea with heavy cream	3 small radishes, sliced
	½ avocado
	¼ cup macadamias

Dinner	
Tilapia Bake (page 251)	Broccoli roasted with avocado oil and garlic

WEEK 2

DAY 8

Breakfast	Lunch
Fast until lunch	Collard Green–Turkey Club Wrap (page 243)
	Veggie sticks with Chive Macadamia "Cheese" (page 222)

Dinner	
Chicken Kabobs (page 238; make extra!)	Herbalicious Shredded Salad with Tahini Dressing (page 270)

DAY 9

Breakfast

Egg Muffins in Ham Cups (page 204; make extra to eat as snacks!)

High-Fat Coffee (page 210), or coffee or tea with heavy cream

Lunch

Bigass Salad (page 259) with leftover chicken

Dinner

Bacon-Wrapped Scallops (page 247)

Creamed Spinach (page 284)

Note: Make Chai Chia Breakfast Pudding (page 205) for tomorrow morning.

DAY 10

Breakfast

Chai Chia Breakfast Pudding (page 205) with:
  1 tablespoon cacao nibs
  2 tablespoons shredded coconut

High-Fat Coffee (page 210), or coffee or tea with heavy cream

Lunch

Crunchy Tuna Salad (page 245), wrapped in collard green

Celery sticks with Chive Macadamia "Cheese" (page 222)

Dinner

Shredded Beef Cabbage Cups with Kimchi (page 248)

Cashew Cream Broccoli Salad (page 282)

DAY 11

Breakfast

Fast until lunch

Lunch

Bigass Salad (page 259), with leftover shredded beef

Dinner

Stuffed Turkey Burgers with Goat Cheese (page 246)

Whole Roasted Romanesco (page 277; substitute cauliflower if not in season)

Note: Make almond milk (see page 218) and use pulp to make Nut Pulp Bread (page 291)

DAY 12

Breakfast

Burger Skillet (page 199)

High-Fat Coffee (page 210), or coffee or tea with heavy cream

Lunch

Greek Yogurt Crunch Bowl (page 201)

Golden Chai (page 215) made with almond milk

Dinner

Cheesy Chicken and Ham Roll-up (page 244)

Lemony Pressure Cooker Artichokes with Aioli (page 281)

DAY 13

Breakfast

Brad's "Ketoatmeal" (page 203)

Lunch

Sandwich on Almond Pulp Bread (page 291):

> 3 ounces sliced roast beef (or meat of choice)
>
> 2 slices raw-milk cheddar cheese
>
> 2 tablespoons Primal Kitchen Mayo
>
> 1 tablespoon Dijon mustard

Small green salad (¼ Bigass Salad, page 259), with 1–2 tablespoons Perfect Vinaigrette (page 221)

Dinner

Spaghetti Squash "Pad Thai" (page 278; make extra Pea-NOT Sauce, page 219)

DAY 14

Breakfast

Katie's Keto Granola (page 207), with ¾ cup plain Greek yogurt

High-Fat Coffee (page 210), or coffee or tea with heavy cream

Lunch

Antipasto Skewers (page 287)

Dinner

Thai Soup with Shrimp (page 252)

Steamed zucchini and yellow squash with Pea-NOT Sauce (page 219)

WEEK 3

DAY 15

Breakfast

Fast until lunch, *or longer if you can*

Lunch

Collard Green–Turkey Club Wrap (page 243)

½ small green apple

2 celery stalks, cut into sticks

3 tablespoons almond butter

Dinner

Pork fajitas:
  Slow Cooker Carnitas (page 229)
  Raw cabbage cups or collard greens

½ cup guacamole or diced avocado
2 tablespoons sour cream
Fresh cilantro

DAY 16

Breakfast

Carnitas Kale Scramble (page 230)

High-Fat Coffee (page 210), or coffee or tea with heavy cream

Lunch

Chicken Liver Pâté (page 225) with vegetable sticks

¼ cup raw salted almonds

Dinner

Chicken and Broccoli Casserole (page 249)

Zucchini Noodles with Arugula Pesto (page 262; make a big batch of pesto!)

Note: Make hard-boiled eggs for tomorrow

DAY 17

Breakfast

Breakfast Egg Salad (page 197)

High-Fat Coffee (page 210), or coffee or tea with heavy cream

Lunch

Next Level Baked Avocado (page 280)

2 ounces raw-milk cheddar cheese, cubed

¼ cup Whoops They're Gone Walnuts 'n Dark Chocolate Snack Bag (page 286)

Dinner

Slow-Baked Salmon with Dill Aioli (page 242)

Massaged Kale Salad with Goat Cheese (page 269; make extra!)

DAY 18

Breakfast

Fast until lunch, *or longer if you can*

Lunch

2 hard-boiled eggs (Marinated, page 290, or plain)

Leftover kale salad sautéed with 1 tablespoon avocado oil

½ avocado

Dinner

Crab-Stuffed Portabello Mushrooms (page 258)

½ cup roasted beets with 2 tablespoons pesto

DAY 19

Breakfast

Waffles with Sausage Gravy (page 209)

High-Fat Coffee (page 210), or coffee or tea with heavy cream

Lunch

Go-to Green Smoothie (page 212)

Dinner

Pan-Fried Cod with Dill Caper Sauce (page 254)

Cauliflower Rice (page 266; use large head and reserve half the riced cauliflower for lunch tomorrow)

Side green salad (¼ Bigass Salad, page 259), with 1–2 tablespoons Perfect Vinaigrette (page 221)

DAY 20

Breakfast

Turmeric Scrambled Eggs (page 206)

Turnip Hash Browns (page 200)

High-Fat Coffee (page 210), or coffee or tea with heavy cream

Lunch

Cauliflower garlic bread

Pizza Bites (page 288)

Dinner

Braised Chicken with Olives (page 255)

Prosciutto-Wrapped Asparagus (page 275)

DAY 21

Breakfast

Fast until lunch, *or longer if you can*

Lunch

Leftover Braised Chicken

English Cucumber Tea Un-sandwiches (page 289)

½ avocado

Dinner

Steak topped with Bacon Chili Butter (page 224)

Massaged Kale Salad with Goat Cheese (page 269)

Perfect Roasted Brussels Sprouts (page 274)

CHAPTER 10

Advanced Strategies to Accelerate Progress

ARE you a driven, competitive, type A who might be reading between the lines of this book's content by this point, wondering how you can fast-track your progress beyond what's been presented so far? Well, there is a way, but you have to be in top shape (diet, exercise, sleep, stress management) if you want to play. If you have progressed steadily to this point through the 21-Day Metabolism Reset and the six weeks of nutritional ketosis, and you still have some excess body fat to lose, you can now unleash some advanced keto strategies to make breakthroughs that were previously not believed to be possible

in losing excess body fat and keeping it off.

For decades, conventional wisdom held health enthusiasts in check. But some basic concepts have been proven to be "pliable." For example, the calories in/calories out law of thermodynamics is *literally* true, but this discounts the critical variable of hormone optimization. You indeed have to burn more calories than you store to lose excess body fat—but what happens when your appetite and fat metabolism are dysregulated by a high-carb/high insulin–producing diet? You are going to eat more than you need and be unable to burn the stored energy, rendering this equation irrelevant. Similarly, we may all indeed have a "set point" of body composition that we drift toward, and some of us were dealt more favorable cards than others. For example, geneticists have validated the obvious observation that those with equatorial ancestry generally have proportionally longer limbs and less body fat (the better to dissipate heat in tropical climates) than those with ancestry distant from the equator, where a stockier body type affords more protection from the elements. However, when we view set points in the context of a carbohydrate-dependency lifestyle pattern, it follows that wherever your set point is at present, breaking free of carb dependency will offer you access to a more desirable set point.

In the fitness world, we have believed for the past half century that carbohydrates are the primary energy source for working muscles. This concept has manifested true in the bodies of real human athletes of the past 50 years, but only because they were locked into high-carbohydrate eating patterns. This led to the aforementioned "furnace will burn" mindset that has—despite our ill-informed protestations to the contrary—compromised our health in pursuit of fitness. In the new metabolic-flexibility paradigm, athletes can leverage hard workouts to teach their bodies to burn cleaner fuel more efficiently—not only during exercise but also around the clock. This means that finally, all that hard work in the gym or on the road can actually promote longevity, disease protection, and weight control instead of constantly be at odds with these goals.

This chapter is going to be a lot of fun—how can you not be tantalized by Dr. Cate Shanahan's concept of "violently recalibrating appetite hormones"? But please remember that these are *advanced* strategies. If you jump into the game of fasted workouts and purposeful glycogen depletion to rewire your appetite hormones when you are not fully fat- and keto-adapted, you are going to make a big mess of things, and possibly tell your sob story to others in the takeout line at the Cheesecake Factory. No kidding, I've lost count of the number of times I've heard people conclude emphatically that they ". . . tried that low-carb stuff—didn't work for me. You see, I need my carbs because . . . [I'm a triathlete], [I'm Italian], I'm [fill in the blank]."

If you're an athlete and you've done the hard work of the 21-Day Reset and a six-week keto stint, you can combine your metabolic fitness with your physical fitness and become leaner, fitter, healthier, and more energetic than you've ever been before.

Targeted Fat Reduction with Keto

If you know your optimal keto carb and protein numbers, it follows that there is a level of fat intake that aligns with your estimated daily caloric expenditure. Eating this amount of fat will predictably help you maintain your current body composition. When you are fat- and keto-adapted and decide to drop some excess body fat, you simply obtain your caloric energy needs from your thighs and your behind instead of from the omelet bar. If you are inclined, you can target a specific fat-reduction goal with corresponding carb, protein, and fat intake levels, and you will lose that amount in your chosen time frame. Even if you aren't interested in such a precise approach, though, it may be helpful to understand the formula for aligning macronutrient intake with estimated daily caloric expenditure, then plugging in a fat-reduction factor to generate a new macronutrient intake pattern to generate fat loss. You can certainly eat intuitively and enjoy fat loss as a natural by-product of metabolic flexibility, but at least you will understand what's happening on a metabolic level when you notice your clothes fitting ever more loosely over time.

This information is presented here because I didn't want you worrying about dropping excess body fat during your initial nutritional ketosis venture. Now, you might have lost a little, or a lot, of body fat during keto, but it's best that this success be incidental instead of purposeful. When you first try going keto, your primary concern is getting through unscathed. You want to hit that delicate three-week checkpoint with good momentum to carry you to six weeks. Consequently, it's best to allow for liberal enjoyment of fat calories to the extent that your carb, protein, and fat calories typically match your estimated daily caloric expenditure. Hey, even if you are eating more fat than you really need to make sure cravings are kept at bay, that's fine, too.

Interestingly, even when you consume more fat than your estimated daily expenditure, it's difficult to add excess body fat when your insulin is minimized by low-carb intake. What happens instead is that your body finds ways to burn those extra calories through *non-exercise activity thermogenesis*—that is, you tend to be more naturally active, alert, and energetic, or perhaps make more ketones that you will burn or excrete (since you can't store ketones like you can fat).

Having succeeded with your initial keto venture, you can then turn your attention to targeted reduction of excess body fat. First, you'll want to estimate your daily caloric expenditure by calculating your basic metabolic rate (BMR) at rest (based on height, weight, and age). You then multiply that by an activity factor called the Harris-Benedict formula. (Review my personal example shortly, then visit bmi-calculator.net/bmr-calculator/ to generate your own numbers, if you are interested.) Knowing your carb and protein goals, you can then back into your estimated break-even daily fat consumption. For example, if you dial back your fat intake to the tune of 300 or 500 calories per day, you will be able to lose 3 to 5 pounds of excess body fat in a single month, or more if you want to be aggressive. Here's how:

466 calorie daily deficit × 30 days = 14,000 calories / 3,500 fat calories per pound = 4 pounds of fat loss.

Let's go through the process with my particulars as follows:

CARBOHYDRATE: My daily carb intake @ 50 grams: 200 calories.

PROTEIN: My total bodyweight 168 pounds, 9 percent fat (15 pounds) = lean body mass of 153 pounds; 153 × 0.7 grams per pound per day = 107 grams of protein: 428 protein calories.

ESTIMATED DAILY CALORIC EXPENDITURE: 5'10", 168 pounds, male age 64 = 1,579 BMR. Harris-Benedict equation "Very Active" category: BMR × 1.725 = 2,724 estimated daily caloric expenditure.

FAT: 2,724 minus 628 (carb and protein calories) = 2,096 fat calories per day / 232 fat grams to maintain current body composition.

MACRONUTRIENT PERCENTAGES: Note that my example aligns with the recommended keto macronutrient profile:

- Carbs (200 calories): 7%

- Protein (428 calories): 16%

- Fat (2,096 calories): 77%

FAT LOSS: Supposing I want to cut up for my role as a wise, benevolent, aging pirate in the spring production at the local high school. I'll target a reduction of 4 pounds of excess body fat in one month, just in time for opening night:

4 pounds × 3,500 calories/pound = 14,000 calories of fat loss. Divide 14,000 by 30 days = 466 calorie fat intake deficit per day. Yes, the caloric deficit always comes from fat, because carbs and protein are already low enough.

ESTIMATED DAILY FAT INTAKE FOR WEIGHT LOSS: Daily caloric expenditure of 2,724 minus 628 (carb and protein calories), minus 466 (stored body fat contribution) = 1,630 dietary fat calories per day.

Make the calculations yourself, use your journaling and an online calculator to confirm you are nailing your goals, and your success will be guaranteed. Notice I didn't mention exercise calories in this story because you don't even need to exercise to drop excess body fat. When you are fat- and keto-adapted and training sensibly, your workouts will pleasantly accelerate your progress. On the other hand, when you are carb-dependent and exercising chronically, your workouts might actually sabotage your progress by stimulating an increased appetite and making you lazier throughout the day. I'll add some parting comments when it comes to exercise and fat loss: be sure you move as much as possible throughout your day, and try some brief, all-out sprints if your progress stalls.

Fasted Workouts

For fitness enthusiasts, conducting fasted workouts, both brief, intense strength sessions and sustained endurance sessions, helps accelerate the process of fat- and keto-adaptation, mitochondrial biogenesis, and autophagy. Since learning of this secret, I conduct almost all of my workouts in an overnight fasted state. I also remain fasted for several hours after my workouts to optimize the flood of adaptive hormones in my bloodstream and the autophagy stimulated by the exercise effort. However, this should be considered an advanced strategy. If you are not fully fat- and keto-adapted and fast aggressively before and/or after workouts, you may compromise your chances at recovery. One safe rule of thumb for fitness enthusiasts to adhere to is to not extend your fast beyond the point of true hunger sensations, as this could generate a fight-or-flight gluconeogenesis response that would compromise the intended benefits of an adaptive hormonal response to exercise and fasting.

Everything that's about to be covered is ill-advised unless you are free from carbohydrate dependency and well down the road to being fat-adapted. If you're a sugar-burner and try an ambitious one-off workout in a fasted state, you'll trigger fight-or-flight gluconeogenesis. Rather than improving your metabolic fitness, it's likely that these bouts, however well intentioned, will further promote carbohydrate dependency over the long term. Once you become fat-adapted, you can promote metabolic and physical fitness adaptations, as well as stimulate mitochondrial biogenesis by demanding that your cells perform with less than the usual supply of fuel. Performing significant physical work (remember, even a casual bike ride or brisk walk gets you up to 6 to 10 Metabolic Equivalents of Task (METs), while a sprint or maximum effort in the gym can go up to 30 METs) without your usual abundance of glucose forces your cells to get better at burning fat much more quickly than just fasting in the morning as you commute or sit at your desk.

However fat-adapted you think you are, you must perform fasted workouts with extreme caution. When you are in the gym or out on the road, keep a carbohydrate drink or convenient energy fuel on hand, just in case you need it. As discussed with regard to the Central Governor Theory in Chapter 2, simply knowing you have a rescue fuel supply available provides a level of psychological comfort that can actually help improve your physical performance. If you feel goofy, dizzy, shaky, hot, or weak, stop the workout immediately to refuel and rehydrate. Ditto if you are trying to sustain a post-exercise fast and start to feel funny. Weak equals WHEN, got it?!

The following is a suggested progression of fasted workout efforts:

12 HOURS (E.G., 8 P.M.–8 A.M.) + BASELINE SESSION + WHEN @ 0–2 HOURS: Conduct these workouts routinely and wait to eat afterward until hunger ensues naturally—it's hopeful that will progress very quickly into longer time frames. If you are competent at fasted mornings but experience hunger soon after even a routine morning workout, your fat burning during exercise needs to improve. This is a possible consequence of chronic exercise patterns, whereby you are still a sugar-burner during exercise even if you are burning fat pretty well at rest.

12 HOURS + BASELINE SESSION + WHEN @ 2–4 HOURS: Now you are getting yourself to midday without any calories, but are including a baseline workout in the mix. Nice progress toward fat adaptation.

12 HOURS + BREAKTHROUGH SESSION + WHEN @ 0–2 HOURS: Conducting a long aerobic session, a high-intensity group workout such as Crossfit, or a personal trainer–guided session in a fasted state—without sipping or slurping any carbohydrate calories during the session—is a great way to emphatically escape carb dependency. Even if you get hungry right away, go ahead and reward yourself. Stay away from refined carbs no matter what.

12 HOURS + BREAKTHROUGH SESSION + KETO WHEN @ 0–2 HOURS: The next progression from the previous would be to make your WHEN meal keto-aligned—for example, a long aerobic run followed by a delicious omelet soon after you get home.

12–14 HOURS + BREAKTHROUGH SESSION + KETO WHEN @ 2–6 HOURS: Delivering a breakthrough effort and making it into early afternoon—again without forcing things or experiencing any overt hunger sensations or food obsessions—gets you into outstanding category as a true fat- and ketone-burning beast!

Violently Recalibrating Your Appetite Hormones

Combining fasting and strenuous exercise offers a purposeful "bonk," where liver and muscle glycogen are half depleted (maybe more), and you get ketone levels up to a minimum of 0.5 mmol/L. If you fast overnight and then deliver a high-intensity workout of 45 minutes, or a sustained aerobic workout of a couple hours, then you fast for a couple hours afterward, you can get to a blood ketone level in one day that might take two to seven days of keto-aligned eating.

When you are in this depleted state after fasted workouts, ghrelin generates rapid and profound sensations of hunger in both the stomach and the brain. "Ghrelin literally gets your stomach growlin'," says Dr. Cate, and you can feel and hear these increased gastric secretions in expectation of the imminent arrival of food. Ghrelin also crosses the blood-brain barrier and stimulates hunger sensations in the hypothalamus. The hypothalamus is the brain's control center for decision making, impulse control, emotions like anger and pleasure, and many other things. A hungry hypothalamus will likely alter the more disciplined and rational behavior patterns you exhibit when ghrelin is not growlin'.

When you answer the intense hunger call with a carbohydrate binge, you trigger a burst of dopamine and endogenous opioids that act on the nucleus accumbens in the hypothalamus to influence neural mediation of food reward; you form a strong connection in the pleasure center of your brain between carbohydrates and intense reward. The fact that sugar and wheat have additional opioid-stimulating properties strengthens this connection. What's more, Dr. Cate asserts that cortisol is a further trigger for habit-forming associations. When you're stressed—whether by exercise-induced depletion or by the hassles of daily life—and you consume sugar, your brain is cementing a connection between stress and sugar.

The incessant burning and refueling of carbs locks you into hormonal and psychological carbohydrate dependency patterns with perhaps greater intensity than a less active person, who neither consumes nor burns as many carbs. This is the premise that has been actualized by sports nutrition companies into a multi-billion dollar business category.

This powerful neural mediation of food reward makes sense from an evolutionary perspective, because our ancestors needed genes that reacted strongly to hunger in order to stay focused on survival. Today, with starvation risk out of the picture, we can imagine an exciting new alternative to a carb binge and engage in what Dr. Cate Shanahan calls "violent appetite hormone rewiring." When you become depleted, your extremely sensitive appetite hormones are primed for rewiring. If you fast for a spell instead of slamming carbs, you will aggressively upregulate your fat burning and ketone production, because your body will strive valiantly to leverage available resources and dump the energy you need into your bloodstream.

Similarly, if you reward yourself after depleting workouts with keto-friendly meals, you will still trigger that dopamine and opioid burst, and this will wire your pleasure center up to high-fat foods. Dr. Cate goes on to suggest that if you hate sardines or olives and make yourself eat them when depleted, you will grow to like them! You may have experienced the influence of neural mediation of food reward if you've over-shopped when hungry or when you dutifully have given up milk chocolate in favor of dark, eventually becoming habituated to the bitter taste of dark, and then find milk chocolate far too sweet when you try it again.

While I've talked at length throughout the book about never struggling, suffering, or going hungry in your quest to ditch carb dependency and become fat-adapted, let's put the soft talk on hold for a moment and get into some type-A straight talk. When you can push the envelope of your abilities to access and burn stored energy instead of default to external feedings, your body will respond quickly to this stimulation by becoming more resilient to hunger, cravings, and willpower cavings. We have a tendency today to constantly take preemptive action against hunger by eating regular meals on the clock, and keeping snack stashes in car, briefcase, backpack, or office drawer. For a carb-dependent eater, getting to the point of hunger is indeed not a great idea, because fight-or-flight gluconeogenesis will be triggered and will increase your overall life stress score.

It's another story when you are partially or fully fat- and keto-adapted. Extending your fasting windows to the point of hunger (or working through a bit of hunger if you're a real *chingon*—Spanish for badass), exerting the discipline to complete a strict nutritional ketosis period of ideally six weeks minimum, or even engaging in a bit of good ol' calorie restriction now and then all help to optimize insulin sensitivity, boost fat and ketone metabolism, enhance your appreciation of food, and get those final 5 pounds off your body once and for all.

These behaviors are considered *hormetic stressors*—positive natural stressors that deliver a net overall benefit and are not too severe to become destructive. Hormetic stressors relating to cellular energy needs will also stimulate mitochondrial biogenesis. When cells are challenged by a lack of caloric energy, via fasting, a challenging workout, or both in tandem, they respond by improving mitochondrial function and building new mitochondria. Hormesis is thus the distinction between the brief fight-or-flight stimulation of a sprint workout that delivers great benefits, and the prolonged fight-or-flight stimulation from a chronic exercise pattern, which is greatly destructive.

You can also put ice baths or sauna sessions in the hormetic stressor category. When your body is temporarily stressed and forced to thermoregulate back to homeostasis, you feel energized and invigorated, and get a boost in immune and metabolic function. If you were to go to unhealthy extremes—fasting, exercising, or staying in a sauna or icy river for too long, these stressors would become destructive instead of hormetic. So, we have a fine line to respect here, since extending too far beyond your metabolic capabilities too often can default you into an overstress pattern with negative health consequences.

The Fanta Strategy—How Speedgolf World Champion Rob Hogan Violently Extinguished His Sugar Habit

Rob Hogan of Galway, Ireland, is world champion in the offbeat sport of Speedgolf. In 2013, he won $10,000 and the world professional title by shooting a 77 on a championship golf course in only 39 minutes (carrying only a handful of clubs and running at high speed between shots). This generated a Speedgolf score (adding strokes and minutes together) of 116. In a quest to improve his endurance for Speedgolf, Hogan, a golf professional by trade, joined a local endurance running club and conducted a series of weekend runs of escalating distance. Over time, Hogan worked up from 13 miles, to 15, and then to 17—a distance he completed four weekends in a row.

Hogan completed these runs without consuming any water or calories! At the finish line, he would enjoy his favorite treat: an ice-cold Fanta orange soda at the local convenience store. On the fourth of Hogan's consecutive weekend 17-mile efforts, he recalls experiencing an intense craving for his Fanta in the latter stages of the run—a vision that popped into his head and would not go away. He could have easily skipped out on his final loop on the four-mile route when this clear and present danger sign of bonking manifested, but Hogan soldiered on, intent on again completing the full distance. By the time he somehow got his body to the finish line by sheer force of will, something extraordinary happened: his desire for the Fanta subsided, as did his penchant for sweets in the weeks and months that followed! Clearly, Hogan violently forced his body into elevated fat and ketone oxidation to get through the last four miles of a run that took him beyond the previously perceived limits of his metabolic abilities. In doing so, he sent a powerful message to his hypothalamus— let's call it the Central Governor, to leverage that descriptor in Chapter 2—to break free from sugar dependency and become a fat-burning beast, forever, in a single day!

The outlandish conclusion to this story required some validation from Dr. Shanahan: "These intense, novel, and unique experiences are powerful signal generators that message the body that it needs to change, and the body responds accordingly. Hogan essentially hacked the typical transition from sugar-burner to fat-adapted—something that might take weeks of gradual dietary transitions and devoted exercise—by pushing his body to the limit while starving it of calories," Shanahan explained.

One of my favorite sayings applies here: "If it were easy, everyone would be doing it." Rewiring your appetite hormones can be done quickly and effectively, but there is a reason Dr. Cate uses the adjective *violent*—it's tough! Your mission, if you choose to accept it, is to stimulate a marked hunger response in your body once or twice a week via the combination of fasting and depleting workouts. When these hunger sensations occur, try holding out for a significant period of time. Perhaps when hunger hits you can keep busy by taking a walk or doing some breathing and stretching exercises—getting the blood flowing to help boost fat oxidation. What you may notice after a few efforts is that you get a bit of a second wind where your hunger spike subsides and you can keep going for another 30 to 60 minutes before you really crack and need to get some nourishment. Be sensible in your approach, make sure your exercise, sleep, and stress-management behaviors are in top shape, and push the envelope once in a while!

CHAPTER 11

The Finish Line and Beyond

AFTER six weeks of sustained nutritional ketosis, congratulations are in order! You should be feeling great—rarely feel hungry, with increased mental clarity, loss of excess body fat if desired, and better stress management. At this point you can decide to continue your keto experiment for a defined longer period of time or indefinitely, or to transition out of ketosis by adding back more carbs (and/or perhaps even a bit more protein). Please understand that the world's leading experts strongly assert that there are precious few definitives in this game, and there appears to be a huge amount of personal variation in defining the best strategy. Not only

that, the best strategy for you might evolve from one season or year to the next!

A growing number of people, including some of the most respected experts like Dr. Phil Maffetone, Nora Gedgaudas, nutritional and neurofeedback healer and author of *Primal Fat Burner*, and the keto athlete and trainer Luis Villasenor, are proponents of staying in nutritional ketosis, all the time, indefinitely. Others, like Dr. Cate Shanahan, advocate for both continuing the benefits of fasting/ketogenic eating periods and enjoying high-nutrient-value carbs in sensible doses—ideally in and around strenuous workouts. Even

Dr. Peter Attia, who was in strict nutritional ketosis nonstop for three years from 2011 to 2014, now follows a more relaxed eating strategy. He suggests that carbs are only problematic when they are excessive enough to disturb homeostasis.

It's really looking like $n = 1$ (a scientific notation meaning "an experiment of one") trumps everything: test, evaluate, and retest to establish your own guiding principles that promote metabolic flexibility. Unfortunately, especially in the diet and fitness world, we seem to crave and respond strongly to absolutes. An incessant stream of regimented diets or workout programs touted as the latest, greatest thing rolls out without pause and each has its day in the sun.

Right now, skeptics are looking at keto and calling it the latest fad diet that will likely fade over time. From an evolutionary perspective, this observation is objectionable. Robb Wolf, former research biochemist and author of the bestselling *The Paleo Solution* and *Wired to Eat,* makes the observation that keto is very likely the default *Homo sapiens* factory setting. This is because a steady supply of food—especially a high-carbohydrate load—was not part of our experience until civilized times. At the same time, the complex and rapidly evolving human brain desperately needed a massive percentage of our daily calories (20–25 percent) in the form of glucose or the glucose-like substitute of ketones. If we didn't evolve to make ketones, we would have been forced to resort to the highly inefficient process of gluconeogenesis every time our brains ran short of fuel. Stripping down lean muscle to fuel brain function is no fun when you trigger fight-or-flight reactions during the afternoon blues, but it's *really* no fun when you are starving with no guarantee of your next meal.

While we know that doing a sustained stint of nutritional ketosis can reprogram genes away from carb dependency toward fat- and keto-adaptation, Wolf suggests that sustaining keto might have a reset effect on your mitochondria such that it promotes desirable apoptosis, the programmed death of dysfunctional cells. Hence, you can use keto as a tool to help recover from the destructive effects of leaky gut syndrome, hormonal burnout from inflammatory, overly stressful exercise and/or lifestyle patterns, and even things like extended antibiotic use or exposure to environmental pollutants.

On the flip side, Wolf ponders whether a prolonged stint of nutritional ketosis might actually diminish metabolic flexibility in some people by promoting what's known as "physiological" insulin resistance in the muscle cells. We know from Phinney and Volek's work that highly adapted individuals will condition their muscles to

Turnip Hash Browns (page 200)
with Sausage, Kale, and Goat
Cheese Frittata (page 202)

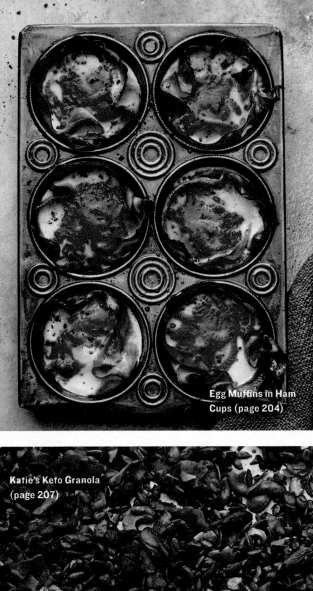
Egg Muffins in Ham Cups (page 204)

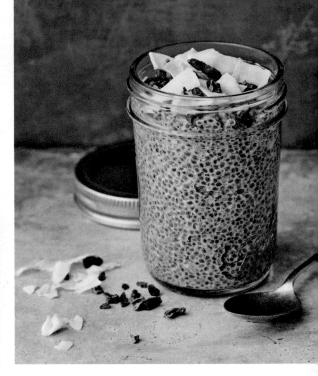
Chai Chia Breakfast Pudding (page 205)

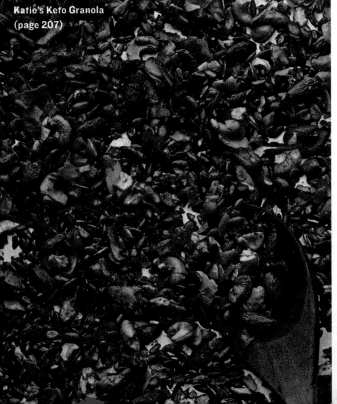
Katie's Keto Granola (page 207)

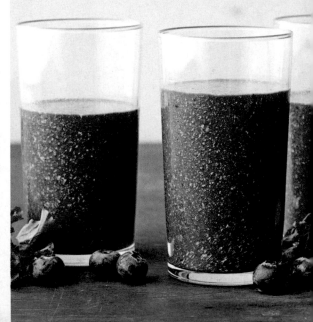
Ginger Beet Smoothie (page 213)

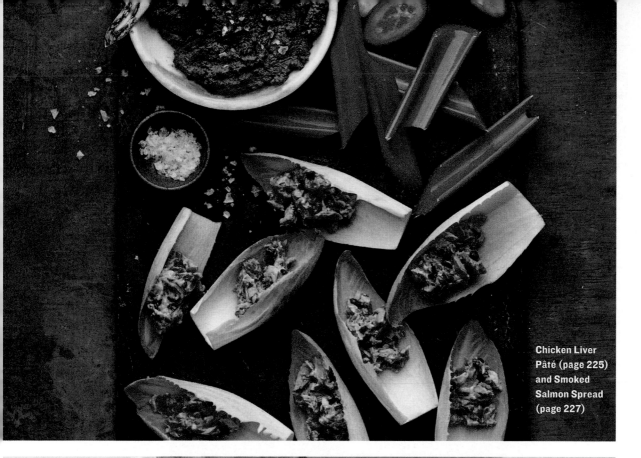

Chicken Liver Pâté (page 225) and Smoked Salmon Spread (page 227)

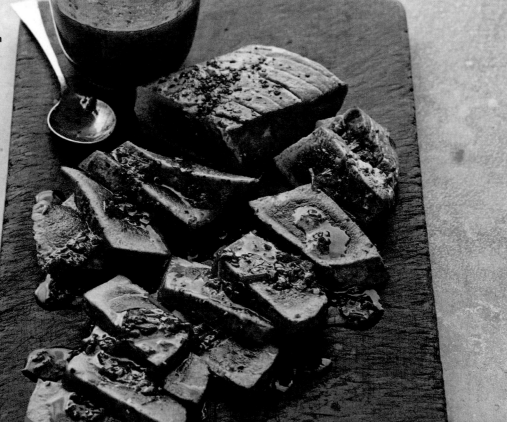

Seared Ahi with Herb + Lime Dressing (page 233)

One-Pan Shrimp and Asparagus (page 239)

Shredded Beef
Cabbage Cups
with Kimchi
(page 248)

Cashew Beef (page 253) with
Cauliflower Rice (page 266)

Pan-Fried Cod with
Dill Caper Sauce
(page 254) and
Primal Coleslaw
(page 261)

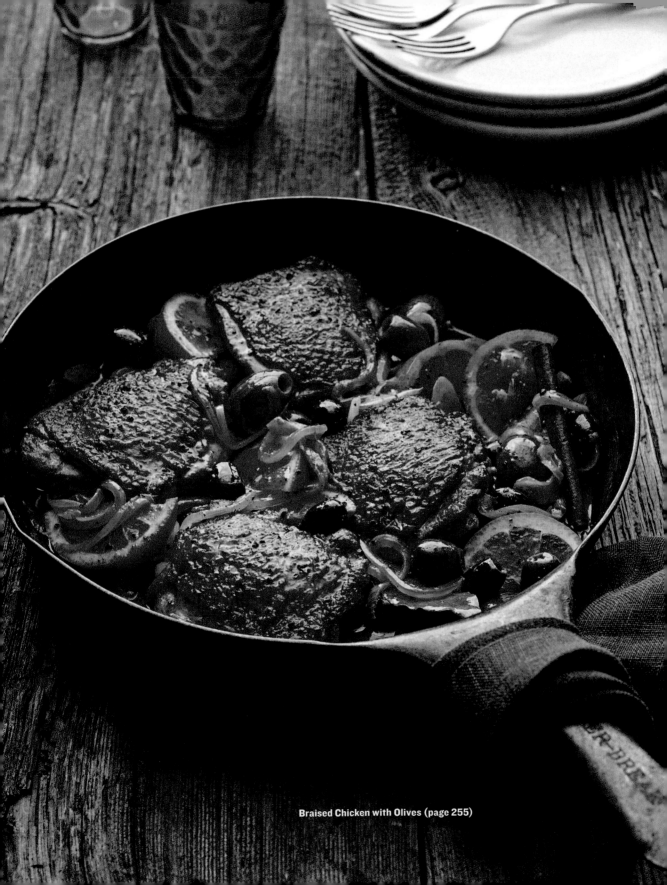

Braised Chicken with Olives (page 255)

Macadamia-Crusted Mahi-Mahi with Browned Butter (page 256)

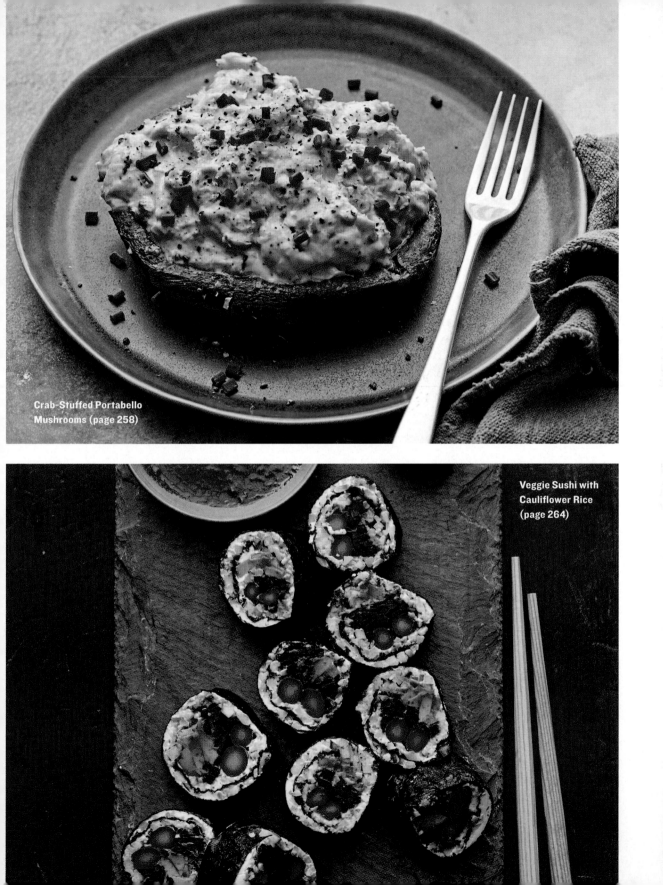

Crab-Stuffed Portabello
Mushrooms (page 258)

Veggie Sushi with
Cauliflower Rice
(page 264)

Perfect Roasted Brussels Sprouts (page 274)

Caesar Salad with Anchovies
and Pancetta (page 276) and
Parmesan Crisps (page 285)

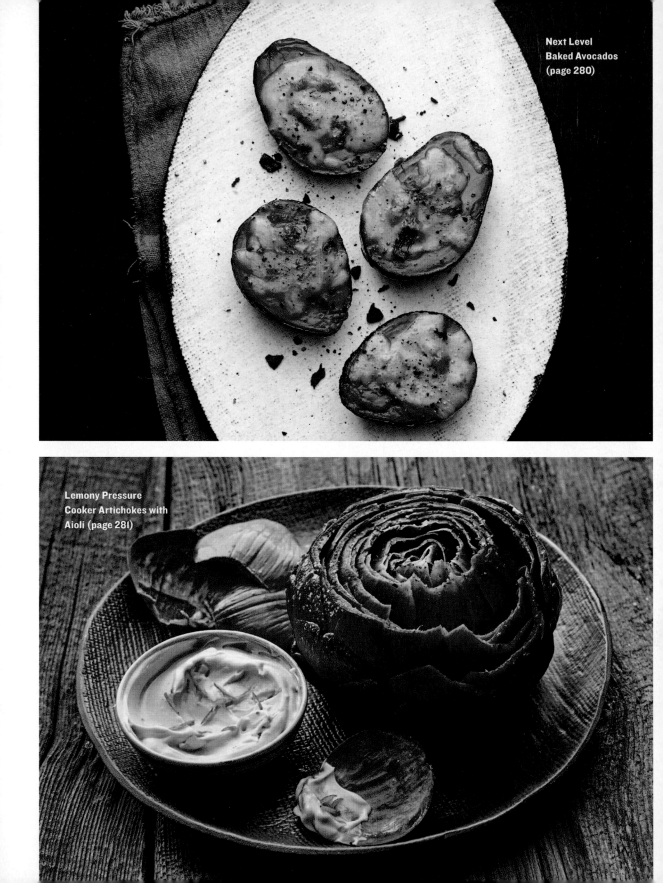

Next Level
Baked Avocados
(page 280)

Lemony Pressure
Cooker Artichokes with
Aioli (page 281)

Antipasto Skewers
(page 287)

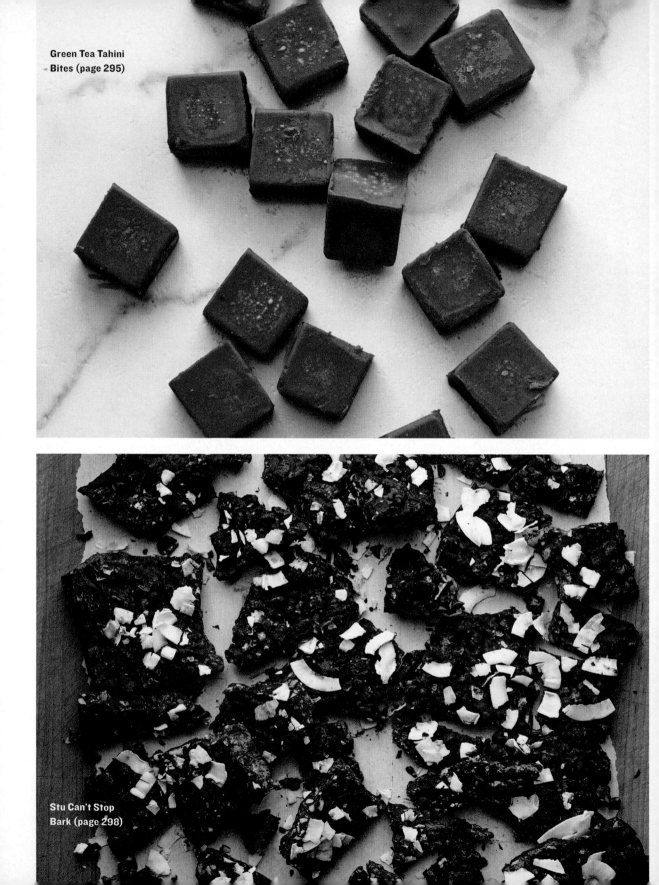

Green Tea Tahini
Bites (page 295)

Stu Can't Stop
Bark (page 298)

Chocolate Avocado Mousse (page 301) with Coconut Milk Whipped Cream (page 302)

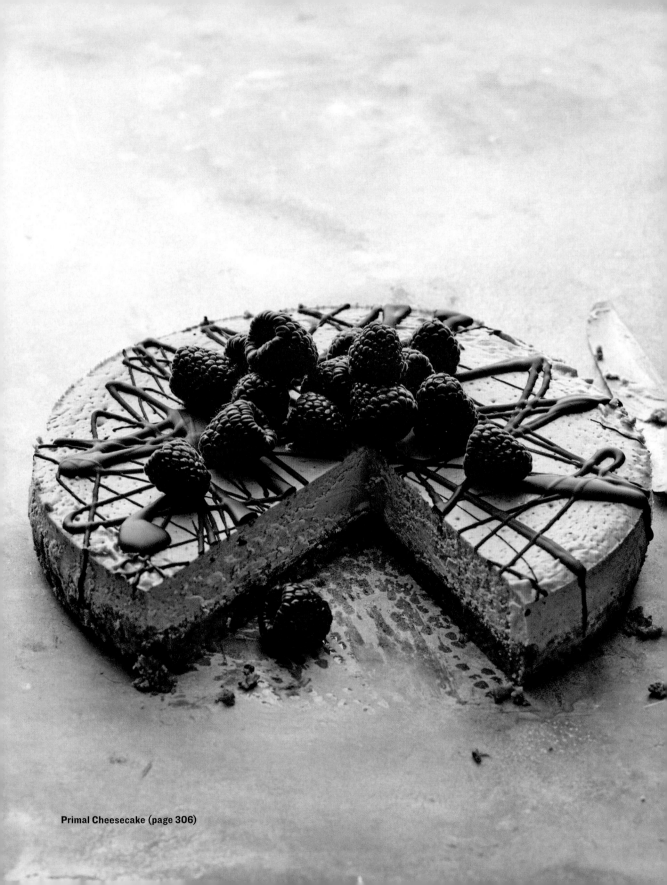

Primal Cheesecake (page 306)

burn primarily fatty acids in order to prioritize ketones for use by the brain. In a highly fat- and keto-adapted metabolic state, a "refeed"—introducing a high-carbohydrate day, weekend, or longer period—might make certain individuals feel like crap (others might feel fine though). Wolf speculates that this could be due to extra insulin being released to drive those now unfamiliar carbs into storage, since your muscles are so used to burning fat instead of glucose or ketones. This is why some experts warn against extreme cycles such as staying in nutritional ketosis during the week and allowing for significant carb binges on the weekend. While the science is not definite, being fat- and keto-adapted and binging on carbs might make you more likely to store those carbs as fat and trigger gluconeogenesis, since your brain suddenly doesn't have the ketones it has come to rely upon (since ketone burning shuts off immediately upon a carb binge).

One as yet unpublished study from Dr. Jacob Wilson had a group following nutritional ketosis during the week and then binging on carbs during the weekend, paired with a control group remaining in nutritional ketosis. The weekend carb bingers not only took almost an entire week to get back into keto but also increased body fat and lost lean muscle mass (likely due to gluconeogenesis). In contrast, a control group staying in keto lost body fat and preserved lean muscle mass.

Being flexible with your eating patterns supports metabolic flexibility—within the context of ancestral-aligned low-carb, moderate protein, and high-fat eating patterns.

At this point in the story, we must take care to heed Dr. D'Agostino's suggestion to be wary of definitives in this game. Interviews with him for this book were characterized by a high frequency of answers like "I'm not sure," and "I don't know," and the sober reminder that "only the mediocre scientists are definitive—they are the ones that make it on TV. The good scientists ask more questions." Actually, the aforementioned observations suggest that being flexible with your eating patterns supports metabolic flexibility! Granted, we are talking about flexibility within the context of a genetically optimal, ancestral-aligned eating style. This means no grains, sugars, or refined vegetable oils; avoiding the all too common chronically excessive protein intake that happens as a result of fat phobia; and making natural, nutritious fats the vast majority of your calories.

Practically speaking, if you want to live a long time and get a gold star from Dr. Attia for optimally low insulin production, your average daily carbohydrate intake will range between 20 and 150 grams for the rest of your life, while your average daily protein intake will be in the neighborhood of 0.7 grams per pound of lean mass, maybe a bit more for certain high-metabolic-demand individuals. When it comes to carbs, be mindful of Dr. Cate's comments that timing is critically important. If your glycogen suitcases are open, you are less likely to disturb homeostasis, immune function, or hormone balance (or even keto efforts if you are active enough), and the aforementioned discussion about developing insulin resistance in your muscles is likely nothing to concern yourself with. In contrast, it is known that eating excessive amounts of carbs and sitting around for sustained periods promotes insulin resistance and fat storage—even if you faithfully conduct your daily workout—per the active couch potato syndrome.

As you chart your course for the future, it may be helpful to review some of the ideas in this book that are virtually undisputed:

‣ Becoming fat- and keto-adapted regulates appetite and hunger such that you are no longer a slave to regular high-carbohydrate meals to sustain energy, mood, and cognitive focus, and can easily maintain ideal body composition.

‣ Becoming calorically efficient/metabolically flexible/insulin sensitive can profoundly benefit general health and longevity.

‣ Becoming fat- and keto-adapted represents the essence of metabolic flexibility, and an escape from the certain doom of carbohydrate dependency (metabolic syndrome, obesity, cancer, heart disease, or at the very least accelerated aging).

‣ A 21-day Metabolism Reset to ditch carb dependency and optimize exercise, sleep, and stress management is the initiator of the journey toward caloric efficiency/metabolic flexibility.

‣ A nutritional ketosis effort lasting a minimum of six weeks avails you of the highest standard of caloric efficiency/metabolic flexibility.

If you agree on the importance of a 21-Day Metabolism Reset and at least one rock-solid six-week nutritional keto effort, where do you go from there? Let's extend out to some more open-ended comments and assumptions, reflecting on your journey to this point in the book:

▸ Personal experimentation and subjective evaluation (via the *The Keto Reset Diet* Midterm Exam in Chapter 8) could be the most important determinants of success.

▸ Those with obesity, metabolic syndrome, metabolic damage from decades of carb dependency, inflammation-related health conditions, or elevated disease risk factors (especially cognitive conditions closely tied to inflammatory high-carbohydrate, nutrient-deficient eating patterns) might be the best beneficiaries of long-term nutritional ketosis.

▸ Athletes/fitness enthusiasts/high-calorie-burners with optimal body composition or those with minimal disease risk factors might benefit less from long-term keto, owing to preexisting metabolic flexibility and a possible increased need for carbohydrates to fuel and recover from strenuous exercise.

▸ Stints of nutritional ketosis can be an extremely valuable lifelong practice to fine-tune fat- and keto-adaptation, reset mitochondria, drop excess body fat quickly, achieve improved athletic performance and recovery, control appetite and craving, and minimize disease risk factors.

▸ It appears that extreme and sudden fluctuations back and forth between nutritional keto and carb binges are not advised. By deduction, it's likely that exiting nutritional ketosis and adding back carbs into a desired higher range is best done gradually. Most people never need more than 150 grams of carbohydrates per day, unless they are extreme exercisers or in growth phases of life (youth, pregnant/nursing mothers).

I'm hoping you have learned along the way some particulars of the keto eating strategy that work best for you. Perhaps, like me, you've discovered that a compressed eating window is the best day-to-day strategy to achieve the benefits of fasting/ketone burning, but allowing for more carb intake flexibility than the rigid keto standard of 50 grams of gross carbs per day, every day.

Long-Term Eating Strategies

Summarizing material that we have covered throughout the book, here are some quick descriptions and rationales for assorted eating strategies:

SUSTAINED NUTRITIONAL KETOSIS: Yes indeed, you can survive, and thrive, eating a minimal amount of carbohydrate and a moderate amount of protein calories for the rest of your life. This is an excellent option to transition out of metabolic syndrome/obesity/Type 2 diabetes status, to recover from metabolic damage caused by decades of high-carb eating and yo-yo dieting, or to minimize disease risk, especially in sensitive/high-risk populations. Compliance may be difficult for many, and it may even be counterproductive for people like athletes or females with thyroid or other hormonal sensitivities.

CYCLIC KETOSIS (A.K.A. CKD—CYCLICAL KETOGENIC DIET): Here, keto periods are balanced with purposeful "refeeds" or "cheat days" in the name of boosting insulin sensitivity and making adherence to keto less arduous. Very popular in bodybuilding circles, it's pitched as a way to have your keto and eat cake, too. Villasenor proclaims that CKD is "the worst of both worlds, based on personal and client experience. It leaves you in a low-carb limbo, where you reap very few, if any, positive effects of keto, and possibly promote metabolic inflexibility and negative protein balance." Villasenor argues that the rationale for refeeds and cheat days comes from the flawed premise that carbohydrates are essential for bodybuilding, and that this flawed premise "has been adopted by soccer moms and weekend warriors, who should never need to load up on carbs."

As yet unpublished research from Dr. Jacob Wilson and Ryan Lowery suggests that extreme departures in and out of keto, such as weekend carb slams and then returning into extreme carb restriction during the week, may be too confusing and disruptive metabolically. You may be more apt to add fat and strip down lean muscle when you are doing extreme cycles. And you may invite risk of developing an eating disorder.

I prefer that you consider keto to be a tool in your arsenal you can unleash any time to obtain targeted metabolic benefits—weight loss, peak athletic or cognitive performance, or simply a hormonal and metabolic reset back to the original human factory wiring. When you are fully fat- and keto-adapted, you can benefit from shorter forays into nutritional ketosis whenever you feel like you need a metabolic tune-up. On your first keto effort, or any other time you are not fully keto-adapted, a minimum of six weeks of nutritional ketosis is essential. It appears that it's best to cycle out of keto with a gradual increase in carb intake (up to a maximum of 150 grams per day), rather than bust out with a make-your-own hot fudge sundae party. On the other hand, it's fine to jump right into a keto phase without concerns for any negative metabolic effects if you are coming from a decent fat-adapted baseline.

ANNUAL KETOSIS: This might be my most enthusiastic blanket recommendation for everyone. Like taking your family on a nostalgic visit to your childhood home, going keto is taking you back to your *Homo sapiens* genetic "factory setting." Keto really is a cleanse from the flawed eating, exercise, sleep, and high-stress patterns of modern life, making it worthwhile for you to set aside six weeks of every year for a keto stint. This will help regenerate mitochondria, do some intra-cellular housecleaning through autophagy, and perhaps help you drop a few extra pounds of body fat that might have shown up. Like getting into a routine of fasted mornings or compressed eating windows, an annual return to keto can have a fantastic impact on your overall metabolic fitness, along with delivering the therapeutic benefits detailed in Chapter 3 for fat reduction, brain function, inflammation control, and athletic performance. Winter is probably the best time for a keto stint, as this aligns with our genetic hard-wiring to reduce carb intake (and carbohydrate expenditure, too) during the shorter days and longer nights of winter.

TARGETED KETOGENIC DIET: This is an interesting option for athletes looking to obtain the big-picture benefits of being fat- and keto-adapted, but ensuring that they perform and recover well during strenuous workouts and training blocks that frequently result in glycogen depletion. If you are a high-calorie-burner, you can establish a baseline pattern of Intermittent Fasting and keto-aligned meals, but allow for targeted carbohydrate intake before and/or after strenuous workouts, or during the most difficult training blocks over the course of a year.

If you bank a ton of hours in a fasted state or eat a string of keto-aligned meals, you will enjoy the fabulous benefits of fat- and keto-adaptation, and your targeted carb intake (around workouts or at the end of the day) is simply honing your metabolic flexibility. Dr. Phinney echoes this sentiment when he says that spending six waking hours a day in ketosis can trigger benefits for a longer period. Realize that six waking hours in ketosis pairs with eight more fasted hours while sleeping, so this is a significant daily commitment to keto. What's more, it's likely that you can officially remain in nutritional ketosis when consuming substantially more than 50 grams of carbs per day if you are burning a ton of calories during workouts.

As Dr. Cate reminds us, "When the glycogen suitcases are open, carbs get prioritized there accordingly, and you don't get a disruptive surge of insulin. Nor will you have that elevated risk of backsliding that a less active person might." While research referenced earlier suggests that both endurance and strength athletes can perform well in long-term nutritional ketosis—even at the elite level—this may not be too easy or effective for many high-calorie-burning fitness enthusiasts to jump right into and maintain indefinitely. As you become more fat- and keto-adapted over time, you may notice your carbohydrate needs diminish accordingly.

When I was an ironman triathlete training virtually all day long, I was most definitely a sugar-burning machine. I estimate that I routinely consumed an embarrassing 600 grams or more of daily carbs (hey, that's only 12 times higher than keto!). However, I also possessed a decent level of metabolic flexibility, because I could easily run for three hours or cycle for six hours with no supplemental calories. Granted, a massive carb refeed was necessary pretty soon after these depleting workouts, or I would have literally passed out. Today, it's amazing to consider that elite fat- and keto-adapted athletes can perform similar feats, and then carry on with their day without eating anything, or eating keto-aligned meals. Witness Zach Bitter setting the American 100-mile-run record, running seven-minute miles *all day* (11 hours, 47 minutes, to be exact)—burning some 900 calories per hour while consuming only 156 additional calories each hour, or grinding all night in and out of river canyons on nothing but water and aminos for the last 38 miles of the Western States 100.

COMPRESSED EATING WINDOW: Limiting your caloric intake to an eating window of 10 hours a day (e.g., 10 a.m.–8 p.m.) or 8 hours a day (e.g., 12 noon–8 p.m.) allows you to bank many hours of fasting benefits, even if your macronutrient intake during the eating windows exceeds keto guidelines occasionally or regularly. If you are active in and around your carbohydrate intake, you will greatly reduce the chances of any potential negative effects from excess insulin or the aforementioned shock of refeeding.

METABOLIC FLEXIBILITY/INTUITIVE STRATEGY: Here's a nod to those of you who can't be bothered with a regimented approach—tracking carb and protein macros, measuring blood ketones and glucose, or even minding the clock to reach fasting or eating window goals—but believe in the benefits of fasting and keto, and are willing to align dietary habits accordingly. Forming a close connection with your appetite and satiety sensations and going with the flow can indeed be an effective long-term strategy, especially if you are super busy. If you need a note card for your wallet, here it is: Ditch grains, sugars and bad oils. Emphasize natural, nutritious fats and high fiber vegetables. Dial in exercise, sleep, and stress management. Then, bank as many hours fasting as you comfortably can to enhance cellular, cognitive, and immune function, and ultimately maximize longevity. Know that keto-aligned meals and ketone supplements allow you to mimic the benefits of fasting without having to starve yourself.

21-DAY METABOLISM RESET PLUS NUTRITIONAL KETOSIS: If you or someone you love has really fallen off the wagon and is back in the carbohydrate-dependency camp, the best strategy is to repeat the 21-Day Metabolism Reset, then enter a 3- to 6-week keto phase. This will get you quickly back into metabolic shape, and help you more easily adhere to an ancestral-aligned eating pattern free from grains, sugars, and bad oils.

My Compressed Eating-Window, Live-Awesome Daily Routine

My main health and dietary goal is to enjoy my life, so I never restrict myself from the foods I wish to eat at any particular meal. Hence, getting into ketosis is not an obsession for me but, rather, a natural by-product of an ancestral-style eating pattern—especially a near-complete and permanent restriction of grains, sugars, and refined vegetable oils. Furthermore, I favor a compressed eating-window strategy, whereby I naturally delay my first food meal of the day until at least 1 P.M., sometimes later, and finish eating by 7 P.M. most days. This allows me to experience the hormonal, metabolic, immune, and cognitive benefits of being in a fasted/ketogenic state for some 18 hours every day, and still be able to enjoy incredibly satisfying natural high-fat foods like meat, fish, fowl, eggs, nuts and seeds, high-fat plants like avocados, olives, and coconut products (and their oils), high-cacao percentage dark chocolate, and quality high-fat dairy products.

On the majority of days, my carb intake during my 6- to 8-hour compressed eating window will land comfortably under 50 grams per day. Consequently, I'm commonly stringing together an 18-hour fast, a 6-hour nutritional ketosis period, and another 18-hour fast. Note: Once in a while, I'll put MCT oil in my morning coffee, and also take a ketone supplement before my late morning workout. Hence, I should qualify my liberal use of the term "fasting," which literally means abstaining from *all* kinds of food or drink. In the Appendix, I mention Dr. Satchin Panda's research suggesting that we also possess a circadian clock when it comes to food ingestion. Consequently, lately I've been more mindful to limit my ingestion of all forms of calories or other metabolites (e.g., coffee, vitamin pills) to a 12-hour daily window.

Occasionally my intake of carbs during my eating window will be significant enough to temporarily push me out of ketosis for the rest of that day. When it comes to extra carbs, I've been known to enjoy fresh fruit (with mascarpone cheese and whipped cream!), sweet potatoes, and dark chocolate, but also some indulgences here and there, like my daughter Devyn's incredible dark chocolate–coconut caramel–almond butter cups (check out her cookbook *Kitchen Intuition*), or even a piece of fresh bread dipped in oil and vinegar at a nice restaurant if I feel like it. I'm never troubled by this, because with my strong baseline routine, a single overnight-to-midday-meal fasting period (at least 16 hours) gets my muscles back to preferring fat, my brain to preferring ketones, and my blood levels back up to between 1.0 and 3.0 mmol/L. An intense mid-morning workout definitely hastens my return to keto.

I am well aware of the consequences of my food choices and can make informed decisions driven primarily by pleasure. Hence, when I'm vacationing in

Italy and facing an evening of wine, pasta dishes, and gelato, I realize that I'll get forcefully spun out of ketosis after a few bites, that my sensitive gut will take a hit (gas, bloating, etc.), and that I'll suffer a mild inflammatory/immune suppressing reaction such as a fluttery heartbeat, mild headache, or mildly increased joint stiffness upon awakening. This awareness has me most often making sensible restaurant choices outside of the grain/sugar category, or consuming very moderate amounts when I do choose to indulge.

Mentioning my litany of symptoms associated with hitting a mini gelato might make me sound a bit like a prima donna here, and I'll definitely admit that. My metabolic machinery is calibrated to consume high-octane fuel, I'm definitely more sensitive to grains than the average person, and consequently will have a bit more to complain about when I pump cheap gas into my tank. This increased sensitivity, increased self-awareness, refined decision making, healthy respect for both the short- and long-term consequences of my dietary patterns, and ultimately greater enjoyment and appreciation of eating are all defining elements of metabolic flexibility.

CHAPTER 12

The Keto Reset Diet Recipes

ENJOY this collection of delicious recipes for everything from breakfast to dinner, to what keto folks call "fat bombs" (filling, high-fat snacks), to dessert treats—using the healthiest keto-approved ingredients. Macronutrient calculations are provided for each recipe. These should be considered estimates to help get you into a rhythm of nailing your protein and carbohydrate targets each day. If you are concerned about calculating your macros very precisely, log the specific brands and quantities you are using with a macronutrient tracking app like FitDay.com, MyFitnessPal, or My Macros+.

You will notice that many of the recipes may not conform to the recommended keto macronutrient ranges of 65–75 percent fat, 15–25 percent protein, and 5–10 percent carbohydrate. In many cases, staying on track with your daily keto targets might entail adding more fat to the recipe, or adding more high-fat snacks and meals during the day. For example, the Slow Cooker Carnitas (page 229) can be topped with avocado and sour cream and eaten with a side of roasted yellow squash with olive oil vinaigrette. By adding these high-fat accoutrements, you will dilute the otherwise high protein contribution of the carnitas and get the overall meal macros more in line with keto.

The recipes are placed into categories, but do not feel bound by them. For example, the delicious side dish of Baked Avocados, Two Ways (page 278), is also great for breakfast. Honestly, I would eat any one of these recipes any time of the day. Even many of the treats are great for breakfast because they deliver nourishing fats and don't stimulate an insulin response. Once you are eating primal or keto style, the concept of distinct breakfast meals or dinner entrees goes out the window.

Speaking of treats, I recommend that you not use any sweeteners of any kind (including artificial) for at least the first month or so of ketogenic eating. This helps break the cycle of carb dependency and learned behaviors, such as habitually eating a sweet treat after dinner. Once you are ready to allow the occasional treat back in, don't go overboard. While I am generally okay with using honey or maple syrup in small amounts, you can also experiment with keto-approved sweeteners, erythritol and stevia being the two most common. Erythritol is less sweet than conventional sugar, whereas stevia extract is much sweeter. Commercial stevia blends with maltodextrin or erythritol are often designed to be a 1:1 sugar substitute. Play around to see what you like.

I encourage you to use these recipes as inspiration for your own keto-eating adventure. Feel free to tweak, or completely disassemble and rebuild, the recipes to express your creativity and please your palate.

BREAKFAST

Primal Omelet

Makes 1 Bigass serving

This is the ultimate go-to primal breakfast, and a great way to transition out of your All-American high-carbohydrate breakfast patterns. If you are accustomed to starting your day with oatmeal, toast, and juice, switching over to a delicious omelet will keep you deeply satisfied for hours, and make going primal, and eventually going keto, a breeze.

1. Melt half the butter in a medium skillet over medium heat. Add vegetables and sauté until soft, 5 to 7 minutes. Remove vegetables from pan.

2. In the same pan, melt the remaining butter. In a small bowl, whisk together eggs, cream, salt, and pepper. Tilt and swirl the pan so the butter coats the entire bottom. Add the egg mixture and tilt and swirl the pan in the same manner.

3. Cook without stirring. As the egg around the edge sets, use a silicone spatula to gently push the egg away from the sides of the pan, and tilt the pan so that the egg mixture in the center can get to the edge.

4. When the entire egg mixture is set, add the vegetables on top of one half of the omelet. Sprinkle half of the cheese (if using) over the vegetables, then gently fold the omelet in half to cover the vegetables. Slide the omelet onto a plate and sprinkle with the remaining cheese. Serve immediately.

CALORIES: 610	FAT: 49 G
CARBOHYDRATE: 12 G	PROTEIN: 30 G

1 tablespon (15 ml) salted butter

1 ounce (28 g) chopped mushrooms

1 ounce (28 g) chopped onions

1 ounce (28 g) chopped red bell peppers

4 medium eggs

1 ounce (30 ml) cream

¼ teaspoon (1 ml) salt

$1/8$ teaspoon (0.5 ml) freshly ground pepper

½ ounce (14 g) shredded cheddar cheese (optional)

Breakfast Egg Salad

Makes 4 servings

This tasty egg salad is great eaten by itself or over a bed of spinach, or lightly toast a slice of keto-friendly bread (like the one on page 291) and make an open-faced egg salad sandwich.

CALORIES: 326	FAT: 30 G
CARBOHYDRATE: 3 G	PROTEIN: 13 G

½ medium avocado

⅓ cup (75 ml) Primal Kitchen Mayo, or other primal-approved mayo (see Note)

6 large hard-boiled eggs

4 slices bacon (no sugar added), cooked until crispy

2 tablespoons (30 ml) finely chopped green onion

½ teaspoon (2 ml) Tajin (see Note)

Freshly ground pepper to taste

1. In a medium bowl, mash the avocado with a fork. Stir in the mayo until well combined.

2. Roughly chop the hard-boiled eggs. Add to the mayo mixture and use a fork to combine, mashing the egg (should remain a bit chunky).

3. Chop or crumble the bacon. Add the bacon bits, green onions, and Tajin to egg mixture. Stir well. Taste and adjust seasoning with pepper.

NOTE: Primal Kitchen Mayo is the name of my commercial product made with an avocado oil base instead of the refined vegetable oil from which most mayonaises are made. If you use mayo in any recipe, ever, be sure it's made with healthy oils. Make your own from scratch or purchase Primal Kitchen or another brand made with a healthy oil.

Tajin is a chili lime salt available in many grocery stores or online. You can also omit the Tajin and use Primal Kitchen Chipotle Lime Mayo, or substitute ¼ teaspoon (1 ml) kosher salt (adjust to taste) and up to ½ teaspoon (2 ml) fresh lime juice.

Coconut Flour Macadamia Pancakes

Makes 8 pancakes; serving size = 1 pancake

Coconut flour pancakes are a great substitute for pancakes made with white or whole wheat flour. The macadamias here add healthy fat and an interesting texture; if you leave them in bigger pieces, you get crunchy pancakes! You can substitute more coconut milk for the heavy cream if you want to make the pancakes dairy-free. Serve these hot with butter, almond butter, coconut butter, or Coconut Milk Whipped Cream (page 302).

CALORIES: 154	**FAT:** 14 G
CARBOHYDRATE: 4 G	**PROTEIN:** 4 G

3 large eggs
¼ cup (½ stick; 60 g) *unsalted* butter, melted
¼ cup (60 ml) heavy cream
¼ cup (60 ml) full-fat coconut milk
½ teaspoon (2 ml) vanilla extract
¼ cup (30 g) coconut flour
¼ teaspoon (1 ml) kosher salt
½ teaspoon (2 ml) baking powder
½ teaspoon (2 ml) ground cinnamon
Keto-friendly sweetener of choice, to taste (optional; see Note)
¼ cup (30 g) macadamias, chopped or ground to desired coarseness
Coconut oil to grease griddle

1. In medium bowl, whisk together the eggs, butter, cream, coconut milk, and vanilla.

2. In a small bowl, stir together the flour, salt, baking powder, cinnamon, and sweetener with a fork, breaking up clumps of coconut flour. Stir the dry ingredients into the wet.

3. Add the macadamias to the batter and stir. Batter will be thick. Add water a little bit at a time until it is the consistency of *thick* pancake batter.

4. Heat a large, flat-bottomed skillet or griddle over medium-low heat. When warm, grease lightly with coconut oil. Drop big spoonfuls of the batter onto the griddle. It will not spread like traditional pancake batter, so use the back of a spoon or spatula to gently spread the batter into a thinner pancake.

5. Allow to cook slowly, several minutes per side until bubbles form, then flip. Serve hot.

NOTE: If you omit the sweetener from this recipe, the pancakes will still be delicious, just not as cakey as you are probably used to. Unsweetened pancakes are great bread substitutes. If you opt to sweeten the batter, though, make a single test pancake and adjust the sweetness. Try starting with ¼ teaspoon (1 ml) powdered stevia or 1½ tablespoons (22 ml) erythritol.

Burger Skillet

Makes 4 servings

I'll eat this meal any time of day, but I particularly enjoy it at breakfast. Feel free to throw a couple pieces of cooked bacon on top for a breakfast bacon cheeseburger!

CALORIES: 414	FAT: 30 G
CARBOHYDRATE: 4 G	PROTEIN: 32 G

2 pounds (900 g) ground beef
2 garlic cloves, minced
1 teaspoon (5 ml) dried oregano
1 teaspoon (5 ml) kosher salt
½ teaspoon (2 ml) black pepper
3 cups (85 g) fresh baby spinach
1½ cups (168 g) shredded cheese
   (cheddar or pepper jack)
4 large eggs

1. Preheat the oven to 400°F (200°C).

2. In an ovenproof skillet (cast iron works well), brown the ground beef. When it is just cooked, in about 5 minutes, push the meat to the edges and add the garlic. Sauté for about 1 minute, then stir into the meat. Add the oregano, salt, and pepper, and stir well.

3. Begin adding the spinach one handful at a time, adding more as it wilts. As soon as all the spinach is incorporated, remove the pan from the heat. Stir in ½ cup (120 g) of the cheese.

4. Spread the meat evenly in the skillet, then create four depressions in the top of the meat and gently crack an egg into each depression. Sprinkle the remaining cheese on top.

5. Transfer the skillet to the oven. Bake 10 minutes. The egg whites should be set and the yolks still runny. Leave in oven for a few minutes longer for firmer yolks, if desired. Scoop out each of the servings and transfer to plates.

Turnip Hash Browns

Makes 4 servings

Once you've tried these hash browns, the potato version will seem bland in comparison. Serve them alongside a frittata (see page 202) for a complete keto brunch.

CALORIES: 159   FAT: 14 G

CARBOHYDRATE: 5 G   PROTEIN: 3 G

2 medium turnips (232 g), washed and peeled

1 large egg

1 tablespoon (15 ml) coconut flour (optional)

1 teaspoon (5 ml) kosher salt, plus more to taste

½ teaspoon (2 ml) black pepper

2 tablespoons (30 ml) bacon fat or butter, or more if needed

Sour cream (optional)

Minced chives (optional)

1. Shred the turnips using a box grater or food processor.

2. In a large bowl, whisk the egg, then add the turnips. Stir in the flour, salt, and pepper.

3. Heat a large, flat-bottomed skillet over medium-high heat. When hot, add the bacon fat; when melted, turn the heat down to medium.

4. Give the turnips another stir and drop by approximately ½ cup (120 ml) servings into the hot grease. Press lightly with a spatula to flatten. Let cook 3 to 5 minutes, until edges brown, then flip and cook on the other side.

5. Move to a plate and sprinkle with a little more salt. If desired, top each with a dollop of sour cream and garnish with a sprinkling of chives.

Greek Yogurt Crunch Bowl

Makes 2 servings

If you aren't familiar with cacao nibs, they are simply the roasted beans of the cacao plant from which chocolate is made. Don't expect them to taste like your favorite chocolate bar, though! They are pure cacao—chocolate before it is processed, without sugar and other ingredients added. Cacao nibs have myriad health benefits, including being a great source of magnesium, iron, and antioxidants. Per serving, they contribute 5 grams of carbs but 0 grams of sugar, so you can decide whether and how much to include here.

1. In a small, dry skillet set over medium-low heat, toast the coconut flakes until lightly brown. Repeat for the sliced almonds.

2. Stir together the yogurt, coconut milk, and sweetener, if using. Divide the mixture between two bowls. Add 1 tablespoon (15 ml) almond butter to each, and stir to swirl together (don't worry about combining entirely). Top each with some toasted coconut, sliced almonds, and cacao nibs, and sprinkle with cinnamon.

CALORIES: 481	FAT: 37 G
CARBOHYDRATE: 18 G	PROTEIN: 19 G

¼ cup (15 g) unsweetened coconut flakes
2 tablespoons (14 g) sliced almonds
1 cup (250 ml) plain full-fat Greek yogurt
$\frac{1}{3}$ cup (80 ml) full-fat coconut milk
Keto-friendly sweetener to taste (optional)
2 tablespoons (30 ml) raw almond butter (no added sugar)
2 tablespoons (14 g) cacao nibs
Sprinkle of ground cinnamon

Sausage, Kale, and Goat Cheese Frittata

Makes 6 servings

Every keto enthusiast should know how to make a frittata. You can use any combination of meat, cheese, veggies, herbs, and spices to tailor it to your liking—it is endlessly customizable.

CALORIES: 494		FAT: 38 G
CARBOHYDRATE: 4 G		PROTEIN: 34 G

½ bunch kale (4 or 5 leaves), any variety
1 tablespoon (15 ml) avocado oil
1 pound (450 g) ground pork
1 teaspoon (5 ml) dried sage
1 teaspoon (5 ml) dried thyme
¼ teaspoon (1 ml) ground nutmeg
¼ teaspoon (1 ml) red pepper flakes
1 small or ½ large onion, diced
2 garlic cloves, minced
8 large eggs
½ cup (120 ml) heavy cream
1 cup (90 g) crumbled goat cheese, or more to taste

1. Use a sharp paring knife to remove any thick stems from the kale leaves. Dice the stems and chop the leaves (keep stems and leaves separate).

2. Heat the oil in a large broilerproof skillet over medium heat (cast iron works well). When hot, add the pork. Cook for 5 minutes, stirring occasionally.

3. In a small bowl, combine the sage, thyme, nutmeg, and red pepper flakes. Add to the meat in the skillet and stir well. Continue cooking until the pork is cooked through, about 5 minutes more.

4. Use a slotted spoon to move the meat to a bowl. If there is a lot of grease in the pan, pour some off so that only 1 to 2 tablespoons (15 to 30 ml) remain.

5. Add the onion and kale stems to the skillet. Sauté until the onion softens, about 5 minutes. Add the garlic and stir for 1 minute. If needed, deglaze the pan with a small amount of water, stirring up any browned particles.

6. Add the kale leaves to the pan a handful at a time, stirring to wilt until all the leaves are in the skillet and cooked slightly. Add the meat to the skillet and stir to combine.

7. Whisk the eggs and cream in a medium bowl. Pour the egg mixture evenly over the meat and vegetables in the skillet. Cook without stirring until the egg starts to set, about 5 minutes.

8. Put an oven rack at medium position (about 6 to 8 inches from the top) and turn the broiler on low. Sprinkle the goat cheese over the eggs. Place in the oven/broiler and cook until the egg is set and the goat cheese is lightly browned. Keep an eye on it to make sure it doesn't burn.

9. Remove the skillet from the oven and allow to sit for a few minutes. Cut into wedges and serve.

Brad's "Ketoatmeal"

Makes 2 servings

Here is Brad's answer to the naysayers who proclaim they can't live without their warm morning porridge. He's currently in negotiations with the Ritz-Carlton to add this to their Healthy Start Breakfast buffet line . . . not! Save the egg whites from this recipe and make the macaroons on page 308.

1. Mix the coconut milk, egg yolks, coconut flakes, cinnamon, vanilla, nut puree, almond butter, salt, and cacao nibs (if using) in a medium saucepan. Heat over medium-low heat, stirring continuously, for 3 to 4 minutes.

2. Remove from the heat and scoop into two small bowls. Top each with 2 tablespoons (30 ml) coconut milk and 1 teaspoon cacao nibs (if using). Eat immediately.

CALORIES: 656	FAT: 62 G
CARBOHYDRATE: 16 G	PROTEIN: 15 G

½ cup (120 ml) coconut milk
3 large egg yolks
¼ cup (60 ml) coconut flakes
½ teaspoon (2 ml) ground cinnamon
1 teaspoon (5 ml) vanilla extract
½ cup (60 g) pureed nuts (walnuts, almonds, pecans, macadamias, or a combo)
2 tablespoons (30 ml) almond butter
⅛ teaspoon (0.5 ml) salt (omit if almond butter contains salt)
1 tablespoon (15 ml) cacao nibs (optional)

TOPPINGS
¼ cup (60 ml) coconut milk
2 teaspoons (10 ml) cacao nibs (optional)

Egg Muffins in Ham Cups

Makes 6 servings

These are a perfect grab-and-go breakfast. Make them the night before so you can pop one in the microwave or toaster oven the next day. Be sure to buy good-quality ham, not cheap lunchmeat.

CALORIES: 178   FAT: 13 G
CARBOHYDRATE: 0.5 G PROTEIN: 14 G

1 tablespoon (15 ml) coconut oil, melted
6 slices ham (thin-sliced is better)
6 large eggs
Salt and pepper to taste
3 tablespoons (45 ml) shredded cheddar cheese (optional)

1. Preheat the oven to 400°F (200°C). Brush six cups of a muffin tin with the melted coconut oil.

2. Line each cup with 1 slice of ham. Crack 1 egg into each cup. Season with salt and pepper, then sprinkle ½ tablespoon (7.5 ml) of cheddar cheese on each egg.

3. Bake for 13 to 18 minutes depending on how you like your egg yolks set.

4. Remove from the oven and let cool for a few minutes before carefully removing the "muffins." Refrigerate in a glass or plastic container so they don't get smushed or dried out.

Chai Chia Breakfast Pudding

Makes 2 servings

This simple make-ahead pudding takes only a few minutes to assemble. Throw it in the fridge, and it's ready when you wake up. If you make it in small screw-top jars, you can put a lid on the jars and take them with you on the go. The spice blend makes more than you need for this recipe; store the extra in an empty spice jar.

1. Stir the coconut milk, chia seeds, spice blend, vanilla, and stevia together in a bowl (or use a blender or immersion blender if you prefer a smoother pudding).

2. Divide the mixture equally between two small jars or ramekins.

3. Refrigerate at least 4 hours, preferably overnight, so it can thicken.

4. When you are ready to eat, add the toppings, if using, and enjoy.

CALORIES: 352	FAT: 32 G
CARBOHYDRATE: 12 G	PROTEIN: 4 G

1 cup (250 ml) full-fat coconut milk
¼ cup (20 g) chia seeds
¾ teaspoon (4 ml) chai spice blend
¼ teaspoon (1 ml) vanilla extract
10 drops liquid stevia, or ¼ teaspoon (1 ml) powdered stevia
Chopped nuts (almonds, pecans, walnuts), coconut flakes, or cacao nibs, for topping (optional)

CHAI SPICE BLEND
2 teaspoons (10 ml) ground cinnamon
2 teaspoons (10 ml) ground cardamom
1 teaspoon (5 ml) ground ginger
1 teaspoon (5 ml) ground cloves
1 teaspoon (5 ml) ground allspice

Turmeric Scrambled Eggs

Makes 2 servings

This simple twist on basic scrambled eggs is a delicious anti-inflammatory start to your day. Turmeric is lauded in health circles because it contains the compound curcumin, which studies have shown to have beneficial effects on everything from arthritis to cancer prevention. Don't omit the black pepper! Pepper contains piperine, which increases the body's absorption of the curcumin.

1. In a small bowl, lightly beat the eggs with the cream. Add the turmeric, salt, and pepper.

2. Melt the butter in a skillet over medium heat. When it just starts to bubble, gently pour in the egg mixture. Stir frequently as eggs begin to set, and cook for 2 to 3 minutes.

3. Remove from the heat, taste and add more pepper and salt if needed, and serve.

CALORIES: 213	FAT: 18 G
CARBOHYDRATE: 2 G	PROTEIN: 10 G

3 large eggs
2 tablespoons (30 ml) heavy cream (optional)
1 teaspoon (5 ml) ground turmeric
Salt to taste
Freshly ground black pepper to taste
1 tablespoon (15 g) butter

Katie's Keto Granola

Makes approximately 6 cups; serving size = ½ cup

From *Paleo Cooking Bootcamp* author Katie French comes a quick and easy preparation that can welcome cereal back into your life. Serve with full-fat coconut or almond milk, top with fresh berries, sprinkle over full-fat Greek yogurt, or pack the granola in snack baggies for a great to-go option that holds up in warm temperatures.

1. Preheat the oven to 350°F (180°C). Line a large rimmed baking sheet or 3-quart casserole dish with parchment paper.

2. If desired, roughly chop the nuts with a food processor, hand chopper, or sharp chef's knife.

3. In a large mixing bowl, stir together the coconut oil, honey, and vanilla. Add the nuts, sea salt, coconut flakes, and cacao nibs and stir well.

4. Transfer the granola mixture to the baking sheet. Bake for 20 minutes, stirring halfway, until lightly toasted.

5. Allow to cool for about 30 minutes, then transfer to an airtight container. Store in the refrigerator for up to 3 weeks.

6. When ready to eat, add the add-ins of your choice.

Granola (½ cup)

CALORIES: 453	FAT: 38 G
CARBOHYDRATE: 20 G	PROTEIN: 11 G

Coconut Milk

CALORIES: 487	FAT: 41 G
CARBOHYDRATE: 21 G	PROTEIN: 11 G

Coconut Milk and ¼ cup Fresh Blueberries

CALORIES: 510	FAT: 42 G
CARBOHYDRATE: 22 G	PROTEIN: 11 G

1 cup (112 g) raw almonds
1 cup (112 g) raw cashews
1 cup (120 g) raw pumpkin seeds
1 cup (120 g) raw sunflower seeds
¼ cup (60 ml) coconut oil, softened
1 tablespoon (15 ml) raw honey
1 teaspoon (5 ml) vanilla extract
1 teaspoon (5 ml) Himalayan sea salt
1 cup (60 g) unsweetened coconut flakes
1 cup (60 g) cacao nibs
Optional add-ins: ¾ cup (180 ml) full-fat coconut milk or unsweetened almond milk; ¼ cup (40 g) in-season blueberries

Curley Boys' Eggy Bites

Makes 4 servings

Eggy bites powered a decade of world travel on a dime, including tasty waves and beautiful babes for Brad's old friends Tyler and Connor Curley.

CALORIES: 287   FAT: 21 G

CARBOHYDRATE: 2 G   PROTEIN: 22 G

1 tablespoon (15 ml) coconut oil
¼ onion, finely chopped
¼ pound (230 g) grass-fed ground beef
1 garlic clove, minced
1 teaspoon (5 ml) ground cumin
1 teaspoon (5 ml) kosher salt
½ teaspoon (2 ml) black pepper
¼ teaspoon (1 ml) cayenne pepper (optional)
6 large eggs
½ cup (45 g) shredded cheese blend

1. Preheat the oven to 400°F (200°C). Line a 6-inch (15 cm) square baking dish with parchment paper (or grease well with approximately 1 tablespoon [15 ml] melted coconut oil).

2. Heat the coconut oil in a large skillet and sauté the onion for a few minutes until starting to brown.

3. Crumble in the ground beef, stir well, and cook until almost no pink remains, about 10 minutes.

4. Push the meat and onion to the edge of the skillet. In the center, add the garlic and cook until fragrant. Stir everything together.

5. Add the cumin, salt, pepper, and cayenne (if using). Stir well, and continue cooking until the meat is fully cooked, about 5 more minutes. Remove from the heat.

6. In a large bowl, whisk the eggs. Add a cup of the meat mixture to the eggs, stirring constantly to keep the eggs from scrambling. Add the rest of meat and stir well.

7. Pour the egg and meat mixture into the baking pan. Sprinkle the cheese over the top.

8. Cook for 20 minutes. Test for doneness by inserting a butter knife into the middle; when it comes out clean, remove from oven. Let cool for a few minutes, then cut into bite-size squares.

Waffles with Sausage Gravy

Makes 4 servings

This recipe is a good way to use the pulp left from making a batch of nut milk (see page 218). I prefer to take the time to whip up my own sausage from scratch, but you can start with store-bought ground sausage as long as it doesn't contain added sugar or other objectionable ingredients.

1. Heat a large skillet over medium heat and add the ground pork. Break up with a fork as it cooks.

2. When the pork is mostly cooked, in about 5 minutes, add the spices and stir well. Cook until fully browned, another 2 to 3 minutes. Add the coconut milk and allow to come to a simmer, then turn the heat to low.

3. In a medium bowl, whisk the eggs with the coconut oil and coconut milk. Add the pulp, salt, baking soda, and arrowroot powder, and mix well. The waffle batter will be thicker than a traditional batter; if needed, add a little water a tablespoon at a time until it is pourable.

4. Pour some batter into a waffle maker set on medium-low heat. (Alternatively, use a lightly greased pan or griddle and make pancakes.) Remove the waffle from the waffle maker when cooked through and continue to make waffles with the remaining batter.

5. Serve the waffles with the gravy on top.

CALORIES: 644	FAT: 56 G
CARBOHYDRATE: 7 G	PROTEIN: 28 G

SAUSAGE GRAVY
1 pound (450 g) ground pork (or ground beef or turkey)
1 teaspoon (5 ml) dried sage
½ teaspoon (2 ml) dried thyme
½ teaspoon (2 ml) garlic powder
¼ teaspoon (1 ml) kosher salt
¼ teaspoon (1 ml) black pepper
About 1¼ cups (300 ml) full-fat coconut milk (See Note)

WAFFLES
2 large eggs
1 tablespoon (15 ml) melted coconut oil
½ cup (120 ml) full-fat coconut milk
¾ cup (80 g) almond flour or nut pulp (see Note)
¼ teaspoon (1 ml) salt
½ teaspoon (2 ml) baking soda
1½ teaspoons (7 ml) arrowroot powder

NOTE: You will need 1 can of full-fat coconut milk in total to make both the gravy and the waffles. Measure off ½ cup of coconut milk for the waffles and use what remains for the gravy. This recipe also works with other types of nut pulp—for example, hazelnut. If you don't have a batch of nut pulp, use almond meal and add a little water at the end to achieve the desired consistency.

BEVERAGES AND SMOOTHIES

High-Fat Coffee

Makes 1 serving

If you used to indulge in a sugary coffee treat every morning, you won't even miss it once you start enjoying this coffee, which is filled with delicious fats that support ketone production. Many keto folks drink a high-fat coffee in place of breakfast and then cruise until lunch or dinner. Start with 1 tablespoon each of butter and MCT oil, and increase as tolerated.

Blend the coffee, butter, and oil in a blender, or use an immersion blender, until frothy. Enjoy.

CALORIES: 358	FAT: 38 G
CARBOHYDRATE: 3 G	PROTEIN: 1 G

1 cup (250 ml) good-quality coffee

1 to 2 tablespoons (15 to 30 ml) unsalted butter

1 to 2 tablespoons (15 to 30 ml) MCT oil (or coconut oil, but MCT preferred)

OPTIONAL ADD-INS

½ teaspoon (2 ml) vanilla extract

¼ teaspoon (1 ml) unsweetened dark cocoa powder

1 tablespoon (15 ml) collagen hydrolysate powder

Dash of ground cinnamon

NOTE: The inimitable Dr. Phil Maffetone makes a version of High-Fat Coffee with a raw egg yolk included. The recipe is available on his website, philmaffetone.com. Give it a try!

Keto Protein Mocha

Makes 1 serving

Try this after a morning workout, or when you have a craving for an overpriced sugar bomb from the local coffee shop.

1. Blend the coffee, butter, oil, coconut milk, protein powder, and cocoa powder in a blender (or use an immersion blender) until frothy. If the drink is too thick, add a little hot water a tablespoon at a time until it is the desired consistency.

2. Pour into a warm mug and top with a dash of cinnamon. If desired, add a bit of whipped cream.

CALORIES: 432	FAT: 40 G
CARBOHYDRATE: 7 G	PROTEIN: 11 G

½ cup (120 ml) strong coffee, or 1 shot espresso

1 tablespoon (15 ml) unsalted butter

1 tablespoon (15 ml) MCT oil (or coconut oil, but MCT preferred)

¼ cup (60 ml) full-fat coconut milk, warmed or steamed

1 scoop (21 g) Chocolate Coconut Primal Fuel meal replacement powder (see Note)

¼ teaspoon (1 ml) unsweetened cocoa powder

Hot water

Dash of ground cinnamon

Whipped Cream (page 305) or Coconut Milk Whipped Cream (page 302) (optional)

NOTE: Primal Fuel is a commercial meal replacement product made with coconut milk solids and whey protein. You can substitute any straight high-quality microfiltered whey protein powder.

Go-to Green Smoothie

Makes 2 servings

When you only have a minute, this is a great, simple option. Don't miss the opportunity to get a large serving of greens!

1. Blend the coconut milk, vanilla, greens, oil, and ice in a high-powered blender.

2. Add the protein powder and blend on low until incorporated. Serve.

CALORIES: 558	FAT: 50 G
CARBOHYDRATE: 13 G	PROTEIN: 14 G

1 can (398 ml) full-fat coconut milk

1 teaspoon (5 ml) vanilla extract

Large handful of greens, such as kale and/or spinach (approx. 2 cups)

1 tablespoon (15 ml) MCT oil or coconut oil

2/3 cup (150 g) crushed ice

2 scoops (42 g) Primal Fuel meal replacement powder (Vanilla Coconut, or try Chocolate Coconut; see Note, page 211) or straight whey protein powder

Ginger Beet Smoothie

Makes 1 serving

This smoothie is absolutely packed with antioxidants, vitamins, and minerals, making it a great recovery drink on days you've done a hard workout. The addition of the macadamias and MCT oil delivers a boost of healthy fats.

1. Blend the beet, blueberries, almond milk, greens, macadamias, ginger, oil, and stevia in a high-powered blender. You might need to run a second cycle if you are using raw beet or if the macadamias aren't fully blended.

2. Add the ice and blend until smooth.

CALORIES: 589	FAT: 53 G
CARBOHYDRATE: 20 G	PROTEIN: 8 G

½ medium beet (roasted beet blends better; if raw, chop small before blending)

¼ cup (110 g) blueberries, fresh or frozen

1 cup (250 ml) unsweetened almond milk or other nut milk

Large handful of greens, such as kale and/or spinach (approximately 2 cups)

10 macadamia nuts

1 inch (3 cm) piece of peeled fresh ginger, diced

2 tablespoons (30 ml) MCT oil or coconut oil

5 to 10 drops liquid stevia, or to taste (optional)

²/3 cup (150 g) crushed ice

Bangin' Kitchen Sink Smoothie

Makes 1 serving

This smoothie is inspired by the smoothie that renowned triathlete and coach Ben Greenfield says is one of his go-to breakfasts. I call it the kitchen sink smoothie because I throw everything but the kitchen sink in there! Feel free to adapt this recipe to include any nuts and herbs you have around. This is a calorie- and nutrient-dense meal in itself, so you might even choose to split it into two servings.

1. Place a steamer basket in a small pan with an inch or so of water in the bottom. Bring the water to a boil and steam the kale for 5 minutes.

2. Transfer the kale to a high-powered blender. Add the coconut milk, avocado, nuts, and herbs. Blend on high for 30 seconds.

3. Add the protein powder, cocoa powder, cinnamon, salt, peppermint extract, and ice and blend until smooth. Add water if needed to achieve desired consistency.

CALORIES: 927	FAT: 67 G
CARBOHYDRATE: 53 G	PROTEIN: 41 G

3 cups (50 g) kale leaves

½ cup (120 ml) full-fat coconut milk

½ medium avocado (approximately ¼ cup; 60 g)

¼ cup (28 g) raw almonds

3 Brazil nuts

½ cup (30 g) loosely packed fresh herbs (see Note)

2 scoops Chocolate Coconut Primal Fuel meal replacement powder (see Note, page 211) or straight whey protein powder

1 tablespoon (15 ml) cocoa powder (dark chocolate preferred)

1 teaspoon (5 ml) ground cinnamon

1 teaspoon (5 ml) Himalayan sea salt

2 or 3 drops peppermint extract (optional)

1 to 2 cups ice cubes

NOTE: My favorite mixture is to use ¼ cup fresh mint leaves and ¼ cup fresh cilantro. Parsley also works well. Use whatever fresh herbs you have on hand.

Golden Chai

Makes 1 serving

Because it contains anti-inflammatory turmeric and ginger, many people believe golden milk has therapeutic properties. This version has classic chai spices added. A warm mug is a great way to help you wind down in the evening.

CALORIES: 219	FAT: 19 G
CARBOHYDRATE: 5 G	PROTEIN: 7 G

1½ cups (375 ml) nut milk (see page 218)

1 teaspoon (5 ml) ground turmeric

1 teaspoon (5 ml) Chai Spice Blend (see page 205)

½ teaspoon (2 ml) black pepper

½ teaspoon (2 ml) vanilla extract

1 tablespoon (15 ml) coconut oil or MCT oil

1 tablespoon (15 ml) collagen powder (optional)

5 to 10 drops liquid stevia, or to taste

1. Warm the nut milk, turmeric, chai spices, and pepper in a small saucepan until hot, but do not boil. Simmer lightly for a few minutes.

2. Stir in the vanilla, coconut oil, collagen powder (if using), and stevia.

3. Using an immersion blender, carefully blend until lightly frothy. Taste and adjust sweetness with stevia (don't make it too sweet).

Chicken Bone Broth

This recipe makes from 8 to 12 cups, depending on what you use, your cooking method, and the size of your pot. Serving size = 1 cup.

Broth, especially chicken soup, is the basis of every great-grandma's home remedy for whatever ails you. Bone broth has enjoyed a resurgence in popularity lately owing to its anti-inflammatory and immune-supporting benefits, and because it is an excellent source of collagen and minerals. Plus it's a great way to use food scraps, so nothing goes to waste. This recipe is flexible—you can throw in just about any vegetable scraps and herbs and spices you want. You won't believe how much better your favorite soup tastes when made with homemade broth. Enjoy a mug of warm broth on a cold morning or as part of your bedtime ritual.

Method 1: Place the bones, vegetable scraps, garlic, ginger, peppercorns, and bay leaf in a large stockpot with enough water to completely cover. Bring to a boil over high heat, then lower the temperature so water is just lightly simmering. Simmer for several hours—the longer the better—keeping an eye on the water level and adding more water if it gets too low.

Method 2: Place the ingredients in a 6-quart slow cooker with enough water to completely cover. Cover and set heat to low. Let cook undisturbed for at least 8 hours, but longer is better. You can cook it for 24 hours or more.

Method 3: Place all ingredients in an Instant Pot or other countertop pressure cooker and fill with water (do not exceed maximum line). Secure the

CALORIES: 50	FAT: 1 G
CARBOHYDRATE: 0 G	PROTEIN: 10 G

4 cups (300 to 400 g) chicken bones or carcass from a 3-pound (1.4 k) chicken

2 to 3 cups (150 to 300 g) vegetable scraps (see Tip); *or* 1 large onion, roughly chopped, including skin and root end if organic, and 2 celery stalks and 2 carrots, roughly chopped, including leaves

2 garlic cloves, crushed

1 tablespoon (15 ml) minced fresh ginger

10 whole black peppercorns

1 dried bay leaf

Fresh herbs, such as thyme or rosemary sprigs (optional)

lid, and cook using the manual setting for 2 hours (120 minutes). Let the pressure release naturally before opening.

2. When the broth is done, strain through a fine-mesh strainer and cool rapidly. The easiest way to do this is to place a stopper in your kitchen sink and fill the sink halfway with ice water. Place a metal bowl or clean metal pot in the ice water and strain the broth into it.

3. When the broth is cooled, transfer to clean containers (mason jars work well) and refrigerate immediately, or freeze if you do not intend to use the broth in the next couple days.

TIP: Keep a large zippered plastic bag in your freezer, and whenever you have vegetable scraps such as the leaves and bottoms of celery, leaves and ends of carrots, broccoli stems, and so on, add them to the bag. You can do the same with leftover chicken bones.

Basic Nut Milk

Makes 4 cups; serving size = 1 cup

Nut milk is delicious, and it can be a great option for keto enthusiasts who want to avoid eating a lot of dairy. However, store-bought nut milks often contain objectionable ingredients and sweeteners. Luckily, making your own is incredibly easy, and you can use whatever nuts you have on hand!

1. Place the nuts in a glass bowl or jar and cover entirely with filtered water. Allow to sit at room temperature for at least 4 hours, but preferably 8 hours or overnight (up to 24 hours).

2. Drain and rinse the nuts. Place the nuts in a high-powered blender with 4 cups of fresh filtered water. Blend on high until very smooth.

3. Strain the nut milk through a nut bag or a clean kitchen towel. Squeeze the pulp to release as much milk as possible (see Tip).

4. If you are adding any of the optional ingredients, rinse out the blender, add the milk and optional ingredients, and blend until smooth.

5. Transfer the nut milk to an airtight container and refrigerate. Use within 5 days.

CALORIES: 35	FAT: 3 G
CARBOHYDRATE: 1G	PROTEIN: 1 G

1 cup (112 g) raw nuts (almonds, hazelnuts, cashews, pecans, or macadamias)

4 cups (960 ml) filtered water, plus more for soaking

1 teaspoon (5 ml) vanilla extract (optional)

¼ teaspoon (1 ml) salt (optional)

½ teaspoon (2 ml) ground cinnamon (optional)

Keto-approved sweetener, to taste (optional)

TIP: Save the nut pulp to use in smoothies, bread, or pancake/waffle batter such as the Waffles with Sausage Gravy (page 209) or the Nut Pulp Bread (page 291).

SAUCES, DRESSINGS, AND DIPS

Pea-NOT Sauce

Makes approximately 1 cup; serving size = 2 tablespoons

I love peanut sauce as a topping for vegetables, chicken, and shrimp, but many primal and keto enthusiasts try to avoid peanuts due to allergenic concerns and the fact that technically they are a legume, not a nut. They also deliver a bit more carbohydrate than your typical nut or seed. Luckily, this Pea-NOT Sauce (see what I did there?) made with almond butter is every bit as good as the original, and without added sweeteners. Try not to eat it all in one sitting!

Mix all the ingredients in a medium bowl, or use a small food processor or an immersion blender. Store in an airtight container in the refrigerator. Finish within 2-3 weeks.

CALORIES: 153	FAT: 13 G
CARBOHYDRATE: 5 G	PROTEIN: 4 G

½ cup (120 ml) raw almond butter

½ cup (120 ml) full-fat coconut milk

2 large garlic cloves, finely minced

Juice of 1 small lime

2 tablespoons (30 ml) tamari (gluten-free soy sauce)

1 tablespoon (15 ml) grated fresh ginger

½ tablespoon (7.5 ml) toasted sesame oil (see Note)

½ tablespoon (7.5 ml) avocado oil

¼ teaspoon (1 ml) red pepper flakes (optional)

NOTE: If you enjoy the taste of toasted sesame oil, you can use 1 tablespoon (15 ml) sesame oil and omit the avocado oil. Some people find the taste of sesame oil overpowering.

Primal Kitchen Mayo Blue Cheese Dressing

Makes approximately 1 cup; serving size = 2 tablespoons

I might be biased, but Primal Kitchen Mayo is a favorite pantry staple in the Sisson household. The tanginess of this mayonnaise is perfect for this recipe, too. You can also use homemade mayo or another store-bought mayonnaise if you can find one without polyunsaturated oils, but you might need to adjust the seasoning to get the desired flavor in your dressing.

1. Whisk together the mayo, lemon juice, coconut milk, and pepper.

2. Add the blue cheese and stir well. Taste and add salt, if desired, and more pepper, if needed.

CALORIES: 71	FAT: 7 G
CARBOHYDRATE: 1 G	PROTEIN: 1 G

½ cup (120 ml) Primal Kitchen Mayo (see Note, page 187)
Juice of ½ lemon
¼ cup (60 ml) full-fat coconut milk or heavy cream
¼ teaspoon (1 ml) black pepper, or more as needed
¼ cup (60 ml) crumbled blue cheese
Salt (optional)

TIP: This recipe is pretty forgiving. You can just guesstimate when you have about ½ cup (120 ml) of mayo left in the jar, then add the other ingredients and shake really well to make this dressing!

Perfect Vinaigrette (with Variations!)

Makes approximately 1 cup; serving size = 2 tablespoons

Most commercially available salad dressings contain polyunsaturated, pro-inflammatory oils. Luckily, making your own salad dressing is quick and easy, and it's a great way to add some healthy fat to a meal.

1. In a small jar with a lid, stir together the shallot, vinegar, salt, and pepper. Allow to sit for 10 minutes.

2. Add the mustard and olive oil. Place the lid securely on the jar and shake vigorously.

Variations

Lemon Vinaigrette: Omit the vinegar; replace with an equal amount of fresh lemon juice and add 1 tablespoon (15 ml) of lemon zest.

Greek Dressing: Add 1 teaspoon (4 ml) each dried oregano, dried basil, and garlic powder.

CALORIES: 182	FAT: 20 G
CARBOHYDRATE: 0.5 G	PROTEIN: 0 G

1 small shallot, very finely chopped
3 tablespoons (45 ml) apple cider vinegar
¼ teaspoon (1 ml) kosher salt
¼ teaspoon (1 ml) black pepper
½ teaspoon (2 ml) Dijon mustard
¾ cup (180 ml) extra-virgin olive oil

Chive Macadamia "Cheese"

Makes approximately 1½ cups; serving size = 2 tablespoons

Nut "cheese" is a great option for keto enthusiasts who can't tolerate a lot of dairy in their diets but who still long for the creamy deliciousness of cheese. This recipe uses macadamia nuts, but you can also use other nuts. Cashews are particularly versatile but they are higher in carbohydrates. (See the recipe for Basic Cashew Cream, page 283.) Always start with raw nuts, as roasted varieties often contain objectionable oils.

CALORIES: 347	FAT: 34 G
CARBOHYDRATE: 7 G	PROTEIN: 4 G

2 cups (240 g) raw macadamia nuts
2 tablespoons (30 ml) fresh lemon
  juice
¼ teaspoon (1 ml) fine sea salt
¼ teaspoon (1 ml) black pepper
¼ teaspoon (1 ml) onion powder
¼ teaspoon (1 ml) garlic powder
1 to 2 tablespoons (15 to 30 ml)
  warm water
3 to 4 tablespoons (45 to 60 ml)
  minced fresh chives

1. Using a high-powered blender or food processor, blend the macadamias, lemon juice, salt, pepper, onion powder, and garlic powder until it becomes a thick, chunky paste. Scrape down the sides as needed.

2. With the blender or food processor running, slowly add the water until mixture is desired consistency. You can stop when the "cheese" is still slightly textured or continue blending until very smooth.

3. Add in the fresh chives and pulse a few times to combine.

Carrot Top Pesto

Makes approximately 1½ cups; serving size = 2 tablespoons

The leafy green part of the carrot is so underappreciated. I usually save mine for adding to a pot of simmering bone broth, but if I'm stocked up on broth (no pun intended), I'll whip up a quick batch of pesto like this one.

1. In a small food processor, pulse the carrot leaves, nuts, garlic, and cheese until combined well. Scrape down the sides of the bowl.

2. With the food processor running, slowly drizzle in the olive oil until the pesto reaches desired consistency. Taste and adjust seasoning with salt and pepper.

CALORIES: 166	FAT: 18 G
CARBOHYDRATE: 1 G	PROTEIN: 2 G

1 cup (30 g) loosely packed carrot leaves and stems
¼ cup (30 g) raw macadamia nuts
¼ cup (30 g) raw walnuts
1 small garlic clove, smashed
¼ cup (25 g) grated Parmesan cheese
¾ cup (180 ml) extra-virgin olive oil
Salt and pepper

Bacon Chili Butter

Makes approximately ¾ cup; serving size = 2 tablespoons

Yes, you read that right; this recipe combines two of our favorite things, bacon and butter. This recipe for a compound butter has the flavors of your favorite chili and is perfect for melting over a juicy steak or a plate of scrambled eggs. For variety, try it on shrimp kabobs, roasted Brussels sprouts, or a piping hot sweet potato on a higher carb day.

CALORIES: 229	FAT: 25 G
CARBOHYDRATE: 1 G	PROTEIN: 2 G

2 slices bacon (not thick-cut)
½ cup (1 stick; 112 g) unsalted butter, at room temperature
1 garlic clove, very finely minced
½ teaspoon (2 ml) sweet paprika
½ teaspoon (2 ml) chili powder
½ teaspoon (2 ml) crushed dried oregano
¼ teaspoon (1 ml) ground cumin
⅛ teaspoon (0.5 ml) onion powder
½ teaspoon (2 ml) kosher salt
¼ teaspoon (1 ml) black pepper

1. Cook the bacon in a skillet until crispy, about 3 minutes. Transfer to a paper towel to drain. Reserve the bacon grease to use for another recipe.

2. Cut the butter into pieces and place in a small bowl. Mash with a fork.

3. Add the garlic, paprika, chili powder, oregano, cumin, onion powder, salt, and pepper and combine well.

4. Crumble or chop the bacon into small pieces. Stir the bacon bits into the butter.

5. Scoop the butter mixture onto a 12-inch (30 cm) piece of parchment paper. Shape into a log and roll up tightly. Twist the ends to secure.

6. Transfer to the refrigerator until ready to use. (The butter can also be frozen.)

Chicken Liver Pâté

Makes approximately 2 cups; serving size = 2 tablespoons

Liver is one of the healthiest foods you can eat, so it's a real shame that it gets such a bad rap. Let's hope this flavorful spread will change your mind about this nutritional superstar. The pâté can be eaten with any raw veggies—try it on celery sticks, cucumber slices, or red bell peppers—or even on sliced apples.

1. Remove any stringy or membranous parts from the livers. Melt 2 tablespoons (30 ml) of the butter and the bacon fat in a medium skillet over medium heat. Add the onion and the livers and sauté for 6 to 8 minutes, until the onion is soft and the livers are browned.

2. Add garlic and sauté for 1 minute more. Turn the heat down slightly and add both vinegars, the mustard, and rosemary. Cook until the liquid is mostly evaporated and livers are cooked through, about 5 more minutes.

3. Transfer everything in skillet to a food processor. Pulse a few times to combine. Scrape down the sides of the bowl and add 2 tablespoons (30 g) of the butter. Process until mostly smooth. Scrape down the sides again. Add the remaining 2 tablespoons (30 g) butter and process until very smooth.

4. Taste and add salt and pepper as necessary. Transfer the paste to individual ramekins and cover with plastic wrap, then refrigerate. Before serving, sprinkle each ramekin with a little bit of flaked sea salt.

CALORIES: 322	FAT: 28 G
CARBOHYDRATE: 2 G	PROTEIN: 14 G

½ pound (225 g) chicken livers
6 tablespoons (85 g) butter
2 tablespoons (30 ml) bacon fat
½ small onion, minced
1 large garlic clove, minced
2 tablespoons (30 ml) red wine vinegar
1 tablespoon (15 ml) balsamic vinegar
1 teaspoon (5 ml) Dijon mustard
½ tablespoon (7.5 ml) minced fresh rosemary
Salt and pepper to taste
Flaky salt (like Maldon), to garnish

Coconut Butter

Makes approximately 1 cup; serving size = 2 tablespoons

If you've never tried coconut butter, you are in for a treat! This versatile butter can be added to coffee or smoothies, mixed into mashed root veggies, used in curries, or eaten spread thickly on apple slices or a piece of extra-dark chocolate. It is also the main ingredient of fat bombs (see page 292). You'll definitely want to keep a jar of this on hand!

CALORIES: 210	FAT: 21 G
CARBOHYDRATE: 8 G	PROTEIN: 2 G

4 cups (360 to 400 g) unsweetened dried flaked coconut (see Note)

If using a food processor: Place the coconut flakes in a food processor and blend for up to 15 minutes, scraping down the sides as needed (some food processors take slightly longer).

If using a high-powered blender: Place *half* the coconut flakes in the blender and blend for 1 minute. Add the remaining coconut flakes and continue blending for up to 10 minutes, scraping down the sides as needed. Make sure your blender does not become too hot!

With either method, expect your coconut butter to go through three stages: First, it will become finely shredded, then it will become a grainy liquid, and finally it will form a smooth butter. This takes a while. If you aren't sure if it is done, give it a taste. The finished product should be mostly smooth with a slight grainy texture, like freshly ground nut butter.

2. Transfer the coconut butter to an airtight container until ready to use. (Coconut butter can be stored at room temperature.) If needed, microwave for 5 to 10 seconds to soften before using.

NOTE: Only dried coconut works in this recipe. You can use shredded in place of flakes, but the result might not be as smooth. Do not use desiccated, sweetened, reduced-fat, or fresh coconut.

Smoked Salmon Spread

Makes approximately 2½ cups; serving size = ¼ cup

This recipe originally appeared on my blog, Mark's Daily Apple. It's a great way to use leftover salmon (like the salmon on page 242). Loaded with healthy fats, this preparation can be eaten as breakfast, lunch, or dinner, or as a healthy snack. It whips up in a matter of minutes, but tastes fancy enough to impress guests at the nicest dinner party. Scoop a few spoonfuls into individual radicchio or endive leaves for an elegant preparation.

1. In a medium bowl, mash the butter and olive oil together with a fork. Stir in the chives, capers, and lemon juice.

2. Use a fork to flake the cooked salmon and add it to the butter mixture. Add the smoked salmon and mix well, mashing slightly. Pack into a bowl, cover, and refrigerate until ready to use.

CALORIES: 83	FAT: 6 G
CARBOHYDRATE: 1 G	PROTEIN: 7 G

4 tablespoons (½ stick; 60 g) butter, at room temperature

1 tablespoon (15 ml) extra-virgin olive oil

2 tablespoons (30 ml) minced fresh chives

2 tablespoons (30 ml) drained capers

2 tablespoons (30 ml) fresh lemon juice

8 ounces (225 g) boneless, skinless salmon fillet, cooked

4 ounces (115 g) smoked salmon, diced small

Salt and pepper to taste

Nutty Tapenade

Makes approximately 1½ cups; serving size is 2 tablespoons

Traditional tapenade is a mixture of olives, capers, anchovies, and onions ground together with a mortar and pestle, and is often served on crostini. It's a great way to get some omega-rich, small, oily fish into your diet. The addition of nuts in this recipe adds some crunch to make up for the missing crostini. Serve this tapenade on slices of cucumber or bell pepper, use as a topping on baked chicken, or mix a tablespoon with additional olive oil to use as a salad dressing.

1. In a small food processor (or using a large mortar and pestle), combine the ingredients and pulse 10 times. Scrape down the sides of the bowl and continue to pulse until the tapenade reaches the desired consistency.

2. Pack into a bowl, cover with plastic wrap, and refrigerate until ready to serve.

CALORIES: 39	FAT: 4 G
CARBOHYDRATE: 1 G	PROTEIN: 1 G

1 cup (250 ml) pitted olives (use a mixture of green, black, and Niçoise—whatever you like)

2 anchovy fillets, packed in olive oil (see Tip)

¼ cup (60 ml) walnut pieces

1 garlic clove, crushed

1 tablespoon (15 ml) drained capers

1 tablespoon (15 ml) chopped fresh basil

3 tablespoons (45 ml) extra-virgin olive oil

TIP: Use the remaining anchovies in the can to make Caesar salad and dressing (see page 276).

Slow Cooker Carnitas

Makes approximately 10 servings; serving size = 1 cup

If I know I have a busy week ahead, I'll often make carnitas on Sunday and eat them throughout the week in different dishes. The best way to reheat this is on a rimmed sheet pan under the broiler.

1. In a small bowl, combine the salt, cumin, oregano, and pepper. Trim excess fat from the roast (you want some fat, just remove any big chunks). Press the seasoning mixture into the roast on all sides.

2. Pour broth into the bottom of a slow cooker. Place the roast inside and arrange the orange slices over the top. Cook on low for 8 to 10 hours (preferable) or on high for 6 hours.

3. Carefully remove the roast from the slow cooker and discard the orange slices. Use two forks to shred the meat.

4. If desired, place the shredded meat on a heavy, rimmed baking sheet or broiler pan. Turn the oven broiler to low and position an oven rack about 4 inches below the heat. Place the tray of meat under the broiler and allow some bits to get crispy, but watch carefully so it does not burn.

5. Divide into serving portions and serve with optional toppings. If desired, place in lettuce or cabbage leaves to make primal-style tacos.

CALORIES: 336	FAT: 19 G
CARBOHYDRATE: 1 G	PROTEIN: 32 G

1 teaspoon (5 ml) kosher salt
1 teaspoon (5 ml) ground cumin
1 teaspoon (5 ml) dried oregano
½ teaspoon (2 ml) black pepper
1 boneless pork shoulder roast
    (4 to 5 pounds; 1.8 K)
1 cup chicken or beef broth
    (250 ml)
1 orange, thinly sliced

OPTIONAL TOPPINGS/SIDES
Finely chopped white or red onion
Minced fresh cilantro
Cubed avocado
Thinly sliced radishes
Lime wedges
Jalapeño rings
Lettuce or cabbage leaves

Carnitas Kale Scramble

Makes 2 servings

This is a great way to use leftover carnitas (page 229) for something different. I love this for breakfast when I'm not in the mood for eggs.

CALORIES: 592	FAT: 41 G
CARBOHYDRATE: 12 G	PROTEIN: 39 G

1. Heat the bacon fat in a large skillet over medium heat. Add the onion and bell pepper. Cook for 5 minutes, until the vegetables start to soften. Add the garlic and cook 1 minute more.

2. Stir in the tomatoes, then stir in the meat. Cook until warmed through.

3. In a small bowl, combine the salt, oregano, cumin, and pepper. Add to the skillet and stir well.

4. Add the chopped kale (might need to do this in two batches, depending on how big your skillet is). When the kale begins to wilt, add the lemon juice and stir well.

5. Sprinkle the cheese evenly over all, turn the heat to low, and cover. Cook a few minutes until the cheese melts. (If your skillet is heatproof, you can also put it under the broiler to brown the top.)

6. Divide into two portions and serve.

2 tablespoons (30 ml) bacon fat or avocado oil
¼ cup (50 g) chopped red onion
¼ cup (40 g) chopped red bell pepper
1 garlic clove, minced
1 tablespoon (5 g) sun-dried or oven-dried tomatoes (see Note)
2 cups (475 g) shredded Slow Cooker Carnitas
1 teaspoon (5 ml) kosher salt
1 teaspoon (5 ml) dried oregano
¾ teaspoon (4 ml) ground cumin
Freshly ground black pepper
2 cups (30 g) roughly chopped kale leaves (approximately ½ bunch)
Juice of ½ lemon
1/3 cup (30 g) grated raw cheddar cheese

NOTE: Be sure to find sun-dried tomatoes that have been packed only in olive oil, not safflower, canola, soybean, or another polyunsaturated oil. If you can't find an acceptable choice, substitute diced fresh tomatoes or ½ tablespoon tomato paste.

Cuban Un-sandwich

Makes 6 servings

Here's another great idea for using leftover carnitas (page 229)! This twist on a traditional Cuban sandwich throws out the bread and leaves you with what matters most—those delicious sandwich fillings. Eat it with a knife and fork, or wrap it in collard greens (see page 243).

1. Place an oven rack 4 to 6 inches below the broiler heat and set the broiler at its lowest temperature. Use the avocado oil to lightly grease a heavy rimmed baking sheet or broiler-safe pan. Place the shredded pork on the sheet so it is in a layer about ¾ inch thick (a half-sheet pan works great for this). Sprinkle with salt, pepper, and lime juice. Place under the broiler and broil until top starts to brown, about 2 minutes.

2. Remove the sheet from the broiler but keep the broiler on. Arrange the pickle slices on top, followed by the ham. Use the back of a spoon or a spatula to carefully spread the mustard on the ham slices. Sprinkle the cheese in an even layer over the ham.

3. Return the sheet to the broiler to brown the top, about 1 to 2 minutes. Keep a close eye on the cheese; you want it to melt and start to bubble and brown, but definitely not to burn.

CALORIES: 426	FAT: 26 G
CARBOHYDRATE: 8 G	PROTEIN: 36 G

1 teaspoon (5 ml) avocado oil
4 cups (950 g) shredded Slow
    Cooker Carnitas
1 teaspoon (5 ml) kosher salt
Freshly ground black pepper
Juice of ½ lime
1 cup (250ml) dill pickle slices
    (regular or spicy; avoid sweet
    pickles!)
6 thin slices ham (make sure you buy
    the cleanest possible)
3 tablespoons (45 ml) Dijon
    mustard
2 cups (180 g) shredded Swiss
    cheese

Curley Caveman Raw-Energy Almond Butter Ground Beef

Makes 4 servings

With a recipe this simple, the quality of ingredients matters! I recommend wagyu-style ground beef (if you can't find this at your local store, it's available to order at MarxFoods.com). At first glance this recipe probably seems odd, but give it a try next time you need serious staying power. This concoction will deliver raw energy and stick-to-your-bones satisfaction for a six-hour hike in a tropical forest.

1. In a medium skillet, brown the ground beef over medium heat until cooked through, 6 to 8 minutes. Add the salt, pepper, and cinnamon and stir well.

2. Stir in the almond butter by the spoonful and stir vigorously. When almond butter is completely incorporated, remove from the heat. Divide into four bowls and serve immediately. If it's your turn to cook at the fire station, quintuple the recipe to keep the crew going for a full weekend shift.

CALORIES: 616	FAT: 46 G
CARBOHYDRATE: 6 G	PROTEIN: 46 G

1½ pounds (675 g) ground beef
1 teaspoon (5 ml) Himalayan pink salt
½ teaspoon (2 ml) ground pepper
½ teaspoon (2 ml) ground cinnamon
½ cup (120 ml) raw almond butter

Seared Ahi with Herb + Lime Dressing

Makes 2 servings

Seared ahi tuna is a dish that might seem difficult, but once you try it, you won't believe how easy it is to make. If you want a quick and easy dish to impress guests, this is it! Serve the tuna with a simple green salad.

1. Slice the tuna steak into 2 or 3 long rectangular portions. Season each side of each slice generously with salt and pepper.

2. Place the cilantro and parsley in a small food processor (see Note). Pulse to chop finely. Add the lime zest, lime juice, tamari, sesame oil, garlic, and ginger. Pulse several times to combine. Scrape down the sides of the bowl.

3. With the food processor running, slowly pour in ¼ cup of olive oil. Scrape down the sides again and pulse a few times. If the sauce is too thick, add more oil until the sauce reaches desired consistency.

4. In a large skillet, heat the avocado oil over medium-high heat until quite hot. Gently place the tuna in the oil and sear for 1 minute without moving. Sear each side in same manner. The tuna will still be pink in the middle, or cook slightly longer for more well-cooked fish.

5. Remove the fish to cutting board and slice approximately ½ inch (13 mm) thick.

6. Drizzle the tuna generously with the dressing and serve.

CALORIES: 551	FAT: 49 G
CARBOHYDRATE: 7 G	PROTEIN: 24 G

6 ounces (168 g) sushi-grade ahi tuna steak
Sea salt
Freshly ground black pepper
2 tablespoons (30 ml) avocado oil

HERB + LIME DRESSING
1 cup (150 g) loosely packed fresh cilantro
1 cup (150 g) loosely packed fresh parsley
1 teaspoon (5 ml) grated lime zest
Juice of 2 small limes (1½ to 2 tablespoons; 25 ml)
2 tablespoons (30 ml) tamari (gluten-free soy sauce)
1 tablespoon (15 ml) toasted sesame oil
1 garlic clove, finely minced or pressed
A 1-inch (2.5 cm) piece of fresh ginger, finely minced or grated
¼ to ½ cup (60 to 120 ml) extra-virgin olive oil or avocado oil
Dash of red pepper flakes (optional)

NOTE: If you don't have a food processor, chop the herbs finely by hand and mix the dressing ingredients in a bowl.

Cabbage Rolls

Makes 6 servings

Traditional stuffed cabbage uses rice to thicken the filling, but of course that won't work for keto folks. This recipe uses riced cauliflower instead to give substance to the filling. It can be cooked on the stovetop or in a slow cooker.

CALORIES: 233	FAT: 14 G
CARBOHYDRATE: 7 G	PROTEIN: 21 G

1 head napa cabbage

1 small cauliflower

2 tablespoons (30 ml) bacon fat or avocado oil

¼ cup (40 g) diced onion

¼ cup (40 g) diced green bell pepper

1 cup (250 ml) beef broth

1 large egg

1 can (14.5 ounces; 411 g) diced tomatoes, drained and with liquid reserved

1 teaspoon (5 ml) kosher salt

½ teaspoon (2 ml) black pepper

1 pound (450 g) ground beef

1. Remove 12 outer leaves from the cabbage. Bring a large pot of water to a boil and drop in the cabbage leaves. Boil for 2 minutes, until softened, then lay flat on a kitchen towel to drain and cool.

2. Use a food processor fitted with a shredding blade (or use a box grater) to grate the cauliflower florets. Measure 2 cups (300 g) of the grated cauliflower and reserve the remainder for another recipe (for example, see Veggie Sushi rolls on page 263).

3. In a medium skillet, heat the bacon fat over medium heat. Add the onion and green pepper, and sauté 2 minutes. Add the cauliflower and ½ cup (120 ml) of the broth. Cook, stirring occasionally, for about 5 minutes, until the cauliflower is cooked but still firm. It should still have some texture to it. Remove from the heat and allow to cool slightly.

4. In a large bowl, lightly beat the egg. Mix in the drained tomatoes, salt, and pepper. Crumble in the meat and mix well. Add the cauliflower mixture and stir to combine.

5. Divide the mixture evenly among the cabbage leaves, placing the filling in the center of each. Fold the sides and roll each one up tightly. Secure with a toothpick.

6. Mix the reserved tomato juice with the remaining ½ cup (120 ml) broth.

7. *If cooking on the stovetop:* Place the cabbage rolls in a single layer in the skillet used to cook the cauliflower. Pour the broth mixture over the top and cover the skillet. Heat over medium high until the liquid boils, then reduce the heat to low. Cook about 40 minutes, occasionally spooning liquid over the rolls.

If cooking in a slow cooker: Place the cabbage rolls in a small slow cooker. Pour the broth over the top, cover, and cook on low for 7 to 8 hours.

8. Using an instant-read thermometer, check the cabbage rolls to see if the meat is fully cooked; the internal temperature should reach 160°F (70°C).

Stuffed Tomatoes

Makes 6 servings; serving size = 1 tomato

This simple recipe is best made with summer tomatoes fresh from the garden. You can use ground turkey or chicken, or even ground lamb, in place of the beef, if you prefer.

CALORIES: 204	FAT: 12 G
CARBOHYDRATE: 5 G	PROTEIN: 18 G

6 medium tomatoes
½ pound (225 g) ground beef
1 teaspoon (5 ml) dried basil
½ teaspoon (2 ml) kosher salt, plus more as needed
¼ teaspoon (1 ml) black pepper, plus more as needed
6 medium eggs

1. Preheat the oven to 400°F (200°C). With a sharp paring knife, cut the stem ends off the tomatoes. Gently cut the seeds out of the middle, scoop out with a spoon, and discard.

2. Place the tomatoes in a small oven- and broiler-proof pan, or use a muffin tin with large cups. Bake for 5 minutes.

3. Brown the meat in a medium skillet until cooked through, about 25 minutes, then season with the basil, salt, and pepper.

4. Remove the tomatoes from the oven and switch the oven to broil (on low heat if adjustable). Divide the meat into six portions and spoon evenly into the tomatoes.

5. Crack one egg into each tomato and sprinkle with additional salt and pepper.

6. Place stuffed tomatoes under the broiler 4 to 6 inches (10 to 15 cm) from the heat for about 5 minutes, watching closely, until the egg whites are cooked completely and the yolks are still runny.

The Best Grilled Chicken

Makes 4 to 8 servings; serving size = 5 ounces (140 g)

I bet this flavorful chicken will quickly become a family favorite. It is delicious placed atop a colorful garden salad, wrapped in collard greens with a dollop of Primal Mayo, or simply served with a side of your favorite roasted veggies. The secret is the initial brining step, which makes the chicken both flavorful and tender.

CALORIES: 245	FAT: 6 G
CARBOHYDRATE: 0 G	PROTEIN: 44 G

4 boneless, skinless chicken breast halves (approximately 2½ pounds; 1.1 k)

3 tablespoons (45 ml) kosher salt

Ice cubes

2 tablespoons (30 ml) avocado oil

2 tablespoons (30 ml) poultry seasoning (make sure there is no added sugar)

1. Cut each chicken breast on the diagonal into 3 long portions.

2. Bring 1 cup (240 ml) of water to a boil. Combine the boiling water and salt in a large glass or metal bowl. When the salt is dissolved, pour in a quart of cold water and add enough ice cubes to cool. Add the chicken slices and enough cold water so that the chicken is covered by 1 to 2 inches. Put in the refrigerator for 15 minutes.

3. Drain the chicken. If you don't want the chicken to be salty, rinse it now, but it's not necessary. Mix the oil and poultry seasoning in the empty bowl, then toss the chicken in the oil. Let sit for a few minutes.

4. Heat a grill to medium-high heat. When hot, place the chicken slices on the grill and close the lid. Cook for about 4 minutes, flip, and continue cooking until internal temperature reaches 165°F (75°C), another 3 to 4 minutes.

5. Remove the chicken from the grill and serve.

Chicken Kabobs

Makes 8 servings; serving size = 1 kabob

Kabobs are my favorite go-to main course when we are having people over for a casual summer barbeque. You can assemble them ahead of time, or you can even allow guests to assemble their own. Because they cook quickly, you won't be stuck manning the grill while your guests have all the fun.

1. Cut each chicken breast into 8 to 10 chunks of approximately equal size and place in a glass bowl. Wash the mushrooms and trim off the stems. Cut the onion and peppers into large chunks. Place vegetables together in a second bowl.

2. Mix the oil and seasonings. Pour half the mixture into each bowl and stir well to coat. Put both bowls in the refrigerator and allow to marinate for 20 minutes.

3. Assemble the kabobs by alternating the chicken and the vegetables on the skewers. Preheat the grill to medium high.

4. Place the kabobs on the grill (or under a broiler) for approximately 3 minutes per side, rotating to make sure every side gets browned, about 10 to 12 minutes total. Check the chicken with an instant-read thermometer to make sure it is cooked through (internal temperature should be 165°F or 75°C).

5. Transfer the kabobs to a platter and serve.

CALORIES: 286	FAT: 12 G
CARBOHYDRATE: 14 G	PROTEIN: 32 G

2 pounds (900 g) boneless, skinless chicken breast halves
24 small button mushrooms (approximately 8 ounces; 225 g)
1 large yellow onion
2 bell peppers (any color you prefer)
¼ cup (60 ml) avocado oil
1 teaspoon (5 ml) dried oregano
1 teaspoon (5 ml) dried basil
½ teaspoon (2 ml) garlic powder
½ teaspoon (2 ml) kosher salt
½ teaspoon (2 ml) black pepper
8 short kabob skewers (soaked in water if wooden/bamboo)

One-Pan Shrimp and Asparagus

Makes 6 servings

I hate washing pots, so a one-pan meal is right up my alley. Plus, this simple dish can be made in less than 20 minutes, start to finish. Gotta love that!

1. Preheat the oven to 400°F (200°C). In a small saucepan, heat the avocado oil over medium heat. Sauté the garlic until fragrant but not brown, about 3 minutes. Add the butter and cook until it starts to bubble, then remove from the heat.

2. Trim the tough ends off the asparagus and place the spears on a large rimmed baking sheet. Spoon 2 tablespoons (30 ml) of the garlic butter over the top and toss to coat. Spread out in a single layer and sprinkle with half the salt and pepper. Place in the oven for 5 minutes, until tender and lightly roasted.

3. Arrange the asparagus on one half of the baking sheet. Place the shrimp on the other half. Pour the remaining garlic butter over the shrimp and toss to coat. Spread out in a single layer and sprinkle with the remaining salt and pepper, adding the red pepper flakes, if using. Squeeze the lemon over the shrimp, then cut the juiced lemon into quarters and place on the baking sheet among the shrimp.

4. Sprinkle the Parmesan cheese over the asparagus only, then place the baking sheet in the oven for 5 to 8 minutes, or until the shrimp is just opaque. Sprinkle the parsley over the shrimp, if using, and serve immediately.

CALORIES: 267	FAT: 17 G
CARBOHYDRATE: 2 G	PROTEIN: 28 G

2 tablespoons (30 ml) avocado oil

3 garlic cloves, minced

4 tablespoons (½ stick; 60 g) butter

1 bunch asparagus (approximately 1 pound; 450 g)

2 teaspoons (10 ml) kosher salt

1 teaspoon (5 ml) freshly ground black pepper

1½ pounds (680 g) shrimp, peeled and deveined

¼ to ½ teaspoon (1 to 2 ml) red pepper flakes (optional)

1 medium lemon, cut in half

1 cup (90 g) finely shredded Parmesan cheese

2 tablespoons (30 ml) chopped fresh parsley (optional)

Sausage and Kale
Makes 4 servings

If you have friends or family members who think they don't like kale, start them with this dish! This recipe is totally customizable—you can add any vegetables you want, and any type of sausage works. Play around with different combos to see what you like. However, make sure you choose sausage that contains only clean ingredients—no added sugars, nitrates, or the like.

1. Use a sharp paring knife to cut the thick kale stems from the leafy portions. Keep stems and leaves separate. Chop the stems approximately the same size as the diced onion. Cut the kale leaves into thin strips.

2. Cut the sausages into ½ inch (2.5 cm) slices. Heat 1 tablespoon (15 ml) oil in large skillet. Add half the sausages in a single layer, cooking 2 to 3 minutes until browned, then flip and cook 2 minutes on the other side. Remove and repeat with other half of the sausages. Remove from the skillet.

3. Melt the remaining tablespoon (15 ml) of oil in the same skillet over medium heat. Add the onion and diced kale stems and cook until vegetables begin to soften, about 5 minutes. Push the vegetables to the edge of the skillet and melt the butter in the middle. Add the mushrooms and sauté for a few minutes. Add the salt and pepper, and stir well.

4. Add the kale leaves and stir to combine. Cook until leaves are wilted, 3 to 5 minutes. Add the sausage back to the skillet along with the chicken broth and red pepper flakes, if using. Turn the heat to medium high. When the liquid begins to boil, reduce the heat to low and simmer until the liquid is mostly evaporated. Taste and add salt if needed. Serve immediately.

CALORIES: 276	FAT: 21 G
CARBOHYDRATE: 5 G	PROTEIN: 21 G

1 bunch kale, any variety

½ medium onion, diced

1 package chicken sausage (like Trader Joe's Garlic Herb Chicken Sausage)

2 tablespoons (30 ml) coconut or avocado oil

2 tablespoons (30 g) butter

8 button mushrooms, trimmed and sliced

1 teaspoon (5 ml) kosher salt, or more as needed

½ teaspoon (2 ml) black pepper

1 cup (250 ml) chicken broth (preferably homemade, see page 216)

¼ teaspoon (1 ml) red pepper flakes (optional)

Turkey Fajita Salad with Chipotle Lime Dressing

Makes 4 servings

This recipe uses ground turkey, but you could also throw this together quickly with leftover grilled chicken (like The Best Grilled Chicken, page 237). The raw green cabbage provides a satisfying crunch to replace the taco shells and tortilla strips that are often part of fajita salads.

1. In a small bowl, combine the Fajita Seasoning ingredients.

2. Make the dressing by whisking together the mayo, coconut milk, lime juice, and ¼ teaspoon Fajita Seasoning. If the dressing is too thick, add water a little at a time until it reaches desired consistency.

3. In a small bowl, mix the sour cream and 1 teaspoon (4 ml) of Fajita Seasoning.

4. Heat 1 tablespoon (15 ml) of the oil in large skillet over medium-high heat. Add the onion and green pepper and sauté 3 to 5 minutes, until crisp-tender. Remove from the skillet.

5. Reduce the heat to medium and add the remaining tablespoon (15 ml) of the oil to the skillet. Add the turkey and cook, breaking apart large chunks, until only a little pink remains. Add the remaining 5 teaspoons (25 ml) Fajita Seasoning and stir very well. Add the tomatoes and cook another few minutes, until turkey is no longer pink.

6. Cut the cabbage into quarters and cut out the core. Use a sharp knife to cut each quarter into very thin strips.

7. Evenly divide the raw cabbage and spinach into 4 wide, shallow bowls. Top each bowl with the onion and peppers, turkey, a dollop of the seasoned sour cream, the shredded cheese, and the diced avocado. Drizzle the dressing over everything and serve with lime wedges to squeeze on top.

CALORIES: 645	FAT: 48 G
CARBOHYDRATE: 19 G	PROTEIN: 40 G

FAJITA SEASONING
1 tablespoon (15 ml) chili powder
1 teaspoon (5 ml) ground cumin
1 teaspoon (5 ml) salt
½ teaspoon (2 ml) sweet paprika
½ teaspoon (2 ml) dried oregano, rubbed
¼ teaspoon (1 ml) black pepper

CHIPOTLE LIME DRESSING
¼ cup (60 ml) Primal Kitchen Chipotle Lime Mayo (see Note, page 197)
3 tablespoons (45 ml) full-fat coconut milk
1 teaspoon (5 ml) fresh lime juice
¼ teaspoon (1 ml) Fajita Seasoning

SALAD
½ cup (120 ml) sour cream
2 tablespoons (30 ml) Fajita Seasoning
2 tablespoons (30 ml) avocado oil
1 small yellow onion, sliced
1 green bell pepper, seeded and sliced
1 pound (450 g) ground turkey
1 can (14.5 ounces; 411 g) diced tomatoes with chiles, drained
1 small head of green cabbage
2 cups (56 g) baby spinach
½ cup (56 g) shredded cheddar jack cheese
1 avocado, diced
Lime wedges

Slow-Baked Salmon with Dill Aioli

Makes 4 servings

Slow baking produces a velvety, melt-in-your-mouth salmon fillet. When you cook it this way the salmon remains quite pink, so don't be alarmed when you remove it from the oven and it still looks raw. On the contrary, it will be the most perfectly cooked piece of fish you've ever eaten!

1. Preheat the oven to 275°F (135°C). Place the salmon fillets in a casserole dish or baking pan. Mix the oil with half the lemon zest and brush over the top of the fish. Sprinkle with salt and pepper. Bake the salmon for 16 to 18 minutes, until you are just able to flake it with a fork.

2. While the salmon is baking, combine the mayo, garlic, lemon zest, lemon juice, dill, salt, and pepper.

3. Serve the salmon with the aioli on the side.

CALORIES: 462	FAT: 36 G
CARBOHYDRATE: 1 G	PROTEIN: 33 G

4 skin-on salmon fillets, approximately 6 ounces (168 g) each (see Note)
½ tablespoon (7.5 ml) avocado oil
Zest from ½ large lemon
Kosher salt
Freshly ground black pepper

DILL AIOLI
½ cup (120 ml) Primal Kitchen Mayo (see Note, page 197), or other primal-approved mayo
2 small garlic cloves, finely minced
Zest from ½ large lemon
2 teaspoons (15 ml) fresh lemon juice
1 tablespoon (15 ml) chopped fresh dill
¼ teaspoon (1 ml) kosher salt
¼ teaspoon (1 ml) freshly ground black pepper

NOTE: When selecting seafood, always check seafoodwatch.org for up-to-date recommendations on the healthiest varieties.

Collard Green–Turkey Club Wraps

Makes 2 servings

After experimenting with several options, I have found collard greens to be the best replacement for flatbread and tortillas. They have a surprisingly mild flavor, and the leaves are big enough and thick enough to keep your fillings secure. This sandwich is a little messy to eat, but so good!

CALORIES: 364	FAT: 26 G
CARBOHYDRATE: 10 G	PROTEIN: 23 G

2 collard green leaves, the bigger the better
4 slices organic sliced turkey breast (no added sugar or nitrites)
4 slices bacon, cooked until crispy
2 slices Swiss cheese, cut in half
½ cup (120 ml) Primal Coleslaw (page 261)

1. Use a sharp paring knife to remove the thick center stem from the collard greens. (You will probably have to cut up the leaf a bit, leaving you with a heart-shaped leaf.)

2. In the middle of each leaf, layer 2 slices of turkey, 2 slices of bacon, and 2 half-slices of cheese, leaving a margin of leaf on the edges. Spoon ¼ cup (60 ml) of the slaw across each leaf nearer to the top (away from the stem end).

3. Beginning at the top end, pull the leaf over the slaw and roll the sandwich up, tucking in the edges like a burrito. Secure the rolls with 2 toothpicks each and cut in half to serve.

Cheesy Chicken and Ham Roll-ups

Makes 4 servings

This is a spin on traditional chicken cordon bleu, a dish in which chicken is wrapped around ham and cheese, then breaded and pan-fried. Of course, the breading is a no-no on a keto eating plan, but you won't miss it with this recipe!

1. One at a time, place the chicken breasts between two slices of wax paper or parchment paper and use a flat meat hammer or rolling pin to pound the chicken until each piece is ½ inch (13 mm) thick. Try to pound so that the chicken ends up in a long rectangular shape instead of a circle.

2. Cut the sliced prosciutto in half lengthwise. Place ½ slice of prosciutto and 1 slice of Swiss cheese on each piece of chicken, then roll up. Secure with toothpicks.

3. Mix the salt, pepper, and thyme in a small bowl, then use the mixture to generously season the outside of each roll.

4. Heat the oil in a skillet large enough to fit the 4 rolls. Brown the rolls on all sides, starting with the side with the seam.

5. Once browned, place ½ slice of prosciutto on top of each roll and sprinkle with Gruyère. Pour in the broth, cover the pan with a tight-fitting lid, and cook over medium-low heat for 30 minutes, or until the chicken is cooked through (see Note).

6. Use tongs to remove the chicken rolls to a broiler pan or heavy rimmed baking sheet and let rest. Preheat the broiler (on low heat if adjustable).

7. Heat the liquid left over in the skillet over medium heat. Add the mustard, then the butter,

CALORIES: 507	FAT: 40 G
CARBOHYDRATE: 4 G	PROTEIN: 33 G

4 boneless, skinless chicken breast halves (approximately 2½ pounds; 1.1 k)

4 slices prosciutto

4 slices Swiss cheese

1 teaspoon (5 ml) salt, or more as needed

1 teaspoon (5 ml) black pepper, or more as needed

2 teaspoons (10 ml) dried thyme

Avocado oil

1 cup (250 ml) shredded Gruyère cheese

½ cup (120 ml) chicken broth, preferably homemade (see page 216)

1 tablespoon (15 ml) Dijon mustard

2 tablespoons (30 g) butter

½ cup (120 ml) heavy cream

½ cup (120 ml) grated Parmesan cheese

then the cream, whisking constantly. Finally, add the Parmesan cheese and whisk until melted. Taste and adjust salt and pepper as needed.

8. Place the chicken under the broiler for a minute to give the cheese a nice golden-brown color. Pour the sauce over the chicken and serve immediately.

NOTE: This recipe can also be made in an Instant Pot pressure cooker. Brown the chicken roll-ups using the sauté function, then cook using the manual setting for 7 minutes. Release the pressure and switch back to the sauté function to make the sauce.

Crunchy Tuna Salad
Makes 4 servings

Here's another idea for something to roll up in collard greens (see page 243). You can also eat this salad on greens, atop sliced radish or cucumber "chips," or just by itself. Be sure to select tuna that is sustainably caught and packed in water or olive oil. One favorite brand is Wild Planet, widely available in stores.

CALORIES: 407	FAT: 35 G
CARBOHYDRATE: 4 G	PROTEIN: 19 G

2 (5 ounces; 142 g each) cans of tuna (do not drain)
½ cup (120 ml) Primal Kitchen Mayo (see Note, page 197), or other primal-approved mayo
2 tablespoons (30 ml) drained capers
1 celery stalk, diced
1 small carrot, diced
4 radishes, diced
Salt and pepper to taste
½ cup (60 g) slivered almonds
2 tablespoons (15 g) sunflower seeds

1. Empty the tuna along with the canning liquid into a bowl. Flake with a fork, then stir in the mayo, capers, celery, carrot, and radishes. Taste and season with salt and pepper.

2. Run a chef's knife over the almonds to roughly chop. Just before serving, stir the almonds into the tuna salad and sprinkle with the sunflower seeds.

Stuffed Turkey Burgers with Goat Cheese

Makes 4 servings

The addition of this one simple ingredient transforms an average turkey burger into something special!

CALORIES: 510	FAT: 37 G
CARBOHYDRATE: 1 G	PROTEIN: 43 G

1. Mix the salt, oregano, thyme, and pepper in a small bowl.

2. Cut 4 slices of chevre approximately ¼ inch (6 mm) thick (you will use the remaining chevre in step 5).

3. Divide one portion of meat in half and form into 2 thin patties approximately 3 to 4 inches (8 cm) in diameter. (If the turkey is sticky, it helps to wet your hands.) Sandwich 1 slice of goat cheese between the 2 patties, pressing the edges together and gently flattening. Repeat with remaining 3 portions.

4. In a large skillet set over medium heat, heat enough avocado oil to lightly cover the surface. Season the top of each burger with some of the spice mixture and place seasoned side down in the skillet. Cook until lightly browned on the bottom, about 5 minutes.

5. Season the tops of the burgers with the remaining spice mixture, then flip the burgers. Crumble or slice the remaining goat cheese over the tops of the burgers evenly. Place a lid on the skillet and cook another 5 to 8 minutes, or until the burgers are cooked through.

6. If desired, place the burgers under a broiler to lightly toast the goat cheese.

1 teaspoon (5 ml) kosher salt
¾ teaspoon (4 ml) dried oregano
¾ teaspoon (4 ml) dried thyme
¼ teaspoon (1 ml) black pepper
11 ounces (320 g) chevre (goat cheese), in a log
1½ pounds (680 g) ground turkey, divided into 4 portions
Avocado oil

Bacon-Wrapped Scallops

Makes 2 servings

Bacon-wrapped scallops are so good...unless the bacon is soggy. This method of cooking ensures that you end up with crispy bacon and perfectly cooked scallops.

CALORIES: 288	FAT: 12 G
CARBOHYDRATE: 9 G	PROTEIN: 36 G

6 slices thick-cut bacon
12 large sea scallops (about
   10 ounces; 280 g)
Salt and pepper
Juice of ½ lemon

1. Preheat the oven to 400°F (200°C). Place an ovenproof wire rack on a rimmed baking sheet. Arrange the bacon on the wire rack so the pieces don't overlap and bake for 8 to 10 minutes, depending on thickness. The bacon should be about half cooked. Remove from the oven but do not turn the oven off.

2. Rinse the scallops and pat dry with paper towels.

3. Cut the bacon strips in half lengthwise (kitchen scissors work well). Wrap one half-piece of bacon around each scallop and secure with a toothpick.

4. Pour off the excess bacon drippings from the baking sheet (save to use for other recipes). Arrange the scallops on the same baking pan and sprinkle with salt and pepper. Place the scallops in the oven and bake for 12 to 15 minutes, flipping halfway through.

5. Squeeze lemon juice over the scallops and serve.

Shredded Beef Cabbage Cups with Kimchi

Makes 10 servings

Kimchi is a staple of Korean cuisine. Similar to sauerkraut, it is a mixture of fermented vegetables and spices. Like all fermented foods, it is great for your gut health. It can be found in the refrigerated section of most grocery stores and certainly in all Asian markets.

1. Season all sides of the roast with salt and pepper. Heat the oil in a heavy skillet over medium-high heat. When hot, sear the roast on all sides, about 5 minutes per side.

2. Mix the broth, both kinds of onion, ginger, tamari, fish sauce, garlic, and honey in a high-powered blender until mostly smooth.

3. Place the roast in a slow cooker. Pour the liquid from the blender over the top, cover, and cook on high for 5 to 6 hours, until the roast is very tender. Remove from the slow cooker and shred the meat with 2 forks, discarding the bone.

4. To serve, carefully remove 10 outer cabbage leaves and place them on a platter in a single layer so they resemble small bowls. Fill each with ½ cup (120 ml) of the shredded meat and 2 tablespoons of the kimchi.

CALORIES: 226	FAT: 12 G
CARBOHYDRATE: 9 G	PROTEIN: 19 G

A 5-pound (2.25 k) bone-in beef roast

2 tablespoons (30 ml) kosher salt

2 teaspoons (10 ml) black pepper

2 tablespoons (30 ml) avocado oil

1 cup (240 ml) beef broth

½ yellow onion, roughly chopped

3 green onions, roughly chopped

A 1-inch (2.5 cm) piece of fresh ginger, peeled and chopped

¼ cup (60 ml) tamari (gluten-free soy sauce)

2 tablespoons (30 ml) Thai or Vietnamese fish sauce

6 garlic cloves, smashed

1 tablespoon (15 ml) honey

1 small head of green or red cabbage

1 jar prepared kimchi, any flavor

Chicken (or Turkey) and Broccoli Casserole

Makes 6 servings

This recipe is great if you are craving something that tastes of traditional home cooking. You can also use leftover broccoli and rotisserie chicken to make this meal in a flash.

1. Preheat the oven to 425°F (220°C). Toss the broccoli florets with 1½ tablespoons (22 ml) avocado oil and spread on a rimmed baking sheet. Sprinkle with 1 teaspoon (5 ml) salt. Bake for 10 minutes, until just tender.

2. Melt the butter in a medium skillet and add the mushrooms. Sauté over medium heat until soft, about 4 minutes, then add the garlic and cook for 1 minute. Stir in the chicken and artichokes. When warmed through, remove from the heat.

3. Reduce the oven temperature to 350°F (180°C). Stir the broccoli into the chicken.

4. In a small bowl, whisk together the coconut milk, broth, eggs, remaining 1 teaspoon salt, the pepper, and nutmeg.

5. Use the remaining ½ tablespoon avocado oil to lightly grease a small casserole dish. Place the chicken and vegetables in the dish, spread out evenly, and pour the egg mixture over the top, making sure to get it into all the spaces and gaps.

6. Bake the casserole for 30 minutes. Sprinkle the cheese evenly over the top and cook for 10 minutes more. Let rest 5 to 10 minutes before serving.

CALORIES: 453	FAT: 33 G
CARBOHYDRATE: 9 G	PROTEIN: 31 G

2 cups (300 g) broccoli florets
2 tablespoons (30 ml) avocado oil
2 teaspoons (5 ml) kosher salt
2 tablespoons (30 g) butter
8 ounces (225 g) button
    mushrooms, sliced
1 garlic clove, minced
3 cups (approximately 750 g) diced
    cooked chicken or turkey
1 small jar (approximately 6 ounces;
    170 g) artichoke hearts packed
    in water (not oil), drained and
    roughly chopped
1 cup (250 ml) full-fat coconut milk
1 cup (250 ml) chicken broth,
    preferably homemade (see
    page 216)
2 large eggs
½ teaspoon (2 ml) black pepper
½ teaspoon (2 ml) ground nutmeg
1 cup (90 g) grated Parmesan
    cheese

Dirty Cauliflower Rice

Makes 6 servings

You might already know how great cauliflower rice is, but I bet you've never had it like this! The chicken livers blend nicely with the strong flavors of the sausage and the spices without delivering too "livery" a taste for those who aren't the biggest fans of chicken liver (but you can omit the liver, if you must).

1. Heat the oil a large skillet over medium-high heat. Add half the sausage slices in a single layer and brown on both sides, about 5 minutes; repeat with remaining sausage slices. Place cooked sausage in a bowl and set aside.

2. Remove any stringy or membranous parts from the livers and roughly chop them into bite-size pieces. Melt the butter in the oil already in the pan. Add the chicken livers and cook until browned, 2 to 3 minutes per side. Remove from pan.

3. Add the onion, celery, and bell pepper to the pan and sauté about 5 minutes, until vegetables start to soften. Add the garlic and sauté another minute.

4. Add the grated cauliflower to the pan. Combine the paprika, oregano, thyme, salt, and pepper in a small bowl, then add to the cauliflower, mixing well. Reduce the heat to medium and cook 3 to 4 minutes.

5. Add the liver and sausages back to the pan. Stir in the broth, and cook until the cauliflower is just tender but not mushy. Taste and adjust salt, if needed.

6. Top each serving with a dollop (2 tablespoons, or 30 ml) of sour cream.

CALORIES: 432	FAT: 33 G
CARBOHYDRATE: 11 G	PROTEIN: 23 G

1 tablespoon (15 ml) avocado oil

4 andouille sausages (approximately 12 ounces; 340 g) sliced ¼ inch (6 mm) thick

8 ounces (230 g) chicken livers

1 tablespoon (15 g) butter

½ cup (120 ml) diced onion

½ cup (120 ml) diced celery

1 green bell pepper, diced

3 garlic cloves, minced

1 medium cauliflower, grated (see page 266), about 4 cups (600 g)

1 tablespoon (15 ml) smoked paprika (or sweet, if you prefer)

1 tablespoon (15 ml) dried oregano, crushed

1 teaspoon (5 ml) dried thyme

1 teaspoon (5 ml) salt

½ teaspoon (2 ml) black pepper

½ cup (120 ml) chicken broth, preferably homemade (see page 216)

Sour cream

Tilapia Bake

Makes 4 servings

Cheese and fish aren't two things you necessarily associate with each other, but this combo really works.

CALORIES: 318	FAT: 20 G
CARBOHYDRATE: 5 G	PROTEIN: 27 G

1. Preheat the oven to 425°F (220°C). Season the tilapia fillets with ½ teaspoon (2 ml) each of the salt and pepper.

2. In a large skillet, melt 2 tablespoons (30 ml) of the butter over medium-high heat. Add the leeks and sauté a few minutes, until soft but not brown. Add the spinach a handful at a time; the spinach will reduce in volume by a lot. Add the cream and the parsley, oregano, and red pepper flakes, as well as the remaining ½ teaspoon (2 ml) each salt and pepper. Reduce the heat to medium low and simmer, stirring frequently, until the mixture thickens a bit.

3. Use the remaining 1 teaspoon (5 g) butter to lightly grease a small glass baking dish. Transfer three-fourths of the spinach mixture to the baking dish and arrange the fish in a single layer on top. Layer the rest of the spinach on top. Sprinkle the feta evenly over and bake for 20 to 25 minutes, or until the fish is cooked through.

3 medium or 4 small tilapia fillets (approximately 1 pound total; 450 g)
1 teaspoon (5 ml) kosher salt
1 teaspoon (5 ml) black pepper
2 tablespoons plus 1 teaspoon (35 g) butter
1 medium leek, white part thinly sliced (¾ cup; 175 ml)
10 ounces (284 g) baby spinach
¼ cup (60 ml) heavy cream
½ teaspoon (2 ml) dried parsley
½ teaspoon (2 ml) dried oregano
¼ teaspoon (1 ml) red pepper flakes
1 cup (250 ml) crumbled feta cheese

Thai Soup with Shrimp

Makes 4 servings

I love the slight spiciness of this soup paired with the lime and the creamy coconut milk. If you are one of those people who thinks cilantro tastes like soap (did you know that's a genetic trait?), simply omit it from the recipe.

1. In a small bowl, combine the salt, pepper, turmeric, cumin, and cinnamon.

2. In a stockpot, melt the coconut oil. Add the green onions and ginger and sauté until fragrant, about 2 minutes. Add the spice mix and stir. Cook about 30 seconds.

3. Slowly pour in the chicken broth, stirring continuously. Add the tamari, fish sauce, and red pepper flakes. Bring to a boil, then reduce to a simmer. Simmer for 5 minutes.

4. Whisk in the coconut milk. Bring to simmer again, then add the shrimp and simmer approximately 5 minutes, or until the shrimp is just cooked through.

5. Remove from the heat. Stir in the lime juice and cilantro. Ladle into 4 individual bowls and top each bowl with one-fourth of the diced avocado.

CALORIES: 464	FAT: 40 G
CARBOHYDRATE: 15 G	PROTEIN: 11 G

1 teaspoon (5 ml) kosher salt

1 teaspoon (5 ml) black pepper

1 teaspoon (5 ml) ground turmeric

½ teaspoon (2 ml) ground cumin

¼ teaspoon (1 ml) ground cinnamon

2 tablespoons (30 ml) coconut oil

4 green onions, trimmed and chopped

1 tablespoon (15 ml) grated or finely minced fresh ginger

3 cups (700 ml) chicken broth, preferably homemade (see page 216)

2 tablespoons (30 ml) tamari (gluten-free soy sauce)

1 teaspoon (5 ml) Thai or Vietnamese fish sauce

½ teaspoon (2 ml) red pepper flakes

1 can (14 ounces; 400 ml) full-fat coconut milk

12 medium shrimp (60 g), peeled and deveined

Juice of 1 lime

¼ cup (75 g) fresh cilantro leaves (optional)

1 large avocado, diced

Cashew Beef

Makes 4 servings

This simple, satisfying version of cashew beef is easy to whip up when you're hit with a craving for Chinese food. Serve over Cauliflower Rice (page 266).

1. In a small bowl, whisk together the tamari, almond butter, sesame oil, and red pepper flakes.

2. Heat the avocado oil in a large wok or pan over medium-high heat. Add the steak strips and cook 2 minutes; flip, add the zucchini, and cook 2 minutes more.

3. Add the garlic and green onions. Cook for about 1 minute.

4. Add the sauce and stir to coat. Cook 2 minutes more, or until the zucchini is soft but not mushy.

5. Remove from heat. Stir in the cashews and serve immediately.

CALORIES: 429	FAT: 25 G
CARBOHYDRATE: 6 G	PROTEIN: 44 G

½ cup (120 ml) tamari (gluten-free soy sauce)

¼ cup (60 ml) raw almond butter

1 tablespoon (15 ml) toasted sesame oil

½ teaspoon (2 ml) red pepper flakes (optional)

2 tablespoons (30 ml) avocado oil

1½ pounds (680 g) flank steak, cut against the grain into thin slices

2 medium zucchini, cut into ¼-inch (6 mm) slices

1 garlic clove, minced

3 green onions, trimmed and thinly sliced

1 cup (150 g) raw cashews, whole or chopped

Pan-Fried Cod with Dill Caper Sauce

Makes 6 servings

I like to keep a homemade sauce on hand—whether it's this minty dill caper sauce, the Pea-NOT Sauce (page 219), a pesto, or a chimichurri—to add to meats and vegetables so meals don't become monotonous. This sauce keeps well in the fridge, so you can make a big batch ahead of time and have this dish done in five minutes. Leftover sauce is great over roasted carrots, too.

1. Prepare the sauce first, even a day or two before. Combine the capers, dill, olive oil, and lemon juice in a jar with a tight-fitting lid. Shake vigorously. If you want to make it more of a sauce than a dressing, you can also pulse the mixture a few times in a food processor or with an immersion blender. Taste and add salt and pepper as needed.

2. Season both sides of the fish with salt and pepper. Heat a large skillet over medium heat. Add the butter and avocado oil, and heat until the butter bubbles; swirl the pan to combine. Add the fish and cook about 2 minutes, depending on thickness. Carefully flip to brown the other side and squeeze the lemon juice over the fish. Cook for 1 to 2 minutes more. Do not overcook.

3. Remove the fish from pan, transfer to a serving platter, and spoon 2 tablespoons sauce over each serving.

CALORIES: 336	FAT: 24 G
CARBOHYDRATE: 10 G	PROTEIN: 19 G

DILL CAPER SAUCE
¼ cup (60 ml) drained capers
1 tablespoon (15 ml) chopped fresh dill
¼ cup (60 ml) extra-virgin olive oil
Juice from 1 small lemon
Salt and pepper to taste

FISH
1½ pounds (680 g) cod fillets, or any other mild white fish
Salt and pepper to taste
1 tablespoon (15 g) butter
2 teaspoons (10 ml) avocado oil
Juice of ½ lemon

Braised Chicken with Olives

Makes 6 servings

You can use any cuts of chicken in this recipe, but I really think bone-in, skin-on chicken thighs (or thighs and drumsticks) are best. Chicken thighs braise beautifully, whereas breasts can become dry. Bone-in cuts will be the most flavorful, plus you can save the bones to use in bone broth (see page 216); just freeze the bones if you aren't making a batch of broth very soon.

CALORIES: 368	FAT: 26 G
CARBOHYDRATE: 7 G	PROTEIN: 27 G

6 bone-in, skin-on chicken thighs (approximately 2 pounds; 900g)

2 teaspoons (10 ml) kosher salt

Freshly ground black pepper

3 tablespoons (45 ml) avocado oil, or more as needed

1 small onion, halved and thinly sliced (approximately ½ cup; 70 g)

4 garlic cloves, chopped

2 teaspoons (10 ml) ground cumin

1 teaspoon (5 ml) smoked paprika

1 teaspoon (5 ml) ground ginger

1 teaspoon (5 ml) ground cinnamon, or 2 cinnamon sticks (optional)

2 cups (500 ml) chicken broth, preferably homemade (see page 216)

1 dried bay leaf

2 lemons, preferably Meyer lemons

1 cup (250 ml) pitted olives (any kind—green, black, kalamata, or a mix)

1. Season the tops of the chicken thighs with 1 teaspoon (2 ml) salt and some pepper. In a large skillet, heat the oil over medium-high heat until quite hot. Place the chicken skin side down in the hot oil and let cook for 3 to 5 minutes without moving. Season the chicken with more salt and pepper, then flip and sear the underside for another 3 minutes or so.

2. Remove the chicken to a plate. Add more oil if the pan is too dry and reduce the heat to medium. Add the onion and sauté for 5 minutes, until soft. Add the garlic and sauté for 1 minute. Add the cumin, paprika, and ginger, as well as the ground cinnamon, if using, and stir well. (If using cinnamon sticks, add them later.)

3. Slowly add the broth, scraping up any browned particles. Turn the heat to medium high, return the chicken to the pan, and pour back in any juice that collected on the plate. Add the bay leaf and cinnamon sticks, if using, to the broth.

4. Cut one of the lemons into wedges and nestle those wedges among the chicken thighs. Scatter the olives evenly over the top of the chicken. Squeeze the juice from the other lemon over everything.

5. Allow the liquid to come to a boil, then reduce to a low simmer. Cover and simmer 30 minutes. Discard the bay leaf and cinnamon sticks. Serve the chicken thighs with sauce from the pan spooned over.

Macadamia-Crusted Mahi-Mahi with Browned Butter

Makes 4 servings

Whenever you eat seafood, check out seafoodwatch .org to find the most up-to-date recommendations for selecting the healthiest and most eco-friendly options. Mahi-mahi is a relatively mild white fish that is thicker than cod or tilapia, so it is perfect for this treatment. If you can find opah in your local market, that also works wonderfully in this dish.

CALORIES: 852	FAT: 74 G
CARBOHYDRATE: 8 G	PROTEIN: 43 G

1 cup (120 g) raw macadamias
3 tablespoons (45 ml) coconut flour
½ teaspoon (2 ml) kosher salt
½ teaspoon (2 ml) black pepper
½ teaspoon (2 ml) garlic powder
½ cup (120 ml) Primal Kitchen Mayo (see Note, page 197), or other primal-approved mayo
4 mahi-mahi fillets, 6 to 8 ounces each (150 g)
½ cup (120 ml) salted grassfed butter, cut into 8 pats

1. Preheat the oven to 425°F (220°C). Lightly grease a glass casserole dish with a little coconut or avocado oil. Place the fish in the casserole dish.

2. Put the macadamia nuts in a food processor and pulse until finely chopped, but do not allow to become a paste. Add the coconut flour, salt, pepper, and garlic powder, and pulse a few times to mix well.

3. Spread the mayo evenly on the fish. Carefully coat each with the nut mixture, gently pressing into the mayo to adhere. Bake for 25 minutes.

4. Place the butter in a small saucepan over medium heat. Cook, stirring frequently, until lightly browned, about 5 minutes.

5. Remove the fish from the oven. Pour the browned butter directly over fish and serve. Alternatively, serve the butter in small ramekins alongside the fish.

NOTE: Browned butter is quite easy to make, but it can burn. After you brown the butter, do not leave it in the hot pan. Pour it into a bowl until ready to serve.

Buffalo Chicken Salad

Makes 4 servings

This salad is super easy to make with leftover or rotisserie chicken. You can serve it over a bed of kale or lettuce, wrapped in collard greens, or on top of a roasted sweet potato if you want some extra carbs.

CALORIES: 487	FAT: 36 G
CARBOHYDRATE: 9 G	PROTEIN: 31 G

8 ounces (225 g) cream cheese

1 cup (90 g) blue cheese crumbles

2 cups (500 g) shredded cooked chicken

2 celery stalks, sliced

1 large carrot, diced small

½ teaspoon (2 ml) kosher salt, or more as needed

¼ teaspoon (1 ml) black pepper, or more as needed

¼ cup (60 ml) hot sauce (see Note)

1. Place the cream cheese in a microwave-safe bowl and microwave 20 seconds. Stir and continue to microwave in 10-second increments until soft but not totally melted. Stir in the blue cheese, then add the chicken, celery, carrot, salt, and pepper. Stir well.

2. Add half the hot sauce and stir well. Taste and, if desired, add the rest of the hot sauce. Adjust salt and pepper as needed. Salad can be served warm or cold.

NOTE: Be sure to look for a hot sauce that doesn't contain objectionable ingredients. Cholula brand is one. Some will be hotter than others, which is why I recommend starting with only a couple tablespoons of hot sauce the first time you make this recipe.

Crab-Stuffed Portabello Mushrooms

Makes 2 servings

Once you know the basics of preparing stuffed portabello mushrooms, you can make any number of variations depending on what you like. For this recipe, if crab isn't your thing, try substituting shredded chicken.

1. Preheat the oven to 400°F (200° C). Grease a small casserole dish with 1 teaspoon (5 ml) of avocado oil. Place the mushrooms gill side down in the dish. Brush the caps with the remaining 2 tablespoons (30 ml) avocado oil and sprinkle with salt and pepper. Roast for 12 minutes.

2. Meanwhile, melt the butter in a small skillet, and sauté the shallot until soft, about 3 minutes.

3. In a medium bowl, combine the crabmeat, cream cheese, mayo, lemon juice, half the Parmesan cheese, the sautéed shallot, chives, ½ teaspoon (2 ml) salt, and red pepper flakes.

4. Remove the mushroom caps from the oven and flip gill side up. Divide the crab mixture evenly between the two caps, mounding the filling and spreading gently to the edges. Sprinkle the remaining Parmesan cheese over the tops. Bake for 10 minutes more.

CALORIES: 796	FAT: 68 G
CARBOHYDRATE: 10 G	PROTEIN: 36 G

2 tablespoons plus 1 teaspoon (35 ml) avocado oil

2 large portabello mushroom caps

Salt and pepper

2 tablespoons (30 g) butter

1 shallot, thinly sliced

½ pound (230 g) lump crabmeat

8 ounces (225 g) cream cheese, softened

¼ cup (60 ml) Primal Kitchen Mayo (see Note, page 197), or other primal-approved mayo

Juice of 1 small lemon (approximately 2 tablespoons; 30 ml)

2/3 cup (165 g) grated Parmesan cheese

2 tablespoons (30 ml) minced fresh chives

¼ teaspoon (1 ml) red pepper flakes (optional)

VEGGIES, SALADS, AND SIDES

Bigass Salad
Makes 1 serving

I eat some version of this salad nearly every day for lunch or dinner. Of course, you can add or subtract elements to customize it to your own taste. I often dress it simply with just a splash of olive oil for a serving of healthy fat, but also try it with one of the salad dressings from page 221.

1. In a large, shallow bowl, layer lettuce, veggies, and cheese in that order. Flake the tuna over the top.

2. When you are ready to eat, sprinkle the nuts and seeds over the top, and drizzle with the olive oil.

CALORIES: 843	FAT: 63 G
CARBOHYDRATE: 24 G	PROTEIN: 54 G

3 to 4 cups (150 to 200 g) lettuce or mixed greens
1 to 2 cups (75 to 100 g) sliced veggies (mushrooms, bell pepper, zucchini, carrots, broccoli, beets)
¼ cup (30 g) shredded cheddar cheese (optional)
1 can (5 ounces; 142 g) tuna packed in water, drained
¼ cup (28 g) nuts (walnuts, pecans, almonds)
2 tablespoons (30 ml) sunflower or pumpkin seeds
2 tablespoons (30 ml) olive oil

Spinach Salad with Warm Bacon Vinaigrette

Makes 1 serving

This simple salad is great as a light lunch or as an accompaniment to a juicy steak dinner.

1. Whisk together the reserved bacon fat and the balsamic vinegar to make the dressing. Taste and season with salt and pepper, if needed.

2. In a medium bowl, toss the spinach and red onion with the dressing until coated. Transfer to a serving plate. Top with the crumbled bacon, mushrooms, and tomatoes. Finish with a pinch of freshly ground black pepper.

CALORIES: 335	FAT: 30 G
CARBOHYDRATE: 9 G	PROTEIN: 7 G

1 slice bacon, cooked until crispy and crumbled, with 2 tablespoons fat reserved

1 tablespoon (15 ml) balsamic vinegar

Salt and pepper to taste

2 cups (56 g) raw baby spinach

1/8 cup (20 g) sliced red onion

¼ cup (18 g) thinly sliced button mushrooms

¼ cup (37 g) cherry tomatoes, halved

Primal Coleslaw

Makes about 4 cups as a side dish; serving size = ½ cup

Most coleslaw recipes use sugar in the dressing, but omitting it yields a wonderful tangy slaw that is satisfying without being sweet. It also allows the natural sweetness of the vegetables to come through.

1. Combine the mayo, sour cream, vinegar, caraway seeds, celery salt, and mustard in a large bowl.

2. Add the cabbage and the carrots to the dressing and stir well to coat completely. Refrigerate at least 1 hour. Taste and adjust with salt and pepper before serving.

CALORIES: 204	FAT: 20 G
CARBOHYDRATE: 5 G	PROTEIN: 1 G

¾ cup (180 ml) Primal Kitchen Mayo (see Note, page 197) or other primal-approved mayo

¼ cup (60 ml) sour cream

2 tablespoons (30 ml) apple cider vinegar

1 teaspoon (5 ml) caraway seeds

1 teaspoon (5 ml) celery salt

½ teaspoon (2 ml) dry mustard

1 medium head of napa green cabbage, shredded (4 to 5 cups; approximately 300 g)

3 medium carrots, grated

Salt and pepper to taste

Zucchini Noodles with Arugula Pesto

Makes 4 side servings

Once you have cut pasta from your diet, it's worth investing in a vegetable spiral cutter—a.k.a. a spiralizer—to make veggie noodles instead. There are several relatively affordable versions on the market. If you don't have a spiral cutter, though, you can julienne the vegetables with a julienne peeler. This recipe calls for zucchini noodles, but you can substitute turnip, rutabaga, or even sweet potato noodles on a higher carb day. To turn this into a complete meal, simply brown 1 pound (450 g) of ground chicken or turkey to toss on top.

1. Place the zucchini noodles in a large mesh sieve and toss generously with salt. Place the sieve over a bowl and allow to stand for 20 minutes to drain. Do not skip this step—it helps keep noodles from turning mushy!

2. Rinse the noodles under running water. Shake off excess water. Place the noodles on a large, clean kitchen towel, roll up, and apply gentle pressure to squeeze out extra moisture. Return the noodles to the sieve and place in the refrigerator uncovered.

3. To make the pesto, put the arugula, macadamias, and garlic in a food processor. Pulse until the mixture resembles coarse sand, scraping down the sides of the bowl as needed. Add the avocado and cheese, along with the salt and pepper, and blend for 15 seconds. Scrape the sides again. With the food processor running, slowly add the olive oil.

4. Remove the noodles from the fridge. If still very moist, roll one more time in a clean kitchen towel. Melt the butter in a large skillet, then add the noodles. Cook without disturbing for 1 minute, stir, and cook for 1 minute more. Remove from the heat. Add the pesto and gently toss to coat. Serve immediately, or refrigerate and serve cold.

CALORIES: 492	FAT: 48 G
CARBOHYDRATE: 10 G	PROTEIN: 5 G

2 medium zucchini, cut into thin noodles
Kosher salt
2 cups (75 g) arugula
¼ cup (30 g) macadamias
2 garlic cloves, roughly chopped
½ small avocado
¼ cup (60 ml) shredded Romano cheese
¼ teaspoon (1 ml) salt
¼ teaspoon (1 ml) black pepper
½ cup (120 ml) extra-virgin olive oil
2 tablespoons (30 g) butter

Sautéed Cabbage with Bacon

Makes 4 side servings

I had you at "bacon," right?

1. With a very sharp knife, cut the cabbage into quarters; cut out and discard the core. Chop the cabbage into narrow strips.

2. Use kitchen shears to cut the bacon into small pieces.

3. Heat a large skillet over medium-high heat. Add the bacon and cook until it begins to crisp. Add the leek and onion. Cook, stirring frequently, until the vegetables are browned, about 3 minutes. Add the garlic and cook for another minute.

4. Stir in the cabbage, salt, pepper, and paprika. Stir and cook about 10 minutes. Serve now, or reduce the heat to low, cover, and cook 30 minutes more, stirring occasionally. The latter option results in much softer cabbage with a deeper bacon flavor.

CALORIES: 149	FAT: 5 G
CARBOHYDRATE: 20 G	PROTEIN: 8 G

1 medium head of green cabbage
6 slices bacon (no sugar added)
1 large leek, white part sliced
½ cup (120 ml) chopped onion
3 garlic cloves, minced
2 teaspoons (10 ml) kosher salt
1 teaspoon (5 ml) black pepper
½ teaspoon (2 ml) sweet paprika

Veggie Sushi with Cauliflower Rice

Makes 4 side servings

These rolls are perfect finger food to bring to a party where you suspect there won't be many keto-friendly options. Just make plenty to share or else you won't get any! The recipe calls for dulse, which is a type of dried seaweed that has a bacony flavor. It is easy to find online, or check your local Asian market. You can wrap up almost any vegetables in these rolls. I picked some of our favorites for this recipe. The beets give the rice a pleasing pink hue.

1. Prepare the cauliflower rice according to Option 2 on page 266. Mix the vinegar and stevia in a small bowl and add to the rice while the rice is still warm. Stir in the dulse. Taste and add salt, if desired. Place in a large metal sieve over a bowl and allow to cool, stirring every few minutes with a fork to keep the rice from sticking to itself. Liquid might or might not drain out.

2. Whisk the ingredients for the dipping sauce in a small bowl.

3. Trim the woody ends off the asparagus and steam for 4 minutes. (You can use the same water and pot you used for the cauliflower.) It should still be a little crunchy.

4. Place 1 sheet of nori shiny side down on a bamboo roller (use wax paper or plastic wrap if you don't have one). Very gently spread ¼ cup (56 g) cream cheese thinly on the nori, leaving at least 1 inch of space at the top and bottom. Make sure to cover all the way across left to right.

5. Add approximately ¾ cup (175 ml) of cauliflower rice and press into a rectangle to cover the nori evenly, leaving the 1-inch space at the top and

CALORIES: 342	FAT: 27 G
CARBOHYDRATE: 23 G	PROTEIN: 11 G

1 small cauliflower, or ½ a large cauliflower

1 tablespoon (15 ml) vinegar (see Note)

2 drops liquid stevia (optional)

1 tablespoon (15 ml) dulse flakes (see Note), minced

Salt

6 asparagus stalks

3 sheets of nori

¾ cup (168 g) cream cheese, softened

1 ripe avocado, cut into thin slices

1 small raw beet, peeled and shredded

3 radishes, shredded

DIPPING SAUCE

¼ cup (60 ml) tamari (gluten-free soy sauce)

2 tablespoons (30 ml) Pea-NOT Sauce (page 219), or raw almond butter plus ½ teaspoon (2 ml) lime juice

⅛ teaspoon (0.5 ml) red pepper flakes

bottom. (If the layer of rice is too thick, remove a couple spoonfuls and smooth it out again.)

6. Add one-third of the asparagus, avocado, beet, and radishes in "stripes" all the way across from left to right. You might need to trim the asparagus to make it fit.

7. Dab water across the top side of the nori, then start with the bottom and roll tightly without tearing the nori. When you get to the top, press the seam gently with damp fingers to seal. Place the roll seam side down on a wooden cutting board. Assemble the other two rolls in the same manner.

8. Slice the rolls into pieces using a sharp knife. Serve with the dipping sauce.

NOTE: If you have coconut vinegar in your pantry, use that here. Or you can use rice vinegar, but make sure there is no sugar added, or use apple cider vinegar.

If you don't have dulse on hand, you can substitute another type of dried seaweed or a seasoning blend that contains seaweed, or add ½ teaspoon salt.

Cauliflower Rice

Makes 4 side servings

When you go primal, paleo, or keto, you should definitely learn how to make cauliflower rice. It's the perfect substitute for white or brown rice in almost any dish. (You can even make cauliflower rice sushi rolls; see page 264.) There are multiple ways to prepare cauliflower rice. Experiment to see which you like best.

Option 1: Start with raw cauliflower and rice it in a food processor before cooking. You can do this using either the shredding blade or, working in small batches, a chopping blade. But for the most consistent, rice-like pieces, use both blades.

1. Cut the raw cauliflower into florets. Attach the shredding blade to the food processor and shred the cauliflower. Transfer to a bowl.

2. Swap the shredding blade for the chopping blade. Working in batches, pulse the shredded cauliflower a few times until pieces are smaller.

3. Cook as directed if you are following a specific recipe. For plain rice, sauté the cauliflower in a large skillet, or spread it on a heavy rimmed baking sheet and cook it for a few minutes under the broiler until toasted. Season as desired.

Option 2: Steam the cauliflower first, then rice it. This creates less mess than the first option, but it also doesn't allow you to flavor the rice as much when you cook it. You can cut the cauliflower into florets first or, for the least messy option, steam the cauliflower whole.

1. Place a steamer basket in a large pot with 1 to 2 inches of water in the bottom. Bring the water to

CALORIES: 53	FAT: 0 G
CARBOHYDRATE: 10 G	PROTEIN: 4 G

1 small cauliflower

a boil. Place the cauliflower in a steamer basket, cover the pot, and steam 3 to 5 minutes, until just becoming tender when you poke it with a fork. It should not be too soft.

2. Remove the cauliflower from the steamer. Allow to cool for a few minutes. If you steamed the whole cauliflower, cut into florets. Working in batches, pulse the florets in a food processor fitted with a chopping blade until it is a rice-like consistency. If you don't have a food processor, you can finely chop the cauliflower with a knife. Season as desired.

Option 3: If you don't have a food processor, you can use a box grater to grate the raw cauliflower. Be advised that this will make quite a big mess, but the finished product will have the right texture. Cook as described in Option 1.

Creamy Gorgonzola "Mac" and Cheese

Makes 6 side servings

Spaghetti squash is a vegetable you should get to know if it's not already a staple in your kitchen. It can be used in endless ways in place of noodles in Italian, Thai, and other cuisines. The easiest way to cook it is in an Instant Pot pressure cooker, but it can also be roasted in the oven or steamed. Either way it's delicious. After it is cooked, use a fork to pull the pulp into strands that you can use like pasta.

CALORIES: 407	FAT: 34 G
CARBOHYDRATE: 9 G	PROTEIN: 17 G

4 ounces (112 g) cream cheese, at room temperature

4 large eggs, lightly beaten

½ cup (120 ml) heavy cream

1 cup (90 g) crumbled Gorgonzola cheese

1 cup (90 g) shredded cheddar cheese, preferably white cheddar

1 teaspoon (5 ml) salt

1 teaspoon (5 ml) black pepper

4 cups (1 k) strands of cooked spaghetti squash

1. Preheat the oven to 350°F (180°C).

2. Place the cream cheese in a large glass bowl and microwave on high in 10 second increments to soften. Add the eggs and cream, and beat together. Add the Gorgonzola and ½ cup of the cheddar cheese, plus the salt and pepper, and mix well.

3. If the spaghetti squash is very wet, place it in a metal sieve and gently press on it with a wooden spoon to squeeze out the remaining moisture or place it on a clean kitchen towel, roll it up, and press gently.

4. Add the spaghetti squash to the cheese mixture and stir very well.

5. Transfer to a casserole dish, smooth the top, and sprinkle with the remaining cheddar cheese.

6. Bake for 40 minutes, or until hot and bubbly. Remove from the oven and let cool for at least 10 minutes before serving.

Massaged Kale Salad with Goat Cheese

Makes 6 side servings

Are you already massaging your kale? If not, you're missing out. Massaging the raw kale helps break down the leaves, making them less tough and bitter. Wear gloves if you have any cuts on your hands, or else the lemon juice and salt will hurt like heck!

1. Use a sharp knife to remove the thick stem from each kale leaf. Cut or tear the leaves into small, bite-size pieces. Place in a large bowl. Squeeze the juice from the lemon over the kale and sprinkle in the salt. With both hands, massage the kale by squeezing, kneading, and rolling it between your hands. Do this for about 1 minute. Be aggressive! You can't hurt the kale.

2. In a small jar with a lid, combine both oils, the vinegar, and a few grinds of black pepper. Secure the lid and shake well.

3. Pour the dressing over the kale and toss. Add the goat cheese and toss again.

4. Heat a small skillet over medium-low heat. Add the pine nuts to the dry skillet and cook, stirring frequently, until lightly browned.

5. Add the warm nuts to the salad and toss well. The nuts will slightly melt the goat cheese. Top with the avocado and serve.

CALORIES: 402	FAT: 35 G
CARBOHYDRATE: 9 G	PROTEIN: 15 G

1 bunch curly kale (green or purple)
1 medium lemon
1 teaspoon (5 ml) kosher salt
3 tablespoons (45 ml) extra-virgin olive oil
1 tablespoon (15 ml) walnut oil
1 tablespoon (15 ml) balsamic vinegar
Freshly ground black pepper
11 ounces (320 g) goat cheese (1 large log), crumbled
½ cup (60 g) raw pine nuts
1 large avocado, cubed

Herbalicious Shredded Salad with Tahini Dressing

Makes 4 side servings

Tahini is a paste made from sesame seeds. It's a staple of Middle Eastern cuisine and is popular in many other regional cuisines as well. You can assemble this flavor-packed salad incredibly quickly if you buy bagged shredded vegetables from the grocery store, but you can also make fresh shredded vegetables very easily if you have a food processor. It's a great way to use broccoli stems you might otherwise toss. Add a small carrot and some radishes, and you're good to go.

1. Make the dressing first by combining all the ingredients in a high-powered blender or food processor. Slowly add warm water until dressing reaches the desired consistency. It should be thick but pourable.

2. Finely chop the cilantro and parsley together. In a large bowl, mix the herbs with the broccoli slaw.

3. Pour in the dressing and stir well. Toss gently with the arugula, top with the avocado, and serve immediately.

CALORIES: 333	FAT: 29 G
CARBOHYDRATE: 12 G	PROTEIN: 6 G

TAHINI DRESSING
¼ cup (60 ml) tahini
¼ cup (60 ml) extra-virgin olive oil
2 tablespoons (30 ml) tamari (gluten-free soy sauce)
2 tablespoons (30 ml) lemon juice
1 garlic clove, pressed or finely minced
¼ teaspoon (1 ml) ground ginger

SALAD
½ cup (75 g) fresh cilantro
½ cup (75 g) fresh parsley
1 small (12 ounces; 340 g) bag broccoli slaw
2 cups (40 g) arugula
1 avocado, cubed

Cheesy Broccoli and Cauliflower Casserole

Makes 4 side servings

Many casseroles have a crunchy breadcrumb topping that obviously doesn't work on keto. This recipe contains a surprise ingredient to get the crunch without the carbs.

CALORIES: 461	FAT: 37 G
CARBOHYDRATE: 12 G	PROTEIN: 20 G

4 cups (600 g) broccoli florets
4 cups (600 g) cauliflower florets
2 tablespoons (30 g) butter
1 cup (250 ml) sour cream
1 cup (90 g) grated Gruyère cheese
1 tablespoon (15 ml) Dijon mustard
1 tablespoon (15 ml) dried thyme
1 teaspoon (5 ml) kosher salt
1 teaspoon (5 ml) black pepper
½ cup (45 g) grated Parmesan cheese
2 cups (180 g) crushed pork rinds or pork rind crumbs

1. Preheat the oven to 375°F (190°C).

2. Chop the broccoli and cauliflower florets into smaller pieces. Melt the butter in a skillet over medium-high heat. Add the broccoli and cauliflower, and let sit undisturbed about 2 minutes. Stir and let sit undisturbed another couple minutes. When the brown bits begin to form, remove from the heat.

3. In a medium bowl, mix the sour cream, Gruyère, mustard, thyme, salt, and pepper. Stir in the veggies. Transfer the mixture to a casserole dish and sprinkle the Parmesan on top.

4. Bake for 20 minutes. Remove from the oven and sprinkle the pork rinds evenly over top. Return to the oven and bake another 10 to 15 minutes, until the top is crunchy and the casserole is bubbling around the edges.

Green Bean Casserole

Makes 8 side servings

This is a healthier version of the traditional Thanksgiving side dish made with canned soup and canned fried onions. If you want to make it dairy-free, omit the sour cream and double the coconut milk.

CALORIES: 334	FAT: 23 G
CARBOHYDRATE: 8 G	PROTEIN: 24 G

1. Preheat the oven to 350°F (180°C).

2. Cut the onion in half and dice half the onion (you will use the other half later). Heat 2 tablespoons (30 ml) of the coconut oil over medium-high heat in a large skillet. Add the diced onion to the skillet and sauté until just soft, about 3 minutes. Add the ground beef and brown, about 5 minutes.

3. Clear a small space in middle of the skillet and sauté the garlic for 1 minute. Stir the garlic into the meat, and add half the salt and pepper. Stir in the green beans and transfer to a large bowl.

4. Turn the heat down to medium. In the same skillet, melt 2 tablespoons (30 ml) of the butter. Add the mushrooms and sauté until soft, about 5 minutes. Season with the remaining salt and pepper.

5. Turn the heat back up to medium high. Deglaze the pan with ½ cup (120 ml) chicken broth. Stir in the rest of the broth and bring to a low boil. Whisk in the coconut milk and sour cream, and reduce the heat to low. Simmer 5 minutes. (If the sauce is still very thin, scoop out about ½ cup [120 ml] of sauce into a bowl, whisk in the arrowroot powder, and then slowly whisk this mixture back into the skillet.)

6. Pour the mushroom sauce over the meat and green beans, and stir to combine well. Transfer to a casserole dish and bake for 45 minutes, or until bubbling.

1 medium onion
4 tablespoons (60 ml) coconut oil
1½ pounds (680 g) ground beef
3 garlic cloves
1 teaspoon (5 ml) salt
½ teaspoon (2 ml) black pepper
1 pound (450 g) frozen green beans, thawed and drained
3 tablespoons (45 g) butter
2 cups (300 g) sliced cremini mushrooms
¾ cup (180 ml) chicken broth, preferably homemade (see page 216)
½ cup (120 ml) coconut milk
½ cup (120 ml) sour cream
1 tablespoon (15 ml) arrowroot powder or tapioca starch, if needed

7. While the casserole is baking, thinly slice the other half of the onion. Heat the remaining 1 tablespoon (15 g) butter in a clean skillet. Place the onion in the butter and do not stir for a minute. Stir gently and let cook undisturbed for another minute. Continue like this until browned.

8. When the casserole comes out of the oven, top with the cooked onions.

Perfect Roasted Brussels Sprouts

Makes 4 side servings

Lots of people think they don't like Brussels sprouts, but that is probably because they have only had boring boiled or steamed sprouts. When it comes to Brussels sprouts, roasting is the way to go. When selecting the sprouts, try to get ones that are similarly sized so they roast evenly.

1. Preheat the oven to 425°F (220°C). If your Brussels sprouts are very large, cut them in half.

2. Toss the Brussels sprouts in the bacon fat and vinegar. Spread on a large rimmed baking sheet and sprinkle with the salt.

3. Roast for 20 minutes, stir, and then roast for 10 minutes more. If the Brussels sprouts are not well browned, roast them for an additional 5 minutes and check again.

4. Melt the butter in a small saucepan. Add the garlic and sauté a couple minutes until soft. Place the roasted Brussels sprouts in a large bowl. Pour the garlic butter over and add the Parmesan. Stir to combine. Serve hot.

CALORIES: 235	FAT: 20 G
CARBOHYDRATE: 4 G	PROTEIN: 8 G

1 pound (450 g) Brussels sprouts, washed and trimmed

2 tablespoons (30 ml) bacon fat, melted (or avocado oil if you don't have any)

1 tablespoon (15 ml) balsamic vinegar

1 teaspoon (5 ml) kosher salt

3 tablespoons (45 g) butter

2 garlic cloves, minced

1 cup (90 g) shredded Parmesan cheese

Prosciutto-Wrapped Asparagus

Makes 4 side servings

This dish is a crowd pleaser and so simple to prepare. It's wonderful at brunch to accompany poached eggs and salmon, or with a steak at dinner.

1. Lightly grease a heavy baking sheet with the avocado oil. Trim the woody ends from the asparagus, cutting the stalks to approximately the same length. Cut the prosciutto slices in half lengthwise to create long strips.

2. Hold 2 or 3 stalks of asparagus together depending on how thick they are. Leaving just the tips of the stalks hanging out, start wrapping one strip of prosciutto diagonally around the asparagus bundle. Wrap tightly, but try not to tear the prosciutto; if it does tear, just overlap the ends and keep wrapping. Place the wrapped asparagus bundles on the baking sheet.

3. Preheat the broiler and place an oven rack about 4 inches below the heat. Grind some black pepper over the asparagus and sprinkle with salt. Place the asparagus in the broiler and watch carefully. After approximately 2 minutes, the prosciutto should be crisp. Flip the bundles, and cook on the second side for another minute.

4. Remove from oven and sprinkle with Parmesan cheese, if desired. Let cool for a couple minutes. These can be served warm or at room temperature.

(with Parmesan)

CALORIES: 191	FAT: 10 G
CARBOHYDRATE: 7 G	PROTEIN: 20 G

1 teaspoon (5 ml) avocado oil

1 bunch asparagus (approximately 1 pound; 450 g)

4 ounces (112 g) prosciutto

Freshly ground black pepper

Salt to taste

1 cup (90 g) shredded Parmesan cheese (optional)

Caesar Salad with Anchovies and Pancetta

Makes 2 side servings

Store-bought Caesar dressing is usually made with ob-jectionable oils, but luckily it's easy to make your own at home. This salad is great also topped with roasted chicken, steak, or shrimp for a main course.

CALORIES: 602	FAT: 53 G
CARBOHYDRATE: 5 G	PROTEIN: 28 G

1. In a high-powered blender, combine the egg yolk, garlic, Dijon mustard, lemon juice, salt, pepper, half the anchovies, and ¼ cup (60 ml) oil. Blend for 10 seconds. With the blender running, slowly pour in the remaining oil in a thin stream so the dressing emulsifies. Add in ½ cup (45 g) of the Parmesan cheese and pulse a few times to combine.

2. Melt the butter in a small skillet and sauté the pancetta until crisp.

3. Toss the lettuce with ½ cup (120 ml) of the dressing. Roughly chop the remaining anchovies and place on top. Sprinkle with the crispy pancetta. Top with Parmesan crisps (see Note) or the remaining grated Parmesan, and additional freshly ground pepper. If desired, drizzle with more dressing.

1 egg yolk, at room temperature

2 garlic cloves, chopped

2 teaspoons (10 ml) Dijon mustard

Juice from 1 large lemon, at room temperature

1 teaspoon (5 ml) kosher salt

½ teaspoon (2 ml) freshly ground black pepper, plus more as needed

1 can (2 ounces; 56 g) anchovies packed in olive oil

1 cup (250 ml) extra-virgin olive oil

1 cup (90 g) grated Parmesan cheese (see Note)

1 teaspoon (5 g) butter

4 ounces (165 g) diced pancetta

4 cups (roughly 400 g) chopped romaine lettuce

NOTE: If you want, whip up a batch of Parmesan Crisps (page 285) to use as "croutons" on the salad.

Whole Roasted Romanesco

Makes 6 side servings

This simple and elegant dish is perfect for highlighting the delicate flavor of romanesco. If you aren't familiar with romanesco, it is a brassica that looks like a spiky green cauliflower, but when you look closely, you'll see the little peaks are fractal in nature. You're most likely to find it in late fall and winter. Check your local farmers' markets.

CALORIES: 148	FAT: 15 G
CARBOHYDRATE: 4 G	PROTEIN: 1 G

1 large or 2 medium romanesco
6 tablespoons (90 g) butter, melted
Salt
Freshly ground black pepper

1. Trim away the bottom stem of the romanesco, but do not cut apart the florets. Place a steamer basket in a large stockpot with a couple inches of water. Bring to a boil, place the romanesco in the steamer basket, cover, and steam for 8 minutes.

2. Preheat the oven to 400°F (200°C).

3. Place the romanesco stem side down in a small casserole dish or cast iron skillet. Pour the melted butter evenly over the top and use a basting brush to make sure every surface is coated. Sprinkle with salt and pepper.

4. Roast for 20 minutes. Test the romanesco by piercing with a sharp knife. It is done if the tip goes easily into the center. If it is not done, baste with the butter in the bottom of the dish and put back in the oven, then test again after 5 minutes.

5. Transfer the romanesco to a platter, and pour the melted butter from the pan on top, then serve.

Spaghetti Squash "Pad Thai"

Makes 2 side servings

Cooked spaghetti squash and Pea-NOT Sauce are two things I often have in my fridge because I use them both in so many ways. This recipe is higher in carbs than some of the others, so I like to eat it on days when I'm very active.

1. In a large wok or skillet, melt the butter. Crack both eggs into the hot wok and quickly scramble. Remove to a small bowl.

2. Add the coconut oil, then the sugar snap peas, to the wok and stir-fry 1 minute. Add the tamari, stir, and place in another bowl.

3. Add the spaghetti squash to the wok and stir-fry until warm. Add the Pea-NOT Sauce and cook until warmed through. Put the sugar snap peas back in the wok and stir.

4. Divide the mixture into 2 serving bowls. Top each with half the scrambled eggs, the beans sprouts, and the raw almonds. Serve hot.

CALORIES: 685	FAT: 53 G
CARBOHYDRATE: 30 G	PROTEIN: 22 G

1 tablespoon (15 g) butter

2 large eggs

1 tablespoon (15 ml) coconut oil

1 cup (150 g) sugar snap peas

½ tablespoon (7.5 ml) tamari (gluten-free soy sauce)

2 cups (500 g) cooked spaghetti squash

½ cup (120 ml) Pea-NOT Sauce (page 219)

½ cup (75 g) bean sprouts

¼ cup (28 g) raw almonds, finely chopped

Baked Avocados, Two Ways

Makes 4 side servings

BASIC BAKED AVOCADOS

Avocados aren't just for guacamole and salads! Baking brings out a whole different side of them that you have to try.

1. Preheat the oven to 425°F (220°C). Cut the avocados in half lengthwise and remove the pits. Use a spoon to scoop approximately 1 tablespoon (15 ml) out of each half to create a bowl.

2. Place the avocados in a baking dish. If they won't stay put without rolling, roll up pieces of aluminum foil to create little holders for them to rest in.

3. Carefully crack one egg into each half, trying not to break the yolk. Sprinkle with the salt and pepper. Bake 15 to 20 minutes, or until the eggs are cooked to your liking. Serve hot.

CALORIES: 194	FAT: 16 G
CARBOHYDRATE: 6 G	PROTEIN: 8 G

2 large ripe avocados
4 medium eggs
½ teaspoon (2 ml) kosher salt or
    Tajin (see Note, page 197)
¼ teaspoon (1 ml) black pepper

NEXT LEVEL BAKED AVOCADOS

Makes 4 side servings

1. Preheat the oven to 425°F (220°C). Cut the avocados in half lengthwise and remove the pits. Use a spoon to scoop approximately 1 tablespoon (15 ml) out of each half to create a bowl.

2. Place the avocados in a baking dish. If they won't stay put without rolling, roll up pieces of aluminum foil to create little holders for them to rest in.

3. Whisk the eggs in a small bowl with the cream. Add the crumbled bacon, salt, and pepper. Spoon the egg mixture into the avocados.

4. Bake approximately 12 minutes or until the egg is just set. Remove from the oven and sprinkle the cheese evenly over the avocados. Bake 5 minutes more to lightly brown the tops.

CALORIES: 269	FAT: 23 G
CARBOHYDRATE: 7 G	PROTEIN: 12 G

2 large ripe avocados
2 medium eggs
1 tablespoon (15 ml) heavy cream
2 slices bacon, cooked until crispy
  and crumbled
½ teaspoon (2 ml) kosher salt
¼ teaspoon (1 ml) black pepper
¾ cup (65 g) shredded Monterey
  jack cheese

Lemony Pressure Cooker Artichokes with Aioli

Makes 2 side servings

Oven-roasted artichokes are delicious, but in the summer I prefer to use my electric pressure cooker to avoid heating up my kitchen. Serve these artichokes with the aioli here or simply with melted butter for dipping.

CALORIES: 257	FAT: 17 G
CARBOHYDRATE: 21 G	PROTEIN: 5 G

2 lemons

4 garlic cloves, pressed or finely minced

½ cup (120 ml) Primal Kitchen Mayo (see Note, page 197), or other primal-approved mayo

Salt and pepper

3 small or 2 medium artichokes (approximately 8 ounces; 225 g)

2 tablespoons (30 g) butter, melted

1. Zest and juice one of the lemons (and save the squeezed lemon). In a small bowl, combine the lemon zest and juice along with ½ teaspoon (2 ml) garlic and the mayo. Taste and adjust the seasoning with salt and pepper. Refrigerate until ready to use.

2. Cut the stems off artichokes to create a flat base. Trim the top leaves. If the leaves are sharp, trim the ends of the remaining leaves with kitchen shears. Rinse the artichokes under running water, gently pulling apart the leaves. Shake off the excess water and squeeze the remaining lemon over the cut sides.

3. Place a steamer basket in your pressure cooker or Instant Pot with about 1 cup water and the squeezed lemons in the bottom. Place the artichokes upright in the basket. Poke the remaining minced garlic between the leaves. Pour the melted butter over top and sprinkle with salt and pepper.

4. Secure the lid and cook at high pressure for 30 minutes using the "Manual" function on the Instant Pot. (For very small artichokes, cook for 20 minutes instead). Let the pressure release naturally for 10 minutes, then open. Do a taste test; if the artichoke is still tough, replace the lid, allow to come to pressure again, and cook for 10 minutes, releasing pressure immediately. Serve with the aioli.

Cashew Cream Broccoli Salad

Makes 6 side servings

This recipe offers an alternative to the traditional broccoli salad. Because it is already egg-free and can easily be made dairy-free by omitting the cheese, this is a great option for keto folks with particular food sensitivities.

1. If the broccoli florets are very large, cut them in half. Bring a large pot of water to a boil. Place the broccoli in boiling water for 1 minute, then immediately transfer to an ice bath. Drain in a colander and shake off extra water.

2. Make the dressing by mixing the cashew cream, vinegar, and pepper in a large bowl. Taste and add sweetener if desired. Taste again and add salt if needed.

3. Place the broccoli, the bacon, onion, and cheese in a bowl and add the dressing; stir to coat very well. Refrigerate for at least 1 hour. Sprinkle the almonds over the top just before serving.

CALORIES: 290	FAT: 21 G
CARBOHYDRATE: 14 G	PROTEIN: 14 G

6 cups (900 g) broccoli florets

1 batch Basic Cashew Cream (recipe follows)

1 tablespoon (15 ml) apple cider vinegar

¼ teaspoon (1 ml) black pepper

Keto-friendly sweetener (optional; see Note, page 283)

Salt to taste

6 slices thick-cut bacon, cooked until crispy and crumbled

½ red onion, diced small

4 ounces (112 g) cheddar cheese, cut into small cubes (approximately 1 cup)

¾ cup (85 g) sliced almonds (or other nut or seed of your choice)

Basic Cashew Cream

Makes ¼ cup

1. Soak the cashews in hot water for at least 4 hours or overnight.

2. Drain and rinse the cashews. Place the cashews, the ½ cup (120 ml) filtered water, and the salt in a high-powered blender and blend until very smooth, scraping down the sides occasionally. This might take several minutes. If the mixture is too thick, add up to ¼ cup (60 ml) more water, a tablespoon at a time.

3. If not using immediately, store in the refrigerator in an airtight container for up to a week.

CALORIES: 143	FAT: 11 G
CARBOHYDRATE: 7 G	PROTEIN: 5 G

1 cup (150 g) raw cashews
½ cup (120 ml) filtered water, plus more for soaking
¼ teaspoon (1 ml) salt

NOTE: The cashew cream is delicately sweet on its own, but those wishing to make a more traditional-tasting broccoli salad might want to bump it up a little. I suggest starting with 1 tablespoon (15 ml) erythritol, or an equivalent amount of the sweetener of your choice, and adjusting as desired.

Creamed Spinach

Makes 4 side servings

This dish goes great with a juicy steak, or you can double the recipe and serve it as a Thanksgiving side dish. To make a lighter, dairy-free version, substitute full-fat coconut milk for the heavy cream and omit the cheese.

CALORIES: 292	FAT: 21 G
CARBOHYDRATE: 11 G	PROTEIN: 15 G

2 pounds (900 g) fresh spinach
2 tablespoons (30 g) butter or ghee
   (clarified butter)
1 small shallot, thinly sliced
Juice of ½ lemon
½ cup (120 ml) heavy cream
1 teaspoon (5 ml) salt
½ teaspoon (2 ml) black pepper
¼ teaspoon (1 ml) ground nutmeg
1 cup (90 g) grated Gruyère cheese

1. Bring a large pot of water to a boil. Dunk the spinach in the boiling water and boil for approximately 2 minutes, until wilted. Pour the spinach into a large colander or strainer and use a wooden spoon to press out excess water.

2. Transfer the spinach to a cutting board and roughly chop. Place on a clean kitchen towel or plate lined with several layers of paper towel and leave to drain.

3. Melt the butter in a skillet over medium heat. Add the shallot and sauté 3 minutes. Add the lemon juice and sauté 1 minute more. Slowly whisk in the cream, then add the salt, pepper, and nutmeg. Cook, stirring constantly, until the sauce thickens.

4. Give the spinach one more squeeze and then add to the skillet along with the cheese. Stir to combine. Cook until the cheese is melted. Taste and adjust salt and pepper.

SNACKS AND BAKING

Parmesan Crisps

Makes approximately 25 crisps; serving size = 5 crisps

These little babies are great when you need a chip fix. They are also customizable—just sprinkle on different herbs and spices before baking. Parmesan works well because it isn't greasy when it melts, but experiment with different cheeses, too!

Heat the oven to 400°F (200°C). Line a baking sheet with a silicone mat or parchment paper. Scoop a generous tablespoon of the cheese onto the sheet and flatten it slightly. Repeat with the rest of the cheese, leaving about 1 inch (2.5 cm) space in between them. Bake for 3 to 5 minutes, until crisp.

CALORIES: 169	FAT: 11 G
CARBOHYDRATE: 6 G	PROTEIN: 11 G

2 cups (200 g) grated Parmesan cheese

Whoops They're Gone Walnuts 'n Dark Chocolate Snack Bag

Makes about 2 cups; serving size = 1/3 cup

For some reason this combo absolutely hits the spot as a go-to snack. If you have a stash nearby, you can skip a meal with no problem. It's great for traveling, too, but it only works in cool temperatures—not a great choice for leaving in your car in the summer. My favorite chocolate for this is Trader Joe's Dark Chocolate Lover's 85% Cacao bar, but any bar with 85% cacao or higher and a good fat-to-carb ratio will do. Check the labels because even some high-cacao dark chocolate bars have objectionable levels of carbs.

CALORIES: 305	FAT: 27 G
CARBOHYDRATE: 9 G	PROTEIN: 7 G

1 3.5-ounce (100 g) bar of dark chocolate
1½ cups (180 g) shelled walnuts
6 tablespoons (30 g) large coconut flakes (see Note) (optional)

1. Break up the bar while it is still in the package, then pour the pieces into a zippered plastic bag. Add the walnuts and shake.

2. If desired, add the coconut flakes to the bag as well.

NOTE: Brands such as Next Organics Dried Raw Coconut Smiles, Let's Do Organic Coconut Flakes, or healthynutfactory.com raw coconut smiles or coconut ribbons are ideal for this use. Note, though, that adding the coconut also adds approximately 37 calories, 3 grams of fat, 1 gram of carbohydrate, and less than 1 gram of protein per serving.

Antipasto Skewers

Makes 8 skewers; serving size = 1 skewer

Go to the party store and pick up some extra-long cocktail toothpicks for this recipe, which can easily be multiplied to serve a large crowd. The Perfect Greek Vinaigrette (page 221) works great here.

1. Cut the mozzarella into 16 small chunks.

2. Skewer 2 pieces each of the mozzarella, basil leaves, salami slices, and coppa slices, along with one artichoke heart, on each skewer. You'll probably want to fold the basil leaves in half and the salami and coppa in fourths (or more depending on size) before skewering.

3. Place the skewers in a small shallow dish and drizzle with the dressing, turning to coat. If possible, let them marinate for 30 minutes or more. Sprinkle lightly with flaky salt and the pepper before serving.

CALORIES: 200	FAT: 15 G
CARBOHYDRATE: 4 G	PROTEIN: 11 G

8 ounces (230 g) fresh whole mozzarella

16 fresh basil leaves

16 slices salami (4 ounces; 112 g)

16 slices coppa or other cured meat like prosciutto (4 ounces; 112 g)

8 artichoke hearts, packed in water (8 ounces; 225 g)

¼ cup (60 ml) vinaigrette made with olive oil or avocado oil and apple cider vinegar

Flaky salt

Freshly ground black pepper

Pizza Bites

Makes 12 pizza bites; serving size = 3 pizza bites

Satisfy your pizza craving with these bite-size treats—they have all the flavors of pizza without the crust. You can add any of your favorite pizza toppings before baking.

CALORIES: 193	FAT: 15 G
CARBOHYDRATE: 2 G	PROTEIN: 11 G

12 large pepperoni slices (see Note; 12 ounces; 84 g)

2 tablespoons (30 ml) tomato paste

12 mini mozzarella balls (approximately 8 ounces; 230 g)

12 fresh basil leaves (optional)

1. Preheat the oven to 400°F (200°C).

2. Line each of 12 cups of a mini muffin pan with one pepperoni slice. To make them sit better, use kitchen shears to make three or four small cuts toward the center of the slice, but do not cut too far in—leave the center intact.

3. Bake 5 minutes, remove from the oven, and allow to cool in the pan for 5 to 10 minutes, until somewhat crisp. Keep the oven turned on.

4. Spoon ½ teaspoon of tomato paste into each pepperoni cup and gently spread to coat the bottom. Place a mozzarella ball and a basil leaf, if using, in each cup. Return muffin pan to the oven and cook another 3 to 5 minutes, until the cheese is melting.

5. Remove pan from the oven and allow the bites to cool for 5 to 10 minutes before serving.

NOTE: Look for large slices of pepperoni in the lunchmeat section, or ask at the deli. If you can't find them, use two or three smaller pepperoni to line each muffin cup.

Sweet Pepper Nacho Bites

Makes 24 bites; serving size = 6 bites

When you need a quick snack, these are just the ticket. You can even skip the baking step if you want to have these ready in less than 5 minutes!

CALORIES: 137	FAT: 12 G
CARBOHYDRATE: 5 G	PROTEIN: 4 G

12 mini sweet peppers (approximately 8 ounces; 230 g)
½ cup (45 g) shredded Monterey jack cheese
½ cup (120 ml) guacamole
Juice of 1 lime

1. Preheat the oven to 400°F (200°C).

2. Carefully cut each pepper in half lengthwise and remove the seeds. Place them cut side up on a rimmed baking sheet so they aren't touching. Place 1 teaspoon of shredded cheese inside each. Bake 3 to 5 minutes, until the cheese starts to melt.

3. Remove from the oven and top each with 1 teaspoon of guacamole. Squeeze the lime juice over top. Serve immediately.

English Cucumber Tea Un-sandwiches

Makes 12 snacks; serving size = 6 snacks

Cucumber sandwiches are a staple of English tea service. They are traditionally served on white bread, but the fillings by themselves make a tasty snack (with or without tea).

CALORIES: 96	FAT: 8 G
CARBOHYDRATE: 3 G	PROTEIN: 3 G

1 large cucumber, peeled (approximately 10 ounces; 285 g)
4 ounces (112 g) cream cheese, softened
2 tablespoons (1 g) finely chopped fresh dill
Freshly ground black pepper

1. Slice the cucumbers into 24 rounds approximately ¼ inch (6 mm) thick. Place in a single layer between two kitchen towels. Put a cutting board on top. Allow to sit about 5 minutes.

2. Mix the cream cheese and dill.

3. Spread 2 teaspoons (10 g) of cream cheese on half the cucumber slices. Grind black pepper over the cheese. Place another slice of cucumber on top of each and secure with a toothpick, if desired.

Marinated Eggs

Makes 6 eggs; serving size = 1 egg

Soy sauce eggs, or *shoyu tamago,* are an umami-licious twist on your basic hard-boiled egg. There are tons of variations on this recipe, but the basic ingredients are soy sauce (salty), sugar (sweet), and vinegar or mirin or sake. I prefer the egg yolks to be *just barely* set, but if soft yolks aren't your thing, go ahead and hard-boil to your liking.

1. Dissolve the sweetener in the water, then add the tamari and vinegar.

2. Peel the eggs and place them in a bowl. Pour the marinade over top. You want the eggs completely submerged, so you might need to weight them down. Nesting bowls can work for this, or place a small plate on top of the eggs.

3. Allow to marinate for at least 2 hours, but you can leave them for longer, even overnight if you wish. (The first time you make this, taste-test one egg after 2 hours.)

4. Drain the marinade and store the eggs in an airtight container until ready to serve.

(See Note)

CALORIES: 94	FAT: 6 G
CARBOHYDRATE: 3 G	PROTEIN: 10 G

1 tablespoon (15 ml) sugar, or 1½ tablespoons (22 ml) erythritol (see Note)

⅓ cup (75 ml) hot water

¾ cup (180 ml) tamari (gluten-free soy sauce)

2 tablespoons (30 ml) sherry vinegar (see Note)

6 large eggs, hard-boiled

NOTE: Because only a negligible amount of the marinade actually ends up in the eggs, I don't feel bad about using real sugar here (either organic cane sugar or coconut sugar), but if you want to be ultra-strict, you can use erythritol. Sherry vinegar is my first choice, or rice wine vinegar as a substitute. Otherwise, use 1 tablespoon (15 ml) white wine vinegar and 1 tablespoon (15 ml) red wine vinegar.

Calculating the macronutrients for these is tricky because you discard most of the marinade. Nutritionally, these are probably minimally different from a plain hard-boiled egg.

Nut Pulp Bread

Makes 1 small loaf; serving size = ⅛ loaf (2 slices, each ½ inch thick)

When I make a batch of nut milk (see page 218), I save the pulp for pancakes or waffles (see page 209) or for this bread. You can make this bread unsweetened or with a keto-friendly sweetener, but I prefer the taste of just 1 teaspoon of honey. It adds only 6 grams of carbs for the whole loaf.

CALORIES: 92	FAT: 59 G
CARBOHYDRATE: 3 G	PROTEIN: 5 G

3 large eggs
Approximately ¾ cup (180 ml) nut pulp, liquid squeezed out (see Note)
¾ teaspoon (4 ml) baking soda
¼ teaspoon (1 ml) kosher salt
1 teaspoon (5 ml) honey
1 tablespoon (15 ml) apple cider vinegar

1. Preheat the oven to 350°F (190°C). Line a small (8 inch x 4 inch or similar; 20 cm x 10 cm) loaf pan with parchment paper.

2. Lightly beat the eggs. Mix in the nut pulp, baking soda, and salt, then add the honey and vinegar.

3. Pour the batter into the pan. Bake for 45 to 55 minutes, or until a toothpick inserted in the center comes out clean. The baking time can vary based on how wet the pulp is.

4. Cool briefly on a rack and then tip out of the pan. Let cool completely and then slice and serve.

NOTE: One batch of homemade nut milk yields about ¾ cup (90 g) of pulp. If you don't have pulp available, you can use ¾ cup (90 g) almond meal plus about 1 tablespoon (15 ml) almond milk or as much as is needed to make a moist batter.

BOMBS, BALLS, AND BITES

Here's a collection of recipes that are great for quick snacks or for fueling your workouts

Fat Bombs

Makes 10 fat bombs; serving size = 1 fat bomb

Fat bombs are a delicious way to get a little extra healthy fat into your diet. The basic recipe can be customized with endless flavor options—just use your imagination. If you want sweeter fat bombs, you can add a keto-friendly sweetener like stevia or erythritol, but try these without sweetener first. Once you have been eating keto for a while, you will probably find that the natural sweetness of the coconut is enough.

Melt the coconut butter and coconut oil in a double boiler or a glass bowl placed over a pan of simmering water. Add the flavoring ingredients of choice (and sweetener if using). Pour into a silicone mini muffin mold. Refrigerate or freeze for at least 10 minutes to harden. Pop the fat bombs out of the mold and place in an airtight container to store in the fridge until you're ready to enjoy one.

CALORIES: 123	FAT: 14 G
CARBOHYDRATE: 2 G	PROTEIN: 1 G

1/3 cup (75 ml) coconut butter, store-bought or homemade (page 226)
1/3 cup (75 ml) coconut oil
Flavoring of choice (see opposite)

Flavoring Possibilities

CHOCOLATE MACADAMIA

CALORIES: 149	FAT: 16 G	CARBOHYDRATE: 3 G	PROTEIN: 1 G

- 2 teaspoons (4 g) dark cocoa powder
- 3 tablespoons (22 g) crushed macadamias

CINNAMON ROLL

CALORIES: 143	FAT: 14 G	CARBOHYDRATE: 3 G	PROTEIN: 1 G

- 1½ teaspoons (7.5 ml) ground cinnamon
- 2 tablespoons (30 ml) almond butter
- ½ teaspoon (2 ml) vanilla extract

SPICY LEMONADE

CALORIES: 123	FAT: 14 G	CARBOHYDRATE: 2 G	PROTEIN: 1 G

- Pinch of cayenne
- ¼ teaspoon (1 ml) ground ginger
- 2 teaspoons (10 ml) grated lemon zest
- 2 tablespoons (30 ml) fresh lemon juice
  Note: Omit the cayenne and ginger for plain Lemon Fat Bombs.

BUTTER PECAN

CALORIES: 147	FAT: 16 G	CARBOHYDRATE: 2 G	PROTEIN: 1 G

- ¼ cup (28 g) finely chopped dry-toasted pecans
- 1 tablespoon (15 ml) unsalted butter

STRAWBERRIES AND CREAM

CALORIES: 128	FAT: 14 G	CARBOHYDRATE: 2 G	PROTEIN: 1 G

- 2 medium strawberries, chopped small (3 to 4 tablespoons; 45 to 60 ml)
- 1 tablespoon (15 ml) heavy cream

Tahini Fudge

Makes 10 pieces; serving size = 1 piece

Mary Shenouda ("the Paleo chef") has a recipe that she calls Phat Fudge that is phantastic. That recipe inspired me to start playing around with my own versions of tahini-based treats. I'm sharing two of my favorite versions here, both of which highlight the delicious flavor of the tahini itself. If you like sesame-based halva, you'll love these.

1. Blend all the ingredients in a food processor until smooth. Pour into a silicone mini muffin mold or silicone ice cube tray. (Alternatively, line a small rectangular loaf pan with parchment paper and pour in the entire mixture.)

2. Freeze until set. Pop the fudge out of the molds or cut the single large piece into bite-size squares. Store in an airtight container in the freezer for the best texture.

CALORIES: 156	FAT: 16 G
CARBOHYDRATE: 3 G	PROTEIN: 2 G

½ cup (120 ml) tahini

½ cup (1 stick; 125 g) butter

½ teaspoon (2 ml) vanilla extract

1 teaspoon (5 ml) ground cinnamon

1 teaspoon (5 ml) dried turmeric

¼ teaspoon (1 ml) black pepper

1 tablespoon (15 ml) erythritol, or to taste (see Note)

1 teaspoon (5 ml) maca powder (optional; see Note)

NOTE: Powdered erythritol will give these a slightly granular texture. If you prefer, use a liquid sweetener. Maca powder comes from the maca root. It has been conferred "super food" status for its antioxidant effects and its purported ability to enhance reproductive hormones, fertility, and libido. The nutty-tasting powder adds an interesting flavor component, but you can omit it.

Green Tea Tahini Bites

Makes 10 bites; serving size = 1 bite

This version of tahini fudge reminds me of those green tea lattes from the trendy coffee shop. (You know the one . . .)

CALORIES: 155	FAT: 16 G
CARBOHYDRATE: 3 G	PROTEIN: 3 G

½ cup (120 ml) tahini
½ cup (120 g) butter
½ teaspoon (2 ml) vanilla extract
5 drops vanilla stevia, or to taste
1 teaspoon (5 ml) matcha green tea
   powder

1. Blend all the ingredients in a food processor until smooth. Pour into a silicone mini muffin mold or silicone ice cube tray. (Alternatively, line a small rectangular loaf pan with parchment paper and pour in the entire mixture.)

2. Freeze until set. Pop the fudge out of the mold or cut the larger piece into bite-size squares. Store in an airtight container in the freezer for best texture.

Turmeric Balls

Makes 8 balls; serving size = 1 ball

Turmeric is popular in health circles because of its purported anti-inflammatory benefits. It is also delicious, but it does have a strong flavor; if you aren't sure you like it, start with less. Definitely do not omit the black pepper! The piperine in the pepper helps unlock the benefits of the turmeric.

CALORIES: 113	FAT: 11 G
CARBOHYDRATE: 5 G	PROTEIN: 1 G

½ cup (120 ml) coconut butter, store-bought or homemade (see page 226)
½ tablespoon (7 ml) coconut oil
⅓ cup (75 ml) finely shredded coconut (see Note)
½ teaspoon (2 ml) ground turmeric
¼ teaspoon (1 ml) ground cinnamon
⅛ teaspoon (0.5 ml) black pepper
1–2 drops liquid stevia (optional)

1. Place the coconut butter and coconut oil in a microwave-safe bowl and microwave on high for 15 seconds. Stir. If they are still too hard to mix, microwave in 5-second increments until they can be stirred. You want the mixture soft but not liquefied.

2. Combine the coconut, turmeric, cinnamon, black pepper, and stevia, if using, and add to the coconut butter mixture.

3. Place a small piece of parchment paper or wax paper on a plate. Scoop out approximately ½ tablespoon of the batter and roll into a ball with your hands, and put it on the plate. If the batter is too soft to roll, place it in the refrigerator for a couple minutes to slightly harden and try again. Continue to make the balls until batter is used up.

4. Refrigerate the balls for 15 minutes to harden, then transfer to an airtight container until ready to enjoy. (The balls can be stored at room temperature unless your kitchen is very warm, in which case keep them in the fridge.)

NOTE: You can chop regular shredded coconut more finely with a knife or nut chopper to achieve the fine chop that is ideal for this recipe.

Vanilla Protein Fudge

Makes 36 squares; serving size = 1 square

This addictive treat packs a punch of healthy fats and protein. One decadent square is enough to satisfy.

CALORIES: 72	FAT: 7 G
CARBOHYDRATE: 1 G	PROTEIN: 2 G

1. In a small saucepan, melt together the cream cheese, butter, and almond butter over low heat, stirring frequently. (You can also do this in the microwave. Combine the ingredients in a microwave-safe bowl and heat for 20 seconds. Stir and, if needed, microwave 10 seconds more.)

2. Scrape the cream cheese mixture into a bowl and add the erythritol, vanilla, and protein powder. Use a hand mixer or immersion blender to blend until smooth. *Do not skip this step!* You will see after 30 seconds or so of mixing that the consistency changes to become smoother and more fudge-like. Keep mixing until thickened and somewhat sticky.

3. Line a 6-inch (15 cm) square baking dish with parchment paper (preferred) or grease with coconut oil. Scrape the mixture into the baking dish and smooth as much as you can with a spatula. Place in the refrigerator for at least 2 hours to harden.

4. Use a sharp knife to cut into even squares. Keep refrigerated until ready to enjoy.

8 ounces (225 g) cream cheese, at room temperature
½ cup (120 g) butter, at room temperature
½ cup (120 ml) raw almond butter (smooth, not chunky)
2½ tablespoons (40 ml) erythritol
1 teaspoon (5 ml) vanilla extract
2 scoops (42 g) Primal Kitchen Vanilla Coconut Primal Fuel or other protein powder (see Note)

NOTE: If you do not have Primal Fuel, you can substitute ½ cup (120 ml) of another whey protein and adjust the sweetness as desired. You can also substitute powdered stevia or another powdered sweetener blend in the appropriate amount for the erythritol.

TREATS

Stu Can't Stop Bark

Makes 24 pieces; serving size = 1 piece

Here's Brad's world-famous recipe for dark chocolate macadamia bark—a delectable tribute to his favorite pooch. Often Stu can't stop barking, and you won't be able to stop eating this delicious treat, which is healthy enough to be your breakfast! An assembly line production team made batches to serve 150 guests at PrimalCon retreats across North America, and were absolutely mobbed every time fresh trays were brought out from the kitchen!

1. Break the chocolate by hand into small pieces. Melt half the chocolate in a double boiler or glass bowl fitted over a small pan of boiling water. Add the coconut oil as the chocolate is melting and stir occasionally.

2. In a big mixing bowl, combine the nuts and the remaining dark chocolate pieces. Pour the melted chocolate mixture into the bowl and stir very well.

3. In a large glass pan (15 x 10 inches; 38 x 26 cm), spread half the mixture thinly across the bottom. Drizzle a thin layer of almond butter over the chocolate, spreading carefully so there are no thick areas. (If your almond butter is too thick to drizzle, you can microwave it for 20 seconds.)

4. Spread the rest of the chocolate evenly over the almond butter. Sprinkle on the coconut or coconut butter, if using. Sprinkle the salt lightly over the top.

CALORIES: 236	FAT: 22 G
CARBOHYDRATE: 9 G	PROTEIN: 3 G

5 bars good dark chocolate (1 pound, or 500 g, give or take), at least 80% cacao content

3 tablespoons (45 ml) coconut oil

2 cups (240 g) macadamia nuts, or a mixture of assorted other nuts, ground into small pieces

3 tablespoons (45 ml) raw almond butter

¼ to ½ cup (25–50 g) finely shredded coconut flakes (optional; see Note, page 226)

2 tablespoons (30 ml) coconut butter (optional)

Sea salt or Himalayan pink salt, to sprinkle on top

5. Freeze for 1 to 2 hours or refrigerate for longer—the mixture must become rock-hard. Remove from chilling, let sit for 5 minutes, then cut into squares. (You'll need a baker's blade or dough scraper or a very large chef's knife to cut successfully; be careful because it will be hard to cut into.)

6. Store the bark in an airtight container in the fridge or freezer and serve cold (but not frozen). When serving, consume immediately because the bark will melt quickly at room temperature.

Blueberries and Cream

Makes 1 serving

Sometimes simple is best.

Place the frozen blueberries in a small bowl. Pour the cream or coconut milk on top and stir quickly. Let sit for a minute. The cream will freeze around the blueberries.

(With Whipping Dream)

CALORIES: 122	FAT: 11 G
CARBOHYDRATE: 6 G	PROTEIN: 0 G

(With Coconut Milk)

CALORIES: 131	FAT: 12 G
CARBOHYDRATE: 6 G	PROTEIN: 1 G

¼ cup (35 g) frozen organic blueberries
¼ cup (60 ml) heavy cream or full-fat coconut milk

Brad's Nutty Bars

Makes 24 pieces; serving size = 1 piece

These are similar to Stu Can't Stop Bark, but nuts are the stars instead of dark chocolate. You can add even more nuts if you want it extra crunchy. A great recipe to try when Trader Joe's occasionally runs out of dark chocolate—which was how the recipe was discovered!

1. Puree the nuts and dark chocolate in a high-powered blender or food processor. Pour into a large bowl, add the almond butter, and stir well.

2. Spread the mixture in a large glass dish (15 x 10 inches; 38 x 26 cm). Sprinkle the coconut flakes and coconut butter over the top, if using.

3. Freeze for 1 to 2 hours or refrigerate for longer—the mixture must become rock-hard in the dish. Remove, let sit for 5 minutes, then cut into squares of bark. (You'll need a baker's blade or dough scraper, or very large chef's knife, to cut into the mixture successfully.)

4. Store the bark in an airtight container in the fridge or freezer and serve cold but not frozen. When serving, consume immediately because bark will melt quickly at room temperature.

CALORIES: 251	FAT: 23 G
CARBOHYDRATE: 8 G	PROTEIN: 6 G

2 cups (240 g) macadamia nuts, or a mixture of assorted other nuts, ground into small pieces

1 to 2 bars (3.5 ounces each; 105 g) dark chocolate, 85% to 90% cacao, broken into pieces

16-ounce (454 g) container of almond butter

¼ to ½ cup (60 to 120 ml) finely shredded coconut flakes (optional; see Note, page 226)

2 tablespoons (30 ml) coconut butter (optional)

Chocolate Avocado Mousse

Makes 4 servings

There are lots of versions of this avocado mousse recipe floating around, but this version beats them all. Because it uses dark chocolate instead of cocoa powder, and has just a bit of cream cheese, it has a very smooth texture and is extra creamy. It is particularly delicious topped with fresh whipped cream and dark chocolate shavings. Substitute coconut milk for a dairy-free version.

CALORIES: 211	FAT: 20 G
CARBOHYDRATE: 7 G	PROTEIN: 2 G

2 ounces (60 g) dark chocolate, 85% cacao content or higher
1 ounce (28 g) cream cheese
1 teaspoon (5 ml) vanilla extract
¼ cup (60 ml) heavy cream
1 avocado (125 g)
Keto-friendly sweetener of choice to taste (optional; liquid works better)

1. In a double boiler or glass bowl fitted over a small pan of boiling water, melt the dark chocolate. Add the cream cheese and stir until combined. Stir in the vanilla and remove from the heat.

2. In a medium bowl, beat the cream until it forms soft peaks. (A hand mixer or immersion blender is ideal for this.)

3. In a separate bowl, smash the avocado with a fork; you should have about ¾ cup. Add the chocolate mixture and stir well (use an immersion blender or hand mixer if you have one). Add the whipped cream and blend well.

4. Taste the mousse. If you want it sweeter, add small amounts of sweetener at a time until it reaches desired sweetness. Divide the mixture among 4 small ramekins. (This dessert is very rich, so small portions are better!) Chill in the fridge until ready to serve.

Coconut Milk Whipped Cream

Makes 8 servings

If you want a break from dairy, or simply love the subtle sweetness of coconut milk, try this coconut milk whipped cream as a topping for any keto treat. It can even be used as a frosting substitute. I prefer not to sweeten mine, but you can add a keto-approved sweetener (liquid works better than powder). Make sure that you buy full-fat coconut milk—none of that lite stuff!

CALORIES: 106	FAT: 10 G
CARBOHYDRATE: 3 G	PROTEIN: 0 G

1 can (13.5 ounces; 398 ml) full-fat coconut milk

½ to 1 teaspoon (2 to 5 ml) vanilla extract (optional)

Liquid stevia or other keto-friendly sweetener, to taste

1. Refrigerate the can of coconut milk overnight or at least 8 hours.

2. When you are ready to make your whipped cream, chill a glass or metal bowl and the beaters from your mixer in the freezer for 10 minutes (see Note). Open the coconut milk gently and scoop out the thickened cream, leaving the liquid behind (you can use this liquid in your next smoothie or iced coffee).

3. Place the cream in the chilled bowl and beat for 30 seconds to 1 minute on medium speed. Add the vanilla and sweetener, if using, then beat again on high speed until desired consistency, another 1 to 3 minutes.

NOTE: You can use a hand mixer or a stand mixer to whip the coconut milk. A high-powered blender or immersion blender will work in a pinch, but the finished product will not be as fluffy.

"Froyo" Bites

Makes 8 bites; serving size = 1 bite

These aren't technically frozen yogurt, of course, but the texture and sweetness will hit the spot if froyo is what you want. I like to make these in individual bites for portioning out easily, but you can also double the batch and freeze in a single container. When you're ready to eat some, let the container sit on the counter for a few minutes, then scoop out like ice cream.

1. Blend all ingredients in a food processor until smooth. Pour the mixture into a silicone mini muffin pan or ice cube tray, or use mini tart cups. (Alternatively, line a small rectangular loaf pan with parchment paper to hold the entire mixture.)

2. Freeze until set. Pop out the individual bites and store in an airtight container in the freezer. Remove from the freezer a few minutes before eating.

CALORIES: 84	FAT: 8 G
CARBOHYDRATE: 1 G	PROTEIN: 1 G

4 ounces (112 g) cream cheese
1 teaspoon (5 ml) vanilla extract
1/3 cup (75 ml) heavy cream
1½ teaspoons (7.5 ml) stevia powder

Lemon Cream "Froyo" Bites

Makes 8 bites; serving size = 1 bite

This is the same idea as the recipe on page 303, but with a lemony twist.

CALORIES: 84	FAT: 8 G
CARBOHYDRATE: 1 G	PROTEIN: 1 G

1. Blend all the ingredients in a food processor until smooth. Pour the mixture into a silicone mini muffin pan or ice cube tray, or use mini tart cups. (Alternatively, line a small rectangular loaf pan with parchment paper and pour in entire mixture.)

2. Freeze until set. Pop out the individual bites and store in an airtight container in the freezer. Remove from the freezer a few minutes before eating.

4 ounces (112 g) cream cheese
1 teaspoon (5 ml) vanilla extract
$1/3$ cup (75 ml) heavy cream
1½ teaspoons (7.5 ml) stevia powder
1 teaspoon (5 ml) grated lemon zest
2 teaspoons (10 ml) fresh lemon juice

Brad's Almond Butter Flan

Makes 8 servings

So delicious, and you can have it for breakfast, too! This treat is easy to make and nutrient-dense with its powerhouse trifecta of egg yolks, full-fat coconut milk, and almond butter.

1. Preheat the oven to 325°F (160°C).

2. Mix all the ingredients a large saucepan, stirring until smooth. Heat for a few minutes on medium heat, stirring well to make sure the almond butter blends.

3. Place 8 ramekins in a large baking dish. Fill the dish two-thirds high with hot water, then pour the mixture into the ramekins.

4. Bake for 30 minutes, or until the mixture has set somewhat; it will still be a bit liquidy. Consume warm if desired, or refrigerate to enjoy cold later.

5. If desired, top with a generous mound of homemade whipped cream when serving.

CALORIES: 379	FAT: 34 G
CARBOHYDRATE: 10 G	PROTEIN: 11 G

2 cans (13.5 ounces; 398 ml each) full-fat coconut milk
8 large eggs
5 tablespoons (75 ml) almond butter
2 tablespoons (30 ml) vanilla extract
1 tablespoon (15 ml) ground cinnamon
1 tablespoon (15 ml) pure maple syrup or keto-friendly sweetener

Whipped Cream (recipe below)

Whipped Cream

Makes 8 servings

Beat all ingredients together using a hand mixer or immersion blender until firm peaks form. (This works better if you chill the mixing bowl in the freezer for a few minutes first.) Use immediately.

CALORIES: 104	FAT: 11 G
CARBOHYDRATE: 1 G	PROTEIN: 0 G

1 pint (475 ml) heavy cream
1 teaspoon (5 ml) vanilla extract
2 to 3 drops liquid stevia

Primal Cheesecake

Makes 10 servings

Is any dessert more decadent than cheesecake? For this version, I use coconut sugar and add a little bit of stevia to bump up the sweetness. It is only a slight indulgence, but you can substitute more stevia or another keto-friendly sweetener for the coconut sugar. For a real treat, add fresh strawberries or raspberries in the summer—yum!!

1. Preheat the oven to 350°F (180°C).

2. Place the crust ingredients in a food processor and pulse until the mixture resembles coarse sand. Press the mixture firmly into the bottom of a 9-inch (23 cm) springform pan.

3. Place the pan on a rimmed baking sheet and bake for 13 to 15 minutes. Remove from the oven when the edges are starting to brown, even though the middle will probably appear underbaked. Allow to cool completely.

4. Keep the oven at 350°F (180°C). Position a rack in the lowest spot, and place a baking dish with 1 inch (3 cm) of water on that rack. Place the other rack in the middle position.

5. With a stand mixer, whip the cream cheese and yogurt. Add the sugar, stevia, and vanilla and beat until smooth. Taste the mixture and adjust sweetness if necessary.

6. Add the eggs and egg yolks and beat on medium speed for about 30 seconds, until all the ingredients are well incorporated.

7. Pour the filling into the prepared crust. Place in the oven on the middle rack and bake 35 to

CALORIES: 455	FAT: 42 G
CARBOHYDRATE: 11 G	PROTEIN: 10 G

CRUST

1 cup (120 g) almond meal
1 cup (112 g) raw pecan pieces
4 tablespoons (½ stick; 60 g) butter
¾ teaspoon (4 ml) powdered stevia

FILLING

2½ cups (560 g) cream cheese, softened
¾ cup (175 ml) plain Greek yogurt
¼ cup (60 ml) coconut sugar
½ tablespoon (7.5 ml) powdered stevia
1 teaspoon (5 ml) vanilla extract
3 large eggs
3 egg yolks

CHOCOLATE DRIZZLE

1 ounce (25 g) 80% or higher cacao dark chocolate
½ teaspoon (5 ml) coconut oil

Whipped Cream (optional; page 305)

40 minutes, until middle is just set but still soft. Turn the oven off and let the cheesecake sit in the warm oven for 30 minutes.

8. Remove the cheesecake from the oven. Run a knife around the edge of the cheesecake and allow to cool in the pan on the counter. Then transfer to the refrigerator to cool for 4 more hours.

9. Just before serving, melt the chocolate and coconut oil together in a small microwave-safe bowl or double boiler. Use a spoon to drizzle the melted chocolate across the top of the cake. Let sit for a minute to harden. Top with whipped cream, if desired.

Keto Macaroons

Makes 10 macaroons; serving size = 1 macaroon

These quick and easy treats are denser than traditional macaroons because they substitute almond flour for white flour, but the flavor is spot on. Enjoy them as a healthier option for your kids' lunchboxes when you want to send a sweet surprise. You can also take these along on a long hike or bike ride as a fueling option; without the optional chocolate drizzle, they will hold up well in your pack.

CALORIES: 59	FAT: 5 G
CARBOHYDRATE: 2 G	PROTEIN: 2 G

3 large egg whites

¼ teaspoon (1 ml) salt

4 tablespoons (60 ml) almond flour

½ teaspoon (2 ml) powdered stevia

1 teaspoon (5 ml) vanilla extract

2 cups (50 g) unsweetened coconut flakes, roughly chopped if very large

½ ounce (25 g) 80% or higher cacao dark chocolate (optional)

¼ teaspoon (1 ml) coconut oil (optional)

1. Preheat the oven to 350°F (180°C). Line a baking sheet with parchment paper.

2. Beat the egg whites until peaks form. In a separate bowl, combine the salt, almond flour, stevia, vanilla, and coconut flakes. Gently fold the egg whites into the coconut mixture.

3. Scoop heaping tablespoons of the mixture onto the baking sheet. Try to make the portions uniform in size and shape. (A cookie scoop is the ideal tool if you have one, but a rounded measuring spoon works as well.)

4. Bake for 20 minutes, or until lightly golden on the edges. Remove from oven and allow to cool completely.

5. If using, melt the chocolate and coconut oil together in a small microwave-safe bowl. Use a spoon to drizzle a few lines of chocolate across the top of each macaroon. Allow the chocolate to cool before serving.

Keto Pie and Tart Crust

Makes enough crust for a 9-inch (23 cm) pie; serving size = ⅛ of crust

Regular pie crust is off the menu now, but you can make a delicious substitute with just nuts, butter, and a little bit of sweetener. It's not the same—it's better! (If you want a recipe to substitute for a graham cracker crust, check out the recipes for Primal Cheesecake on page 306 or the Lime Bars on page 310!)

CALORIES: 197	FAT: 19 G
CARBOHYDRATE: 3 G	PROTEIN: 4 G

1½ cups (180 g) walnuts or pecans
3 tablespoons (45 ml) salted butter, cut into cubes
2 tablespoons (30 ml) erythritol

1. Preheat the oven to 325°F (190°C). Line a 9-inch (23 cm) pie or tart pan with parchment paper by cutting a circle the size of the bottom of the pan.

2. Combine the ingredients in a food processor and pulse until the mixture resembles coarse sand.

3. Press the mixture firmly into the bottom of the pan and up the sides until it is a uniform thickness. Bake for 13 to 15 minutes, until the edges are brown. Do not overbake; the nuts can burn quickly. Once it smells like toasted nuts, it needs to come out. The middle of the crust will probably look undercooked; take it out anyway.

4. Allow to cool completely, then add desired filling and bake again, or fill with no-bake filling. If you bake it again, use a crust shield or aluminum foil to protect the edges of the crust from burning.

NOTE: You can easily scale this recipe to any other size pie or tart pan. Just keep the same ratio of ½ cup nuts to 1 tablespoon butter.

Lime Bars

Makes 16 squares; serving size = 1 square

This tangy desert is nice when you get a little tired of dark chocolate. It's packed with healthy fats from the secret ingredient—avocado. Because avocados turn brown when they are exposed to air, this dessert is best eaten shortly after assembling.

1. Preheat the oven to 350°F (180°C). Line an 8-inch (20 cm) square baking dish with parchment paper. Use a rectangular piece of parchment paper (8 x 12 inches; or 20 x 30 cm) so that the paper comes up two of the sides. You will use these like handles to lift out the bars later.

2. Place the crust ingredients in a food processor and pulse until the mixture resembles coarse sand. Press the mixture firmly into the bottom of the pan, making sure to get it into the corners. Bake for 13 to 15 minutes. Remove from oven when edges start to brown. The crust will probably appear underbaked in the middle. Allow to cool completely.

3. Place all the ingredients for the filling except 1 tablespoon (15 ml) of lime juice in a large mixing bowl and beat with a hand mixer until very smooth. (You can also use a stand mixer, food processor, or immersion blender for this.)

4. Spoon the mixture into the crust and smooth with a spatula. Sprinkle the remaining 1 tablespoon (15 ml) lime juice over the top. Swirl and tip the pan around to distribute; this will help keep the top from oxidizing.

5. Place in the refrigerator for at least an hour to cool, several hours is preferred. When ready to serve, use the parchment paper to carefully lift the cake out onto a cutting board. Cut into squares and serve.

CALORIES: 128	FAT: 12 G
CARBOHYDRATE: 5 G	PROTEIN: 2 G

CRUST
¾ cup (84 g) raw pecan pieces
¾ cup (90 g) almond meal
3 tablespoons (45 ml) salted butter
2 tablespoons (30 ml) erythritol

FILLING
Grated zest of 3 limes
 (2½ tablespoons; 37 ml)
¼ cup plus 1 tablespoon (90 ml) lime juice
1 teaspoon (5 ml) vanilla extract
Pulp of 3 avocados (12 ounces each; 350 grams), mashed with a fork
2 tablespoons (30 ml) coconut sugar
4 drops liquid stevia
¼ cup (60 ml) heavy cream

APPENDIX

THE NITTY-GRITTY DETAILS: SCIENCE, SUPPLEMENTS, TESTING, TROUBLESHOOTING

THE critical assumptions presented at the end of Chapter 11 are the most important things you need to know to succeed with keto. The intent of this appendix is to delve deeper into an assortment of topics that can help increase your knowledge of keto, and aid you in making the best decisions along your personal journey. We'll cover the special considerations for athletes going keto, examine the benefits and best use of ketone supplements—including a list of many products on the market—delve into additional macronutrient and scientific details, review targeted benefits for distinct populations, learn the particulars of testing blood for ketones and glucose, and present a detailed troubleshooting section should you encounter the most common keto pitfalls.

Athletes— Special Concerns

Dr. Dom D'Agostino speculates that elite-level athletes may require an adaptation period of at least six weeks and possibly up to six months during which performance is a little below standard. This is likely attributed in part to the mitochondria reacting to their surprising new fuel source by producing more reactive oxygen species in the short term. A less active individual might not notice this, because his or her metabolic needs are not as exacting. In the athlete, though, this hormetic stressor eventually stimulates the mitochondria to adapt and become more efficient than ever at producing energy from the clean fuel sources of fat and ketones. When you fully adapt to your transition, you will be poised for significant performance breakthroughs due to the awesome athletic benefits of keto detailed in Chapter 3.

Another interesting peculiarity of athletes and keto is a somewhat common pattern of low blood ketone readings in seemingly highly adapted individuals. What's likely happening is that your expertise in manufacturing and burning ketones (due to elevated enzyme activity in comparison to an inactive person, among other reasons) results in your not needing to produce high levels to get the job done. As discussed previously, being fully fat- and keto-adapted means your muscles burn mostly fat, while ketones are prioritized for your brain. Studies from Phinney and Volek reveal that blood ketone levels are higher in the early stages of adaptation when the muscles and brain are both using ketones, and lower in the advanced stages of adaptation when your muscles prefer fatty acids and your brain burns most of the ketones.

This phenomenon is what Dr. Cate Shanahan calls *ketone flux*—you produce and burn through ketones quickly instead of accumulating them in the blood. Cate explains:

> If you're a healthy human with an efficient metabolism, you get really good at producing only what you need and no extra—whatever the hormone or metabolic agent we are talking about. This is why it's important for a healthy athletic person concerned about low readings to consider real-life experience to evaluate metabolic efficiency. Can you skip a meal, or two, and maintain good energy and concentration for hours? Can you perform athletically in a fasted state—whether for a short, high intensity session or a prolonged endurance session? This means that you are fat- and keto-adapted, no matter what your numbers say. Furthermore, there is simply significant variation among individuals when it comes to blood ketone readings—likely for genetic reasons.

More peculiarity comes with the observation that some athletes are reporting high glucose readings even when coming off of extended fasts, adhering to keto macronutrient guidelines, and performing ambitious workouts. My co-author Brad and I have both experienced this phenomenon in our intensive blood- and glucose-testing efforts in the R&D for this book. What's likely happening here is that athletes are flexing their metabolic muscles by making glucose, either in the aftermath of workouts or in reaction to fasting or keto-aligned meals. In contrast, an inactive, metabolically inflexible person would deplete his or her energy stores and either most likely cave in to sugar cravings or pass out in a hypoglycemia-induced exhaustion.

Finally, it seems that a certain percentage of healthy athletic individuals who have minimal body-fat concerns or disease risk factors may not respond well to the macronutrient parameters of a ketogenic diet. Some of this might be attributed to a flawed approach, something we'll address in the "Troubleshooting" section.

Ketone Supplements

The growing interest in the benefits of ketone burning has led to an explosion of scientific studies and laboratory discovery. Consequently, today you can consume exogenous sources of ketones—the same stuff your body works so hard to produce—via a powdered or liquid supplement. Consuming a ketone supplement shoots you into ketosis within 30 minutes of consumption. While you'll burn through the moderate amount of calories provided by a ketone supplement in a short time (a typical supplement serving size is 50–150 calories of beta-hydroxybutyrate), it's believed the supplements can help boost internal ketone production if they are used in conjunction with fasting, keto-aligned eating, or at least low-carbohydrate eating. It's also believed that consuming medium-chain triglycerides (MCTs), even though they are not ketones, will help speed the rate of fat oxidation in the liver and thus increase internal ketone production. Coconut oil is naturally high in MCT, and there are also numerous MCT supplements in both oil and powdered form.

Dr. Dom D'Agostino, who is at the forefront of ketone supplement research, states that "ketone supplements deliver a drug-like antioxidant, anti-inflammatory, signaling molecule effect that is independent of the metabolic effects [burning a clean source of calories]. Pharmaceutical companies are beside themselves with excitement about the anti-inflammatory potency of ketones and the potential broad application for numerous disease pathologies." Ketones' signaling molecule effects can protect against seizures or combat the growth of cancerous tumors, and reduce inflammation as well as or better than prescription anti-inflammatory drugs. Ketone supplements can also deliver targeted benefits for athletic performance and help you get through rough spots in your quest to become fat- and keto-adapted.

The active agent in ketone supplements is beta-hydroxybutyrate. This is one of two forms of ketones your body produces internally, along with acetoacetate. Beta-hydroxybutyrate is used in supplements because it is more stable. Most commercial products are actually compounds known as ketone salts, or beta-hydroxybutyrate salts. They consist of sodium, potassium, and beta-hydroxybutyrate. Some products are purely ketone salts, while others include supporting ingredients, such as electrolytes and amino acids.

When you consider how ketone supplements can short-circuit the hard work it takes with dietary restriction to achieve ketosis, it's tempting to imagine them as a hack method to save the trouble of counting carbs, or even as a magic bullet to right the ship after you binge on carbs. There is even a study from Oxford University suggesting that taking exogenous ketones can moderate a glycemic response after a meal for a true hangover remedy effect; Dr. D'Agostino was conducting a so-called cupcake study in his own lab in early 2017 to validate this.

While it appears that ketone supplements can actually deliver some amazing stop-gap benefits, it's clearly better to view the supplements as a tool to leverage devoted dietary efforts toward keto, or for targeted performance or disease protection applications. Furthermore, it's believed that long-term nutritional ketosis stimulates mitochondrial biogenesis, unlike the more transient benefits of supplements.

I believe the athletic applications for ketone supplements are very interesting—potentially surpassing any performance nutrition supplement ever made. In using ketone supplements before my most difficult workouts (2-hour Ultimate Frisbee matches requiring both endurance and repeated explosive sprints), I notice more explosiveness in my sprinting and jumping, and less muscle tightness and better concentration levels late in the matches. This is likely due to both the metabolic effects in the muscles and perhaps because my central governor is getting more oxygen. In the hours afterward, I notice less fatigue and inflammation, along with reduced next-day muscle soreness. I believe these benefits are real, not imagined, because I have extensive comparative reference from matches with and without ketone supplementation. I believe these benefits accrue from having a fuel source that delivers more oxygen and generates less inflammation and muscle breakdown than glucose.

AFTERNOON BLUES: The greatest potential struggles come during the early stages of nutritional ketosis, when your muscles and brain are starved of their usual glucose offerings and are competing for the precious resource of ketones. At these times when you feel a bit of brain fog or energy lull, a ketone supplement may give you an immediate energy boost and perhaps stave off a backslide carbohydrate binge.

ATHLETIC PERFORMANCE: Taking a ketone supplement 30 minutes before an intense session will give you a clean-burning fuel source, reducing the stress impact of the workout on your brain and body. I believe there is also tremendous potential for endurance athletes to consume a steady supply of ketones during prolonged workouts, perhaps in conjunction with fat fuels and the high-tech super-starch carbohydrate supplements.

DISEASE PROTECTION: Ketone supplements appear to have excellent potential as an adjunct therapy for cancer treatments, as well as to combat drug-resistant seizures. This was Dr. Russell Wilder's original application of the ketogenic diet back in 1924, at the Mayo Clinic.

MORNING BEVERAGE: Preparing a morning hot beverage consisting of MCT oil and/or a ketone supplement may make skipping breakfast easier and deliver a burst of mental clarity for a busy, productive morning.

You can consume ketones directly with the assortment of products containing beta-hydroxybutyrate, or consume a medium-chain triglyceride product (liquid or powder) that will help boost liver ketone production, especially if you are adhering to nutritional ketosis guidelines. The beta-hydroxybutyrate formulations deliver it either straight up or with beneficial agents such as amino acids (to guard against lean tissue breakdown via gluconeogenesis), minerals (calcium, magnesium, potassium, and sodium), fiber (to ease concerns about digestive distress when consuming beta-hydroxybutyrate), caffeine (some believe this helps mobilize free fatty acids, and of course it delivers a stimulant effect for athletic performance), or MCT oil. Some popular brands include Kegenix, KetoCaNa, KetoForce, Keto//OS, Nutricost, and Perfect Keto Base.

MCT oil supplements are popular to mix in coffee, delivering an effect similar to a creamer. This stuff is the real deal, and can serve as a great catalyst to keep your momentum going when you might be struggling to adhere to nutritional guidelines. MCT oil has such a distinct effect on ketone production that in 1971, the late Dr. Peter Huttenlocher, a pediatric neurologist, devised a diet in which 60 percent of the calories came from MCT oil. This allowed his patients to be less restrictive with carbohydrate intake and still experience the therapeutic benefits of ketosis.

There are a fair number of complaints that liquid MCT oil can cause extreme digestive disturbances (as in an impromptu sprint to the bathroom), so powders or capsules seem to be the preferred supplement form. However, the powders may be less stressful to digest in part because many of them are cut with agents that reduce digestive distress, though these agents may be objectionable to some purists. For example, Quest Nutrition's MCT oil (D'Agostino says he uses this brand, as do Brad and I) contains probiotic agents to help with digestion, but also on the label as contents are soluble corn fiber, sodium caseinate, sunflower lecithin, and silicon dioxide. Personally, having been a victim of the MCT oil-induced sprint workout (the bathrooms were locked at the Ultimate Frisbee field, so it was actually an automobile rally plus a sprint to take care of matters back home), I suggest trying Quest or another powder to get some experience using MCTs before dabbling in an oil product. Also, start with small doses to build your tolerance and work your way up.

The MCT products differ in terms of the length of the carbon chains on the fatty acids. MCT oil supplements contain a blend of fatty acids of different carbon chain lengths, mixing C8 (caprylic fatty acids), C10 (capric fatty acids), and C12 (lauric acid). C12 is more biologically similar to a long-chain fatty acid than to a medium-chain fatty acid, and it doesn't contribute to ketone production as significantly as C8 and C10 do (although C12 has other health benefits).

Some popular oil products include Brain Octane Oil, CapTri, Keto8, KetoMCT Oil, MiCkey T Eight, XCT Oil. Brands offering 100 percent MCT oil powder include AMRAP, NutraBio, and Perfect Keto. Brands offering MCT oil powder blended with other ingredients include KetoSports, Phat Fibre, True Nutrition, Quest Nutrition, and Pruvit.

Macronutrient/Scientific Details

LIVER KETONE PRODUCTION: Ketone production happens under special circumstances in the liver when dietary carb intake is low, insulin is low, and liver glycogen stores are low. In these conditions, ketones are manufactured from fatty acids, as well as from the conversion of so-called ketogenic amino acids. Interestingly, glucose is always made in conjunction with ketones and they are released into the bloodstream together. The glucose comes from the conversion of so-called gluconeogenic amino acids, as well as from the fatty acid metabolism, during which the glycerol molecules are split away from the triglyceride and are converted into glucose.

The liver's conversion rate of fat to ketones depends on how much glucose is in the bloodstream. A single liver hormone known as FGF21 is responsible for the oxidation of fatty acids into ketones in the liver. When glucose levels are high, ketone production is suppressed; the body deems it unnecessary to go to the trouble of making ketones because of the abundance of quick-burning glucose. While almost everyone is making a little bit of ketones by the time they awaken—a consequence of not eating overnight, the ingestion of a single high-carbohydrate snack or meal will abruptly shut down the fragile ketone assembly line while glucose takes center stage.

In a state of complete starvation or maximum fat- and keto-adaptation, your muscles will burn mostly fatty acids so that nearly all the ketones you produce get sent on an express train to your highly demanding brain. Unlike fatty acids, ketones are water soluble so they can easily cross the blood-brain barrier and be used as a clean-burning energy source by the brain. After a few days in keto, your brain learns to obtain around 25 percent of its energy from ketones, and it can very quickly ramp up to the estimated maximum—that can range from 66 percent to 80 percent for the highly keto-adapted. With the brain burning around 25 percent of your daily calories, a quick calculation using my personal estimate of 2,700 calories burned per day suggests that my bare-minimum glucose requirement in my highly keto-adapted brain is only around 42 grams per day (675 brain calories per day × 25 percent glucose = 169 glucose calories or 42 grams). Realize that a sugar-burner is at virtually 100 percent glucose in the brain—a whopping 169 grams in my example!

MACRONUTRIENT BREAKDOWN FOR KETO: Dr. Dom D'Agostino suggests that the modern ketogenic diet for general use would come in at 65 to 75 percent fat, 15 to 25 percent protein, and 5 to 10 percent carbs. The leading experts all quote similar macronutrient ratios. For protein intake, Phinney and Volek recommend obtaining 0.6 to 1.0 gram of protein per lean mass per day. Villasenor cites research saying 0.82 grams per pound of lean mass per day delivers maximum performance benefits, with more being unnecessary. He also advocates for getting at least 0.8, especially if you are athletic or elderly. Even if you calculate an even 1 gram per pound of lean mass, this is still only a moderate contribution to total daily calories.

Special Populations

Following are some distinct personal attributes or performance/lifestyle goals and how ketogenic eating can be customized to serve them:

DISEASES/DISORDERS: If you are diagnosed with cancer, cognitive conditions such as Alzheimer's, dementia, ADHD, or autism, or especially seizures, the ketogenic diet has been shown to deliver profound druglike benefits for these and many other health conditions. It's beyond the scope of this book to dispense any message that could be remotely construed as medical advice. Alas, ketogenic eating is a pretty hot topic in medical and pharmaceutical circles these days, and it may benefit you to investigate the current best practices for diagnosed health conditions, as well as talk to your healthcare professional about the potential integration of ketogenic eating into your comprehensive approach to healing or managing conditions.

ENDURANCE ATHLETES: The implications of keto for endurance performance breakthroughs are absolutely mind-blowing. Imagine becoming bonk-proof—even on ultra-distance efforts; minimizing or eliminating the need for on-board calories, and thereby avoiding the minor to major digestive difficulties that virtually everyone suffers from; having all workouts seems easier to your central nervous system; and feeling less inflamed and fried even after long, hard sessions, because your high-octane fuel generates less inflammation and fewer free radicals. Any serious endurance athlete would be well served by giving keto a shot—not just for a potential competitive advantage but also to mitigate the oxidative stress on the body that comes from being in a high-calorie-burning, carbohydrate-dependent pattern.

STRENGTH/POWER ATHLETES: Early into the keto craze, the party line was that this was great stuff for endurance plodders, but that strength/power athletes doing high-glycolytic (glucose burning) workouts needed to fuel with glucose. It was further suggested that one would lose top-end power when transitioning from high-glucose-burning to ketone-burning. This has now been disproven, and even the most explosive, high-intensity training programs can be fueled by keto with great results. Dr. Dom D'Agostino made a nice effort to impress this point on skeptics by deadlifting ten reps of 500 pounds after a seven-day fast! Google some photos of Luis Villasenor and you can see keto is not hampering his maintenance of a high-performance physique.

WEIGHT LOSS: Going keto will resolve any frustration you have had with fat reduction, once and for all. The secret to solving this frustrating puzzle is not calories in–calories out. While that's literally true from a thermodynamic perspective, losing fat and maintaining ideal body composition over the long term is a matter of escaping carbohydrate dependency and becoming fat- and keto-adapted. This calibrates your appetite, metabolic and fat-storage hormones such that you feel completely satisfied after all your meals and snacks because they are naturally nutrient-dense whole foods instead of quick-energy junk foods. You will never be inclined to overeat or crave sugar; won't have to struggle with calorie counting, obsessive exercise, or portion control; and will become expert at burning stored fat, ketones, and glycogen as needed. Your metabolic flexibility status allows you to unleash tools like Intermittent Fasting, nutritional ketosis, and ketone supplements to quickly address and resolve any excess body fat issues, and then to set your cruise control to enjoy your life without obsessing about your diet or your body fat.

If you are shaking your head in dismay, counter-arguing that you have been unfortunately endowed with the "fat gene" from your parents and wondering if it's really possible to shed the final 10 or 20 pounds that have been there for 10 or 20 years, realize that any excess body fat you have today is a function of carbohydrate dependency and chronically excessive insulin production, combined with whatever level of familial genetic predisposition toward fat storage that you possess. To determine your predispositions, you can do genetic testing to determine how many copies of the AMY1 gene you have (a salivary enzyme that breaks down starches; the more copies you have, the less likely you are to accumulate fat)—or you can just look at yourself in the mirror. Regardless, if you become fat- and keto-adapted, your genetic predisposition toward storing fat will become irrelevant because you are calibrated 24/7 to burn fat and ketones.

When you have some weight to lose and have built the metabolic machinery primed for the challenge, you can use tools like Intermittent Fasting, nutritional ketosis, and exogenous ketone supplements to get the job done quickly—and not even struggle while you are dropping weight; you can then relax and enjoy delicious meals and stable appetite, energy, mood, and concentration every day, for the rest of your life.

YOUTH/GROWTH POPULATIONS: If you are in that relatively brief growth phase of life, from infancy to reaching your final height, restricting your intake of nutritious carbs to reach keto is probably not necessary or advised. Youth are much more insulin sensitive than adults as well, so they can handle more carbohydrate intake without the adverse effects we discuss so commonly. Keto might not be advised if you fall into other "growth" categories, such as pregnant/nursing mothers and bodybuilders or athletes looking to acquire and maintain extra muscle mass for specific performance goals who try cyclic keto (CKD) instead of making a full commitment. When you are looking to achieve cellular or muscular growth, insulin is your friend, because it feeds the cells the carbs, protein, and fat they need to grow.

The carbohydrate green light for growth populations applies only to high-nutrient-value carbohydrates, of course. Consuming refined grains and sugars is never justified, for anyone. Consider the ever-growing (pun intended) percentage of youth who are classified as overweight or obese; this is a clear indication that they are getting an excess of carbs and stimulating an unhealthy excess of growth factors like IGF-1 (insulin-like growth factor-1) and mTOR (mechanistic target of rapamycin). Over-activation of growth factors at any time is destructive to health and increases risk of cancer and other metabolic diseases over the long term. Similarly, insulin-resistant or obese mothers can actually pass insulin resistance on to their offspring, giving them a higher risk of obesity and disease throughout their lives.

It's becoming clear that a nutritious ketogenic diet can definitely help you preserve or build lean mass, and even meet the nutritional needs of a little one (as it surely often did for our ancestors). However, those brief periods of life when you are focused on growth (and are not overfat) might not be the most advantageous times to try going keto.

Testing Ketone Levels

As mentioned in the sidebar in Chapter 1 (page 14), testing glucose and ketones with a portable blood or breath meter can be helpful to assess how numerous variables affect your readings. I'm particularly interested to see what happens to my numbers as a consequence of fasting, conducting intense workouts, or ingesting a ketone supplement. Once you get into a good routine with nutritional ketosis, your ketone levels become fairly predictable; most people will land between 0.5 to 1.5 mmol/L, qualifying as mild nutritional ketosis. Those with unique genetics or extreme devotion to keto might get into that 1.5 mmol/L to 3.0 mmol/L range. If you consume a single recommended serving of a ketone supplement and test 15 to 30 minutes later, you may double whatever value you were otherwise sitting at—easily bumping up to 0.5 or higher, even if you were flatlining with ketones before the supplement. By the way, if you're super fat-adapted but not keto, you'll likely post nothing higher than a 0.2 mmol/L.

When you eat even a single moderate- to high-carbohydrate meal, you will quickly drop ketones below 0.5. I find that a single extended fast is sufficient get me back over 1.0, while others seem to take a bit longer to make an official return to 0.5 and above. As stated previously, athletes might deliver readings on the lower end. Brad reports that even deep into an ambitious nutritional ketosis effort and lengthy fasting periods, he'll often deliver numbers under 0.5—perhaps due to the ketone flux described by Dr. Cate Shanahan earlier. This is why subjective testing is perhaps more important than your entire database of blood values. Can you skip a meal without feeling cranky? Can you produce a quality workout in a fasted state, then hang out for a bit afterward before eating anything without passing out? If you can, you're fat- and keto-adapted—period.

Theoretically, the ideal representation of being fat- and keto-adapted is a moderate fasted glucose reading paired with a higher ketone reading. This is representative of your limited dietary carbohydrate intake and a diminished metabolic requirement for glucose. Despite a logical guess, the first thing in the morning might not be a good time to achieve low glucose and high ketones. Morning blood ketone readings can be low because fat oxidation rates are low in the morning (you haven't had to burn many calories for many hours). Morning glucose readings can be high (even after an overnight fast) because of the routine, and desirable, sympathetic nervous system/cortisol response that helps you awaken with energy and alertness. Part of this morning hormonal process is the cortisol spike triggering gluconeogenesis and consequent robust glucose readings. You also might be a little underhydrated in the early morning, which can raise glucose values because your blood is more concentrated.

When testing ketones, it's important to test under similar circumstances each day. Dr. D'Agostino recommends testing in the afternoon, either fasted or a couple hours after a keto-aligned meal. Afternoon is when the highest levels are typically seen in most people. This is even more pronounced when you conduct an intense or prolonged workout in the morning, then stay sedentary for a few hours. In this condition, your body has responded to the workout stimulus by upregulating ketone production, essentially prepping you to continue the workout for as long as possible. However, ending the workout and then becoming inactive results in minimal ketone burning, and consequently high blood values.

With glucose, things get a little more complex and confusing. Glucose levels will fluctuate wildly in response to carbohydrate snacks and meals. Exercise can also cause big swings in glucose numbers. If you are a sugar-burner and conduct a depleting workout, you don't need a blood meter to tell you that your glucose has nose-dived. On the flip side, Brad and I have both had the alarming experience of delivering high glucose readings (over 100—something traditional blood testing designates as pre-diabetic) despite drawing samples on the heels of extended fasting and/or keto-aligned eating. This may be in part due to physiological insulin resistance resulting from advanced fat- and keto-adaptation. Here the muscles are so good at burning fat that they resist insulin's attempt to deliver glucose, leaving more circulating in the bloodstream.

With Dr. Peter Attia's ideal of a moderate fasting glucose (well under 100) and a tight standard deviation even after meals, it's a good idea to take glucose readings frequently and determine if you are generally looking sharp but delivering some outlier readings now and then, or whether you might have a problem with glucose regulation. Fortunately, glucose strips cost only pennies, unlike the scary-expensive ketone strips. It's also important to consider Dr. Cate Shanahan's speculation that these meters (or perhaps your testing circumstances) might be significantly inaccurate. Dr. D'Agostino speculates that the Precision Xtra seems to be some 5 percent higher on glucose than actual laboratory-derived glucose values. If you are concerned about your glucose fitness, consider trying Robb Wolf's recommended sensitivity test of consuming 50 grams at one sitting, then testing glucose two hours later to see if you can deliver a reading below 150 mg/dL.

You may have heard of the urine strips called Ketostix that are commonly used to test for ketone levels. When the Ketostix comes in contact with urine, it turns a certain color over a specified time period. A color spectrum correlating with the level of acetone (one of the ketone bodies) in the urine can then be used to roughly estimate how actively the body is burning ketones. This is far less accurate than testing ketone levels in the blood directly. For example, the Ketostix may reveal low readings because an individual has become keto-adapted to the extent that ketones are being burned instead of excreted in the urine—the Ketostix providing a false negative in this example. Ketostix readings can also be rendered inaccurate owing to excessive hydration. Finally, the Ketostix only measures one of the ketone bodies, acetoacetate. The other ketone body, beta-hydroxybutyrate, is actually the predominant ketone body that is burned for energy in the bloodstream, once an individual is keto-adapted.

Troubleshooting

Dr. Dom D'Agostino cites a statistic that 20 to 30 percent of enthusiasts don't respond well to a ketogenic diet. This is a disturbingly high figure when you consider that humans have been in a fat- and ketone-burning state for the vast majority of the past 2.5 million years. It's likely that this high non-responder figure is largely attributed to those with a flawed approach. Dr. D'Agostino speculates that many enthusiasts, especially females, may be engaging in a disastrous combination of overexercising and other high-stress lifestyle behaviors, combined with fat phobia when they attempt to go low carb or keto. The fat phobia is likely a subconscious remnant that many of us harbor, a result of decades of cultural programming that eating fat makes you fat.

Cutting carbs, protein, and fat to the extent that you get insufficient total calories and overall nutrition is a bad deal. Our genetics are highly averse to overexercising;

the frequent depletion and fatigue is perceived to be a matter of life or death, as it was in primal times. Consequently, our appetite and reproductive hormones rage in response to the extent that we not only overeat, but also that we direct those calories to be stored as fat instead of burned. When you add to the picture the common themes of insufficient sleep and overly stressful lifestyle patterns with insufficient downtime, you have a high-stress approach that puts you at risk of total operating system failure: blowing out your thyroid, frying your adrenal glands, picking up a mysterious auto-immune illness, or landing with other world-of-hurt conditions that often escape the diagnostics of Western medicine.

Other less extreme struggles may come from an assortment of factors or flawed strategies that are important for even the most health-astute to reflect upon, as follows:

- History of significant metabolic damage and trying to progress with carb restriction too quickly.

- Not actually adhering to the macronutrient guidelines, due to not tracking and journaling food intake and/or being inaccurate or delusional with your estimates.

- Choosing foods of inferior nutritional value—even if the macros are keto-approved. Man cannot live on high-fat coffee and pork rinds alone!

- Deficiency in metabolizing certain fatty acids, requiring an emphasis on different fat sources (e.g., less bacon and cheese, more avocado and coconut).

- Adverse microbiome consequences from going keto, requiring an increase and diversification of high-fiber vegetable intake.

- Mineral and electrolyte imbalances. Reduced cellular inflammation and water retention is a good thing, but it might warrant increased intake of water, sodium, potassium, and magnesium—especially during the transition to keto.

A much smaller percentage of enthusiasts might actually be responding poorly to the macronutrient template of 65 to 75 percent fat, 15 to 25 percent protein, and 5 to 10 percent carbs, and can try to tweak these ratios, while always emphasizing the healthiest sources of animal products and produce. For now, have faith that some semblance of evolutionary-based eating and ketone-burning will work for you, and carefully review the entries in this section to see if any corrections that can enhance your progress are warranted.

CALORIC DEFICIENCY: Lingering fat phobia causes insufficient total caloric intake, making compliance difficult, increasing the risk for malnutrition, and making carb binges likely. The quick solution here is to eat more natural, nutritious fats. If you're making eggs and bacon for breakfast, double your portions. Add even more butter to your steamed vegetables or more avocado oil to your salads. Have an extra handful of macadamia nuts at snack time. Make sure that you achieve total dietary satisfaction at every meal while adhering to your carb and protein intake guidelines. Respect the stringent carb and protein guidelines, but make a concerted effort to consume a variety of nutrient-dense, high-fiber vegetables and quality sources of protein as close to their natural state as possible (e.g., eggs instead of soy burgers). Once you become fat- and keto-adapted, you will discover that you require fewer fat calories to feel great and perform and recover optimally. At this point, you can use keto as a secret weapon to become leaner, stronger, and healthier than you have ever been in your life.

CONSTIPATION: While most people experience a dramatic improvement in common digestive issues such as gas and bloating when going low-carb or keto, some experience constipation or other digestive irregularities. Dialing in your hydration, electrolytes, and minerals is critical here—we'll discuss these shortly—as is making a concerted effort to consume a variety of high-fiber vegetables, because your fiber intake will decline when you cut out grains. Some recommend fiber supplements to battle carb restriction–influenced constipation, but others suggest that increasing sodium may be even more effective.

FATTY ACID CONCERNS: Because you are transitioning to a high-fat diet, it's even more important to emphasize healthy natural fats, to completely eliminate unhealthy refined vegetable oils, and to ensure that you obtain an ideal balance of the various kinds of natural fats. This means you'll be emphasizing foods containing saturated, monounsaturated, and/or omega-3s fats. One keto mistake is upping the fat intake indiscriminately, to the extent that refined high-polyunsaturated fatty acids leak into the picture significantly, perhaps from cooking otherwise good stuff with them, consuming nuts roasted in vegetable oils, dining out with high frequency, or overcooking meats—especially meats from conventional feedlot animals. Furthermore, it's thought that certain people have a genotype that results in a deficiency in metabolizing saturated fats, in which case they might want to back off the bacon and cheese in favor of more avocado, coconut, and olive products.

If you have uncomfortable digestive or autoimmune reactions when upping your fat intake or you suspect that saturated fats somehow might not agree with you, consider testing some key lipid values to track if any adverse changes occur in your transition to keto. Dr. Cate Shanahan asserts that one's triglyceride:HDL ratio is perhaps the most important heart disease marker to track. Ideally, you want to achieve a 1:1 ratio. Getting your ratio under 3.5:1 is essential to moderate your heart disease risk, as is getting your total triglycerides under 150 mg/dL. In the vast majority of people going keto, triglycerides will actually decline owing to the reduction in insulin that eases the overtaxed lipid processing system. You are now burning fats in the form of fatty acids instead of transporting them into storage in the form of triglycerides. What's more, HDL levels are likely to rise as a consequence of consuming more saturated fats.

Your total LDL amount may also increase when you go keto, as an expected consequence of increased fat intake. This is most likely nothing to concern yourself with, as recent science strongly validates the concept that total LDL level is not an accurate predictor of heart disease risk. Interestingly, a UCLA meta-study (a collective study of many smaller studies on a particular topic) revealed that 75 percent of patients hospitalized for a heart attack had an LDL of less than 130 mg/dl (widely accepted as "safe"), and that half the victims had an LDL under 100, widely considered "ideal."

Testing your *LDL particle size* is far more relevant to heart disease risk than your total LDL. Small, dense LDL particles are the problematic agents that are small and dense enough to lodge on artery walls, become oxidized, and cause atherosclerosis. Large, fluffy LDL are generally harmless molecules that can increase in number when you increase fat intake. Even if you don't get the specialized and potentially expensive particle size breakdown on your blood tests, you can gain assurance of minimized risk when your triglycerides are low, because this implies that small, dense LDL are low, and whatever LDL number you have is weighted toward large, fluffy. (Note: This is a basic overview of the dynamics and metrics involved in the heart disease process, and should not be construed as medical advice. If your triglycerides elevate significantly when you go keto, consult with your physician and perhaps an alternative health-care practitioner.)

FEMALE CONCERNS: There has been plenty of talk in primal/paleo circles about how females might have a more difficult time with extreme carb restriction than males. After all, female genetics are calibrated to the ultimate evolutionary goal of reproduction. Shedding excess body fat quickly contradicts this hardwiring, so if you are female you may likely not see results as quickly as your male study partner making a similar keto effort. Furthermore, if you have a history of metabolic damage from yo-yo dieting, hormonal irregularities (particularly thyroid or adrenal dysfunction), emotional disturbances relating to eating, or a general difficulty with losing excess body fat or struggling with sugar cravings, you may want to adopt a more gradual approach to carbohydrate restriction and progressing toward ketogenic eating.

Some health experts even contend that vulnerable females taking an aggressive approach to carb restriction may risk compromising adrenal, thyroid, and other hormonal functions. According to Elle Russ, author of *The Paleo Thyroid Solution,* "Going keto can cause appetite suppression to the extent that thyroid hormone metabolism suffers in response to what is perceived as starvation. Maintaining a healthy intake of nutrient dense vegetables, making sure to meet protein minimums, and enjoying ample natural, nutritious fats will support a healthy balance of sex and thyroid hormones." Russ also asserts that if you are on thyroid hormone replacement when you go keto, you should test frequently at the outset to ensure that your levels are optimized. It's been observed that some thyroid patients who go keto become more metabolically efficient to the extent that thyroid function improves and they have a reduced need for medication! "The beneficial effects of keto might entail reducing thyroid dosages to avoid becoming hyperthyroid or igniting a reverse T3 issue," concludes Russ.

While it may be unnerving to envision your keto efforts messing with your sensitive thyroid or adrenals, especially if you are under a doctor's care for such issues, I propose that there might be a bit too much chatter about females having a difficult time with low carb and keto. It's possible that a good percentage of those struggling might have a flawed approach that involves many of the red flags covered in this section. Russ's book provides details about how chronic exercise patterns and yo-yo dieting have a destructive effect on thyroid function—a connection that traditional medical care often fails to recognize.

If you follow a correct approach with great discipline, and it ends up taking three months to completely ditch grains, sugars, and refined high-polyunsaturated vegetable oils instead of three weeks, so be it. We are talking about (relatively) quickly reprogramming your genes to unwind decades of metabolic damage and dysfunction, losing excess body fat and keeping it off, and reducing disease risk for the rest of your life, so patience is necessary to enable steady forward progress and obtaining results that stick. Respect the recommended benchmarks to reach after each step so you don't take on any challenges that you are not ready for.

GUT HEALTH: As mentioned in Chapter 6, transitioning away from a high-carbohydrate diet to a more narrow range of foods might adversely affect the health of your gut microbiome, since many high-carbohydrate foods are also high in the fiber that supports gut health. Furthermore, in some rare cases, starving carb-dependent gut cells can cause them to die, and the debris from these dead cells can release chemicals that stimulate an inflammatory reaction in your gut. This in turn might manifest as nausea or even diarrhea for a short period of time. These conditions will correct as you continue with keto. The best way to support your gut health when going keto is to make a concerted effort to consume a wide assortment of high-fiber, low-glycemic vegetables grown above the ground, such as leafy greens, cruciferous veggies, the onion family, and even herbs and spices.

It's also advisable to supplement your diet with sources of prebiotic fiber—a.k.a. resistant starch. These are indigestible agents that pass through your intestinal tract and take residence in your colon as healthy bacteria. The best sources of prebiotics are raw potato starch (available in the baking section of quality grocery stores, or online— not to be confused with potato flour, which is high in carbs), green bananas, and cooked and cooled white rice and white potatoes. Interestingly, the unripe contents of a green banana are resistant starch, but a yellow banana has ripened into fully digestible carbohydrate form. A green banana has about 5 grams of carbs—trivial even when you are going keto, while a yellow banana has 27 grams—enough to knock you out of ketosis.

When you consume white rice or potatoes in their typical warmed state, you are getting a big dose of high-glycemic carbohydrates—37 grams in a medium baked potato, 45 grams in a cup of white rice. Ditto if you add raw potato starch or green bananas to a recipe and heat them—they convert into digestible carbohydrate. When you consume white rice or potatoes in a cooled state (after being cooked of course), their molecular structure becomes indigestible; they become a form of "resistant" starch. As with the green banana, you get only minimal carbs and mostly resistant starch. While raw potato starch, green bananas, and cooked and cooled white rice and potatoes deliver big-time doses of resistant starch, many other keto-friendly foods contain small doses of resistant starch in their ordinary states, including: almonds, bone broth, dark chocolate, and pistachios.

Strive to obtain 20 to 30 grams of resistant starch per day, but introduce your sources gradually to protect against potential digestive disturbances that might result from a sudden increase. Start by adding a teaspoon of raw potato starch to your smoothies or a bowl of full-fat Greek-style yogurt. Work up to a tablespoon (there are 8 grams of resistant starch per tablespoon) and try to add cold rice, cold potatoes, and green bananas into your game now and then. You can mask the gummy taste of green bananas with almond butter, or throw the banana into a smoothie. It is these prebiotic fibers that you nourish with dietary or supplemental sources of probiotics. Great dietary sources of probiotics include fermented foods (kefir, kimchi, kombucha, pickles, sauerkraut, yogurt), fermented soy products (miso, tempeh), fresh berries, green tea, and high-cacao percentage dark chocolate. High-potency probiotic supplements are a good suggestion to keep your gut happy during keto efforts.

HUNGER: In a word, this is the purported reason that many rudimentary keto efforts have failed. We've talked at length about the ideal strategy and progression to avoid suffering hunger bouts causing carbohydrate binges. Beyond that, Luis Villasenor says point blank, "Hunger is either boredom or a sign of a nutrient deficiency such as magnesium, sodium, or iron."

HYDRATION/ELECTROLYTES/MINERALS: When you ditch refined carbohydrates and vegetable oils, your immune system relaxes its sustained inflammatory reaction against these agents that are so offensive to healthy cellular function. Consequently, you'll notice less swelling and water retention throughout your body—often very quickly and to the tune of dropping a quick ten pounds in the first week of your 21-Day Metabolism Reset. While it's great news to reduce your waste product–laden extracellular fluid (often attributed to leaky gut—undigested foreign particles entering the bloodstream through permeable intestinal walls that have been damaged by gluten), your new, less inflamed, leaner body may have lower than normal accumulations of water, electrolytes, and minerals.

Making a concerted effort to increase water intake and add sodium, potassium, and magnesium-rich foods or supplements may be particularly important if you are making a quick and radical shift from high-carb eating to keto, and/or if you are an athlete who sweats frequently. While it's obviously irresponsible to offer a pinpoint personal suggestion here, some helpful general guidelines are as follows: Dr. D'Agostino recommends adding 4 to 8 grams (1 or 2 teaspoons) of sodium to your diet each day when going keto. Use sea salt or Himalayan pink salt, as they are more nutritious than routine iodized table salt. Himalayan salt contains a full spectrum of 84 minerals, including calcium, magnesium, potassium, copper, and iron. Consider trying a magnesium supplement from a trusted supplier or alternative health-care practitioner. Most capsules or powders deliver between 150–400 mg of this agent that health experts believe most people are deficient in. You can boost your potassium intake with keto-friendly high-potassium foods like avocados (the reigning champ at 1,000 mg—a fifth of your recommended daily intake and twice as much as bananas), wild-caught salmon, and assorted vegetables like Brussels sprouts, chard, kale, mushrooms, and spinach.

It's essential for all keto enthusiasts to pay more attention to hydration, and especially those with devoted workout regimens. While going by thirst is effective for the most part, you may also want to strategically hydrate before and rehydrate after workouts. Since sodium plays a key role in fluid absorption, it's a good idea to add a pinch of salt to every cup of water you drink and to sip your fluids gradually over an extended time period. If you indiscriminately chug plain water in the name of hydration, you may just excrete a lot of it. Never force yourself to drink more than you are comfortable with, as you have likely heard about the serious health consequences of the overhydrated, under-salted state of hyponatremia. Finally, if you continue with keto but fail to optimize your sodium, potassium, and magnesium intake, you can suffer from the same bloating, fatigue, and inflammation as a carb addict.

LIFESTYLE: Own this: stress = sugar. Chronic overstimulation of the fight-or-flight response, through exhausting exercise or lifestyle habits, overrides attempts at fat-adaptation and pushes you back toward carbohydrate dependency. Ditto for insufficient sleep.

METABOLIC DAMAGE: Yo-yo dieting is severely destructive to your metabolism, because it makes you default to fat storage as a fight-or-flight reaction to frequent bouts of starvation while carbohydrate-dependent. Even years later, your body is not too interested in dropping excess body fat, even if you diligently restrict carbs and exercise sensibly. If you are trying to unwind years or even decades of metabolic damage, adopt a more gradual approach to dietary transformation. A 42-day metabolism reset might not be as sexy as the 21-Day, but you are building the foundation for a healthy future and an emphatic departure from the destructive genetic and hormonal patterns that have compromised your health.

MEAL TIMING: Dr. Satchin Panda, a professor at the Salk Institute for Biological Studies in La Jolla, California, asserts that we have a circadian rhythm for calorie consumption and metabolism just as we do for sleeping and waking. Panda's laboratory research suggests that meal timing can optimize the function of the liver, gut microbiome, and other digestive processes to promote efficient fat metabolism, insulin sensitivity, mitochondria function, immune function, and gut microbiome diversity, as well as lower growth factors like IGF-1 to reduce cancer risk. Panda's studies suggest that it's best to confine calorie consumption to an 8- to 12-hour time window each day, and this has generated extraordinary body composition results with mice eating in a restricted time window.

Interestingly, Panda states that any xenobiotic substance (something foreign to the body that it has to metabolize) will start your digestive circadian clock, even if it is noncaloric. So, consuming black coffee in the morning (caffeine has to be metabolized by liver enzymes and your intestinal tract—a morning wakeup call for your digestive tract, too!), herbal tea at night, or even swallowing vitamin pills should respect this 12-hour window.

The time window doesn't necessarily have to correlate with your sleep/wake cycles, as we have discussed the benefits of delaying your morning meal. However, it might be valuable to rethink any justification for late-night snacking, even if it's healthy food. Keep your digestive tract on an 8- to 12-hour shift and don't allow any overtime. Being fat- and keto-adapted makes this a breeze, but it might require some mindfulness to finish eating at a respectable time in the evening, especially on those days when you do eat breakfast.

REFEEDING/BUSTING LOOSE: Refeeding is a popular strategy in the low-carb and keto community to help preserve insulin sensitivity in the face of prolonged suppression of insulin through keto eating. Refeeding strategies are also seen as a way to reduce the psychological stress of adhering to rigid macronutrient standards by allowing for what are often called "cheat days." This is a term I despise, because it implies that your normal dietary patterns are somehow unpleasant. I'd rather your approach to keto be motivated by a deep appreciation for the most satisfying, nutrient-dense foods on the planet, and that instead of longing for grain and sugar treats on occasional cheat days, you habituate away from nutrient-devoid modern foods by replacing them with foods that are deeply nourishing.

The rationale for refeeding is that if you maintain low insulin levels for a long time, your cells may become somewhat resistant to insulin's signals because they don't have to deal with significant amounts of insulin—like a muscle atrophying from lack of use. Consequently, a refeed is conducted to balance prolonged periods of carb restriction with purposeful days or weekends of high carbohydrate intake. This would prompt a heavy insulin response, wake up the receptor sites, and hone insulin sensitivity in the process. A refeed also allows for some dietary indulgences that aren't happening when one is trying to adhere to keto guidelines. As stated previously, it's possible that refeeding can be problematic for certain individuals, and that a gradual reintroduction of higher-than-keto carbohydrate intake is the best strategy.

That said, there are simply and absolutely no health objections to long-term keto (remember, that's our predominant ancestral dietary pattern). Indeed, indefinite keto can be the healthiest strategy for many individuals, especially those with metabolic damage.

What's more, Luis Villasenor—going strong and getting stronger in keto for 16 years and counting—asserts that the complaint of developing insulin resistance from long-term keto is likely due to confusing *pathological* insulin resistance with *physiological* insulin resistance. With the former—the traditional disease definition—chronic overproduction desensitizes cell receptor sites, setting the stage for type-2 diabetes. With the physiological insulin resistance that occurs in highly fat- and keto-adapted individuals, fatty acids accumulate in muscles as the primary fuel source, causing receptor sites to turn away glucose. This can cause glucose to occasionally rise in the bloodstream, giving the appearance of pathological insulin resistance, but without any disease or adverse health consequences. Referencing earlier discussions about athletes having low ketone numbers and occasional high glucose numbers, physiological insulin resistance could provide a good explanation.

ACKNOWLEDGMENTS

THE authors are deeply appreciative of the tremendous interest and support of Celeste Fine of Sterling Lord Literistic and Diana Baroni of Harmony Books, the world's best literary agent and editorial director, respectively. Thanks to Farley Chase of Chase Literary Agency for the introduction! The all-star teams at Sterling Lord and Harmony did an exceptional job to help make this book the best it can be. Dr. Cate Shanahan, Dr. Peter Attia, Dr. Dom D'Agostino, Luis Villasenor, and Dr. Phil Maffetone graciously and patiently assisted the authors in preparing a clear, precise, and scientifically validated message throughout the book. Lindsay Shaw Taylor did a fabulous job spearheading the recipe project; you can thank her on Instagram (@theusefuldish) as you will undoubtedly find a few recipes that will no doubt change your life! Thank you to Andrew and Carrie Purcell for the fabulous food photography. Thanks to Big George and Dr. Steven "E" Kobrine for the writing retreat facilities.

The most important acknowledgment goes to you, the reader, for having an open mind in your quest for health. Exploring the benefits of ketogenic eating is a dramatic departure from a grain-based, high-carbohydrate diet, and you are battling some significant cultural pressures to depart from conventional wisdom. Good luck, and keep making the empowering choice to take responsibility for your health every single day.

Mark Sisson
Brad Kearns
Malibu, California
July 2017

INDEX

Note: Page numbers in *italics* indicate recipes.

ABOUT THE AUTHORS

MARK SISSON is the bestselling author of *The Primal Blueprint* and numerous other books promoting primal/paleo living and cooking. His MarksDailyApple.com is one of the most-visited health information websites on the Internet, lauded for challenging and reshaping flawed conventional wisdom about diet, exercise, and lifestyle. Mark's efforts to promote primal living extend to print and online educational materials, a health coach certification program, a line of healthy kitchen condiments and nutritional supplements, and a chain of fast casual primal-style restaurants. Mark is a former 2:18 marathoner and fourth-place finisher in the Hawaii Ironman Triathlon. He lives in Malibu, California, and holds his own every weekend in high-stakes Ultimate Frisbee matches with hotshots half his age.

BRAD KEARNS is the President of Primal Blueprint Publishing and has worked closely with Mark Sisson for a decade promoting the primal lifestyle. He co-authored (with Sisson) *Primal Endurance,* organized nine PrimalCon weekend retreats across North America, and presented the Primal Transformation Seminar in 22 cities. He is a former national champion and #3 world-ranked professional triathlete, and currently a professional Speedgolfer; he shot 78 on a championship golf course in 47 minutes at the 2017 California championships.